Health
Policy
in Australia

SECOND EDITION

Health Policy in Australia

SECOND EDITION

Edited by
Heather Gardner &
Simon Barraclough

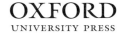

OXFORD
UNIVERSITY PRESS

OXFORD
UNIVERSITY PRESS

253 Normanby Road, South Melbourne, Victoria 3205, Australia

Oxford University Press is a department of the University of Oxford.
It furthers the University's objective of excellence in research, scholarship,
and education by publishing worldwide in

Oxford New York

Auckland Bangkok Buenos Aires Cape Town Chennai
Dar es Salaam Delhi Hong Kong Istanbul Karachi Kolkata
Kuala Lumpur Madrid Melbourne Mexico City Mumbai Nairobi
São Paulo Shanghai Singapore Taipei Tokyo Toronto
with an associated company in Berlin

OXFORD is a trade mark of Oxford University Press
in the UK and in certain other countries

National Library of Australia
Cataloguing-in-Publication data:

Health Policy in Australia.

2nd ed.
Bibliography.
Includes index.

ISBN 0 19 551348 7.

1. Medical policy—Australia. 2. Health planning—
Australia. I. Gardner, Heather. II. Barraclough, Simon,
1952–.

362.10994

Edited by Sandra Goldbloom Zurbo
Text and cover designed by Racheal Stines
Indexed by Max McMaster
Typeset by Kerry Cooke
Printed through Bookpac Production Services, Singapore

Contents

Tables

Figures

Boxes

Acknowledgments

In bringing together this book, the efforts of many people must be recognised. The authors are to be thanked for agreeing to write on topical issues and for their willingness to undertake revisions of their drafts to clarify points and add new information. Many of the authors would have been unable to produce their chapters without the assistance of informants from both the public and private sectors who provided insights and relevant documents— their willingness to assist in the process of research is greatly appreciated. The editors also acknowledge the highly professional of support from those at Oxford University Press, in particular Jill Henry, and Sandra Goldbloom Zurbo, who carefully read and commented upon the various chapters.

Contributors

Simon Barraclough is a senior lecturer in the School of Public Health at La Trobe University. He is a political scientist who has researched and published widely on Australian and Asian politics and health. He is co-editor, with Heather Gardner, of this second edition of *Health Policy in Australia*.

Valerie A. Brown AO is the Foundation Professor of Environmental Health and a director of the Regional Integrated Monitoring Centre at the University of Western Sydney. She is Team Leader of the Local Sustainability Project, which works on decision making towards integrated local, social, and ecological sustainability. She has written and contributed to books on local environmental management for the local government sector, the coastal zone, community landcare, emergency management, and Indigenous communities.

Alice Creelman is Director, Acute Care Development, in the Department of Health and Ageing. She has worked for many years in health and aged care policy development. She has a keen interest in community-based aged care and has contributed to a number of initiatives aimed at supporting older people in their choice to stay at home. One of her areas of focus in her present role is exploring the development of care options for older hospital patients with chronic health-care needs.

Jeanne Daly is an associate professor in the School of Public Health at La Trobe University. She has researched and written extensively on medical technology.

Stephen Duckett is a health economist with extensive experience as a university lecturer, author, and senior public servant in federal and state health departments. Currently, he is Dean of the Faculty of Health Sciences at La Trobe University. Previously, he was Secretary to the Commonwealth Department of Human Services and Health.

Heather Eastwood is a lecturer in the Department of Social and Preventive Medicine at University of Queensland, where she lectures on the health system. She has published widely on complementary medicine.

Heather Gardner is a political scientist who has lectured in health policy to health science and public health students for many years, and teaches policy analysis to postgraduate students and staff from the Commonwealth Department of Health and Ageing. She has published widely on health and politics and on the health professions. Until mid 2000, she was Associate Professor and Foundation Head of the School of Public Health at La Trobe University. Currently, she is an Adjunct Associate Professor in the School of Public Health, La Trobe University, and editor of the *Australian Journal of Primary Health*, and of *Environmental Health*, the journal of the Australian Institute of Environmental Health.

Carol Grbich is an associate professor in the School of Nursing at Flinders University, South Australia, and prior to that at the Lincoln Institute of Health Sciences, Victoria. An acknowledged expert in and author of works on the sociology of health, her teaching and research interests are in gerontology, qualitative research, and palliative care.

Linda Hancock is an associate professor in and Director of the Public Policy and Governance program at Deakin University and was previously a commissioner on the Law Reform Commission of Victoria, as well as a presiding member of the Social Security Appeals Tribunal. She has worked as a researcher, consultant, and tertiary teacher for more than twenty years, and has published widely. Current research includes the Women's Audit-Project and the New Social Settlement Project. International comparative work includes analysis of Australian federal–state intergovernmental relations for the Canadian Social Union Project, work on social policy and regional policy in the European Union, and regional policy at the OECD. She is a Victorian Executive and National Board member of the Women's Electoral Lobby.

Emma Hughes is a lecturer with the Healthcare Education and Research Group, School of Public Health, La Trobe University. She is a health sociologist with research interests in consumer health-care decision-making and the impact of information technologies and telecommunications on healthcare practice.

Vivian Lin is Professor in and Head of the School of Public Health, La Trobe University. Formerly she was the Executive Officer, National Public Health Partnership, and Manager Intergovernmental Relations, Acute Health Services Division, Victorian Department of Health and Community Services. She has extensive experience in public health, and health promotion and policy.

Amanda L. Neil is a senior lecturer in health economics at the University of Newcastle. She teaches various aspects of health economics—primarily clinical economics at a postgraduate level—in Australia and overseas. She has diverse research interests, including the export of health products (the focus of her PhD studies), the benchmarking of pathology laboratories, and the application of economic evaluation, most recently in mental health care. She is a member of the Economic Subcommittee of the PHAC and a member of the Advisory Committee, Benchmarking in Pathology QA program, RCPA QAP.

Rosemary Nicholson is a lecturer in environmental health at the University of Western Sydney, whose teaching interests span health promotion and linkages between the environment and human health and wellbeing. She also has a strong interest in integrating students' academic and professional development at undergraduate and postgraduate levels. She is currently researching the changing role and profile of practitioners in environmental health and is co-author and co-editor of a national handbook on community-based environmental health action.

Debra O'Connor is the health promotion coordinator at Dianella Community Health, Broadmeadows, Victoria. She was until recently the coordinator of Health

Promotion Programs, School of Public Health, La Trobe University. She is the Chair, Consumer Advisory Committee, Health Insurance Commission, the consumer representative of the General Practice Computing Group, and a member of the Telehealth Group at La Trobe University.

Corinne op't Hoog is a haemodialysis nurse at the Royal Melbourne Hospital, where she has developed a critical interest in the use of the term 'noncompliance'. She is currently completing a Master of Public Health at La Trobe University. Her qualitative research is concerned with understanding noncompliance with health advice, from the patient's perspective.

Chris Peterson is a senior lecturer in the School of Public Health, La Trobe University, and is the leader of the Telehealth Group. He is a sociologist who teaches and publishes in occupational health and safety, the evaluation of health services, and primary health care.

Rosemary Roberts is an associate professor in and Director of the National Centre for Classification in Health, Faculty of Health Sciences, University of Sydney. She is an adviser to government on health information classification and policy.

Kerin Robinson is coordinator of the Bachelor of Health Information Management in the School of Public Health, La Trobe University. She is also the editor of the *Journal of the Health Information Management Association of Australia*.

Yvonne Robinson has worked in, taught, and written about health promotion for more than fifteen years. She has a longstanding interest in and commitment to cooperation and intersectoral collaboration as strategies for responsive, flexible, and effective service provision. As Director of the North East Health Promotion Centre, a networking structure in Melbourne, she was involved in bringing together primary and acute health services, local government, and a university to enhance health promotion planning and activity. She is currently Director, Programs, at VicHealth, where she is contributing to the development of VicHealth's role in supporting sustainable partnerships for innovative health promotion.

James Smith is a consultant to government and the community sector in public health management. He is a research associate in local governance, Regional Integrated Monitoring Centre, University of Western Sydney.

Pauline Stanton is a senior lecturer in the Graduate School of Management at La Trobe University. She specialises in human resource management and employment realtions. She has a background in industrial relations, and has also worked in education and training and health services management. She has an honours degree in economics and social science and a masters degree in employment relations. She is currently completing her doctoral thesis on employment relationships in Victorian public hospitals.

Peter Stephenson is a senior lecturer in Environmental Health and is Executive Director of the Regional Integrated Monitoring Centre at the Hawkesbury Campus of the University of Western Sydney, and a qualified environmental health officer, teacher, and researcher. His professional interests include environmental health development work in Australia and overseas. For the past five years he has managed a national education and workforce capacity building program for Indigenous environmental health practitioners of Australia. He has also recently contributed to a national project linking local community environmental health action with environment and public health policy and practice of government.

Hal Swerissen is an associate professor in and Director of the Australian Institute for Primary Care, La Trobe University. Formerly, he was a policy adviser to the federal Minister for Human Services and Health and to the Victorian Minister for Community Services.

Rae Walker is a senior lecturer in Health Promotion at La Trobe University. Her research focuses on issues in interorganisational relations, mainly in the primary care sector in Australia. She has completed a number of studies of collaboration between primary care organisations in community health and general practice. Most recently her work has focused on issues of trust between organisations and how that trust is measured.

Dianne Williamson is a senior lecturer in health information management, School of Public Health, La Trobe University. She has research interests in quality in the management of health databases.

Eileen Willis is a senior lecturer in the School of Nursing and Midwifery at Flinders University. Her research interests are in the sociology of work in the health industry. She has published widely on best practice in health care.

Introduction

Continuity and Change in Australian Health Policy

Heather Gardner and Simon Barraclough

The chapters presented in this book provide insights into diverse aspects of contemporary health policy in Australia and are written by authors working in various fields. Some are academic analysts of the policy process, others are involved in the actual formulation and implementation of policy, and still others are both observers and practitioners. Common to the approach of each author is a concern with the values, institutions, and interests that shape the direction of decisions taken by governments about strategies and the allocation of resources. These chapters chronicle familiar continuities, as well as change. Some aspects of change are due to a rethinking of values and how these should be achieved through policy, others reflect altered domestic and global economic relations, while in some cases it is technological innovation that calls forth new public policy responses. Moreover, as is evident in the chapters that follow, the health policy process is continually shaped and reshaped by a complex interplay of competing values and interests and sub-jectively interpreted by those observing the process.

The emphasis is, as in the first edition, on national policies, not only on how they provide frameworks for health directions in the states and terri-tories,[1] but also on how they are influenced by those states and territories, and by the interests whether of stakeholders or partners. Although strategic direction by the Commonwealth government has increased and developed since the first edition, there has been an attempt to provide states, territories, and local governments with more flexibility in deciding their own health policies and how they use their health resources within the current federal guidelines. Strategic alliances and the development of policy networks are other federal directions that have been encouraged as means of making better use of existing resources, whether they are in centres for medical research, public health, or health promotion in the community.

As the chapters clearly demonstrate, health policy cannot be considered in isolation from broad socioeconomic developments. The health care system is not only an essential element of the social welfare structure of Australian society, but is also a major industry. Efforts by governments to control expenditure on health care and to increase productivity in the health sector are aspects of wider economic policy, partly shaped by international values and pressures. The determinants of health are not restricted to the health care system and biological factors; they extend to environmental, socioeconomic, and lifestyle influences, so that the emphasis in health policy becomes evidence-based with a focus on outcomes—where and how we can make a difference with the most efficient use of resources, referred to colloquially as being 'more bang for your buck'. This approach has been made possible by changes in technology and the ability to manipulate huge data sets collected in Australia and overseas on the health of populations and their burden of disease and injury, so that programs can be strategically focused on particular population and disease groupings. Examples of this approach are the six national health priority areas—cancer, heart disease, injury, mental health, diabetes, and asthma.

The second edition is predominantly new—it has only two revised and updated chapters—so contains chapters on issues that were not covered in the first volume but which are now timely. The chapters largely reflect the themes referred to above: although there are continuities in health as there are in other areas of policy, and as there must be in a stable political democracy, there are also more changes of a substantial nature taking place than there have been in previous periods. Again, these reflect other areas of policy, and the influence of neoliberalism and its emphasis on the market, on those areas and values in health and health care.

Part 1, 'The Australian Health System', contains seven chapters, which together provide an overview of the health system as well as analyses of continuities and change in health and health care. Swerissen and Duckett, in their revised chapter (chapter 1), perceive Australian health policy as buffeted by a variety of political, institutional, and structural pressures, which have brought about a more unstable and unpredictable policy environment than was previously the case. They investigate the ways in which these pressures are reshaping primary, acute, and extended care.

At the governmental level, shared responsibility for health policy variously gratifies and frustrates policy makers and policy analysts involved in Australia's complicated federal system of governance. The federal government remains the major source of funding through Medicare rebates to individuals and through the Australian Health Care Agreements, under which the states and territories are financially assisted to maintain public hospital services. These agreements allow Canberra to use funding to influence health policy at the subnational level. The federal government has also sought to take a leadership role in such areas as bioethics, health information management, research, and public health. Federal and state governments have, through formal and informal processes, developed co-operative practices while still engaging in conflict (often of a ritualistic nature) about health policy, and in particular health care financing. Conflict within the federal political system may be intensified at times by the admixture of competing political parties holding power at the different levels of government. Many of the issues and controversies surrounding the interplay of federalism, party politics, and national health care policy are described and analysed by Hancock (chapter 2), who also explores the tensions between the ideals of autonomy for the states within a federal system and the imperatives of developing national policies.

Australia's universal compulsory national health insurance scheme, Medicare, continues to underpin the health care system. Financed almost entirely from general taxation revenue, but also from a levy on taxable income, Medicare offers free or subsidised access to medical services and free accommodation and treatment in public hospitals, as well as in private hospitals that have been contracted to treat public patients. Approximately three-quarters of consultations with general practitioners are bulk billed, thereby providing care at no direct cost to patients. Not surprisingly, such a scheme has proved highly popular with the general public, a political reality not lost on the major political parties.

Since its introduction in 1948, the Pharmaceutical Benefits Scheme has been a prominent feature of the health policy landscape. Aiming to provide access to effective and necessary medications, the scheme subsidises three-quarters of all prescriptions filled in Australia. Such a scheme has posed continuing problems for medicinal drug policy makers who have increasingly sought to balance the goal of equitable access with the imperatives of cost-effectiveness. The federal government has now extended the evidence-based research approach taken to pharmaceuticals, to medical interventions and their reimbursement. It will take many years before this gains acceptance by the medical profession's various political associations, which see it as challenging the art of medical judgment and medical autonomy.

General practitioners still constitute the bedrock of the health care system, and public policy has sought to strengthen and further 'professionalise' their role. In the 2001 Budget extra funds were allocated to enable general practitioners to conduct longer consultations with their patients.

The Australian Medical Association remains an important player in the health policy process, albeit within a system characterised by increasing plurality in the expression of sectional interests and institutionalisation of consumer participation in many health policy processes. The new Minister for Health, Dr Kay Patterson, appointed after the Coalition's election victory in 2001, will bring health experience and a consensus management style, together with a concern for consumers, to the renamed Department of Health and Ageing. Public hospitals, enlarged in many cases by the process of amalgamation, continue to capture much of the popular policy imagination as they seek to operate in a climate of continuing tight financial control and scrutiny. Waiting lists and their attendant political consequences endure as a policy issue.

Continuity is also evident in the articulation of values about health care. Equity remains as a consensual policy goal, although the devices employed to seek its attainment remain contested. The universality principle of Medicare has been modified by proponents of a residualist view that those who can afford to do so should insure privately, thereby freeing up public hospital services for those who really need them. In a major policy change the Liberal–National Party Coalition government sought to boost the uptake of private health insurance by a carrot-and-stick approach, introducing a 30 per cent premium rebate and a higher premium for those older than 30, which increased progressively by 2 per cent per year. An impost of 1 per cent on the Medicare surcharge for higher income earners if they had not insured privately was also introduced. This was a system of lifetime health cover rather than the previous community rating. As a result of these policies, the number of Australians taking out private health insurance rose sharply. The implications for equity from this shift towards an emphasis upon private health insurance are discussed by Grbich (chapter 3), who sees these developments as part of a continuing ambiguity in the universality of Medicare and as a further weakening of the welfare state in Australia.

Computer and electronic communications technologies offer unprecedented capacities to record, store, manipulate, and transfer health data. The federal government has encouraged the computerisation of health records, even offering subsidies to general practitioners to install such systems in their practices. In their survey of the burgeoning agenda of health information policy in Australia, Roberts, Robinson, and Williamson (chapter 4) identify the huge potential benefits offered by information technology in the health system, but also identify some of the accompanying practical and ethical issues, including the need for the privacy of patients to be safeguarded and the necessity for a national approach to be taken. The speed with which information technology continues to develop has given added meaning to the belief that much public policy is made on the run. This chapter is an important inclusion in the book as, although health information, for example, now provides the data upon which health funding such as casemix is based, it has received very little acknowledgment or detailed treatment outside the profession's own publications.

The National Public Health Partnership represents an attempt to foster effective intergovernmental relationships and develop a broadly based forum of nongovernment organisations. In her account of this innovation, Lin (chapter 5) sees a number of valuable lessons for health policy, including the benefits of a whole-of-system approach, with an emphasis on public health infrastructure and capacity rather than a narrower focus on specific health issues. Walker, Gardner, and Robinson (chapter 6) take up the importance of intergovernmental relationships in public health and health promotion. They analyse the origins of strategic alliances and show them working at different levels of government, including local government, within a network of health and other organisations.

Although it is health care that retains its dominance over the distribution of resources in Australian health policy, as the aforementioned chapters and the one by Brown, Nicholson and Stephenson (chapter 7) demonstrate, environmental health and health promotion have become increasingly prominent in health policy discourse. International influences on Australian health policy are not merely of an economic nature. Multilateral treaties are increasingly cited in policy discourse to advocate particular courses of action, as has been seen in disputes about policy on heroin injecting rooms and assisted reproduction for single women. Conflict in the field of environmental policy came to the public fore as an international issue in the case of the Kyoto Protocol on climate control, with the Australian government weighing the domestic economic and political consequences of accepting lower rates of carbon emissions against Australia's international reputation. But it was prior to this that Australian governments had begun to develop an environmental health strategy, followed by an implementation strategy reaching into the community, with its subsequent action plans. And even prior to these there were many initiatives, such as Healthy Cities. The various and complex strands are traced in this important chapter. Environmental health must take its place as the health direction for the future. We have been, and continue to be, far too slow in recognising its importance.

Many of the themes from part 1 are taken up in depth in part 2, 'Case Studies of the Health Policy Process'. In the biomedical realm conflict persists about a range of ethical issues. Federal and state governments find themselves seeking to accommodate disparate policy pressures about such things as reproductive technology and assisted euthanasia. The Commonwealth government is brokering a national agreement to develop a uniform policy approach to reproductive technology. Several state governments sought to broaden the policy process by holding drug summits, at which diverse views were expressed as to how the growing problem with illicit drugs should be handled. Indeed, the issue of illicit drugs and their control provides a practical example of the ways in which values can engender seemingly insoluble conflict in health policy. Moves to experiment with safe injecting rooms on the part of some state and territory governments faced strong opposition from the federal government, which argued that its policy of being tough on drugs would be compromised by any toleration of illegal drug use. Despite this opposition, at least one state chose to experiment with a policy of harm-minimisation. In mid 2001, Australia's first legally sanctioned injecting room was opened in the inner Sydney suburb of King's Cross.

Alongside these familiar features, change is also evident—changed that calls into question some of the conventional assumptions and conceptual models previously employed to understand the dynamics of health policy in Australia. The chapters in this book suggest that the shifting political economy of health care in Australia calls into question previous assumptions about fundamental policy differences towards Medicare and private insurance on the part of the major political parties. Previous overt hostility towards Medicare on the part of the Liberal–National Coalition has mellowed into a grudging acceptance of the scheme as a continuing institution with wide popular—and hence electoral—support. In the 2001 Budget, the scope of Medicare was actually enlarged for the first time since its inception by allocating funds to subsidise visits to psychologists. For its part, the Australian Labor Party has—equally grudgingly—endorsed public subsidies for private health insurance, a decision that it simultaneously dismissed as bad policy.

The Australian health care system has become considerably more corporatised and subject to market forces in terms of the ownership of health facilities. Commercial investment in the health care system is increasingly evident in the hospital and general practice sectors. Governments appear to have looked favourably on private participation in the public health care system, perhaps believing that it increases competition—a significant factor given that all health legislation is subject to National Competition Policy— although corporatisation in health has mostly occurred through benign neglect: without interference, but also without government involvement. It has been at a distance. The term 'partnership' has sometimes masked a policy predilection for privatisation. Colocations of corporate commercial operations have become commonplace in major public hospitals.

The distinction between the private and public sectors is not clearly discerned; nor has general practice escaped the involvement of big capital. As is evident in the exploration of current research on general practice, large corporations have been buying out general practices and applying managed care techniques with a view to increasing profits, and perhaps decreasing the quality of patient care. The medical profession has also faced policy pressure from the federal government to reduce or eradicate the gap payment faced by privately insured patients. Private insurance agencies have sought contracts with care providers with the aim of pegging prices. Not surprisingly, many in the medical profession have resented what they regard as American-style managed care eroding their historical role as arbiters of the cost and degree of medical care.

Willis (chapter 8) regards citizens, health professionals, the state, and the private-for-profit sector as the major groups of interests that influence Australian health policy. She provides three case studies, each describing the ways in which an interest group can capitalise on state-based reforms. The National General Practice Strategy and the National Rural Health Strategy illustrate the ways in which the medical profession has effectively bargained with the government to maximise its own interests. However, the cost of the struggle to general practitioners is found in recent developments in the corporatisation of general practice. The third case study, women's health policy, provides the opportunity to explore how policy can be influenced by a social movement and then be recaptured by a medical interest group. Willis suggests that the case studies show that, as with any game, there are winners and losers, but the more important issue might be who owns the stadium and who decides what game is being played. Is the game about the health of citizens or the health of the market? Raising these issues is an important factor in understanding the shape of health care policy and the impact of shifts in ideology and practice. Opening up the welfare state to market forces can make it difficult to control.

How, then, do other health professionals fare? What of women in the health sector, not as consumers but as providers? The vast majority of nurses are still women, although in general medical practice the numbers of men and women are more even. There is a strong demarcation in the Australian health care system between those service providers who are self-employed and those working for a salary in the public or private sectors. Although the overwhelming majority of medical and dental practitioners and some allied health professionals are self-employed, most allied health professionals are employees. But it is nurses who constitute the most numerous category of health professionals employed in the health care sector, and who, after decades of attempting to establish their rightful position as an irreplaceable part of that sector, have still not achieved appropriate recognition. A substantial support staff is also employed to provide the 'hotel' side of hospital care, although the free market is also in evidence here in the many functions that are contracted out to the private sector.

Labour relations in the health sector have not been immune from wider influences, such as the decline in trade union membership and the advent of enterprise bargaining. Enterprise bargaining is a federal industrial relations policy, supported by both major political parties as an alternative to the previous system of centralised awards in setting wages and conditions. Labour costs are a major element of public health care expenditure and, since governments (particularly at the state level) are a major employer, they have sought to increase workplace productivity by a number of means. As Stanton's chapter (chapter 9) on workplace reform in the public health care sector explains, in addition to the introduction of enterprise bargaining, workplace reform has included new funding schemes, cost control, and the use of private service providers.

Consumerism is evident in the nature of health services and necessitates a recognition that the use of complementary therapies is a permanent and continuing feature of the health system Their recognition by public policy has, at least in the past, been largely perfunctory and the scientific evidence for the efficacy of many of the therapies remains undemonstrated, such therapies are nevertheless part of the globalisation of health. Although in Australia there is no equivalent in national health policy to Britain's homoeopathic hospitals, some jurisdictions have legislated to regulate traditional Chinese medicine, and a number of private insurance agencies have recognised certain complementary therapies. The federal government, through the Therapeutic Goods Administration, has intensified the monitoring of traditional remedies, while the Office for Complementary Medicine has been established to regulate the industry. As Eastwood argues (chapter 10), complementary therapies continue to gain popular legitimacy and have become a billion-dollar element of the health industry. Yet, despite some regulatory action on the part of governments, public policy has not adequately responded to the manifest demands of consumers who have enthusiastically embraced such therapies, as indeed have some pharmaceutical manufacturers.

The role of big capital and the willingness of the state to subsidise private health care suggest that, after some decades of being unfashionable, the politics and analytical approaches from political economy might make a comeback in the theoretical exploration of Australia's contemporary health care system. Moreover, the developments described by Grbich and Willis, and by O'Connor and Peterson (chapter 11) suggest that the longstanding assumption of medical dominance in Australian health policy literature is no longer tenable. The growth of for-profit ownership of health facilities and services will also require a rethinking of the ways in which structural interests are identified in the Australian health care system.

Corporate rationalists from the commercial sector certainly have a vested interest in promoting rational policies, such as managed care, in the face of professional monopolist resistance. Yet the profit motive will, at times, bring them into conflict with the wider rationality of public policy. There is commercial rationality in the vertical integration of general practice, pathology and radiology services, pharmacies, and hospitals under a single corporation. However, such an arrangement could well lead to over-servicing and the erosion of competition, thereby inviting the intervention of government to restore a wider public policy rationality.

Evidence-based health appears to be completely rational and yet, for consumers of health care, a different rationality might be operating. Daly, Hughes, and op't Hoog (chapter 12) are sceptical of the claims of the proponents of evidence-based health and argue that public policy has failed to evaluate adequately its promised benefits for the clients, for whom non-compliance—or reduced compliance—is both rational and life enhancing. The clients in this chapter speak movingly for themselves rather than being reflected in policy.

The ways in which disease and illness are part of the health policy process are important considerations, since most health policy is directed towards the acute sector, and towards cure rather than care. Creelman (chapter 13) explores the ways in which chronic illness is defined in health policy domains and analyses the policy ramifications of the conflicting perspectives of those living with chronic illness, the health professionals treating them, and, more particularly, the people who care for them. By legislating to provide support for the carers, the federal government is recognising carers' importance to those with a chronic illness, and to the health sector, in that they allow a person with a chronic illness to remain at home as long as possible.

Increasingly, the hitherto largely domestic concerns of health policy have been influenced by international factors, sometimes labelled 'globalisation'. These influences derive from economic and intellectual sources. The Australian health industry is inescapably linked to the global economy. Pharmaceuticals, therapeutic devices, consultancy services, even health professionals, are international commodities, but many of the technologies imported from Europe and North America are proving increasingly costly for an Australian economy suffering a longstanding adverse balance of payments and a currency declining in value against the developed nations.

In a chapter devoted to export issues, Barraclough and Neil (chapter 14) explore the manifest potential of the Australian health industry to sell its goods and services internationally. They trace policy on the promotion of health industry exports from its origins to concerns about Australia's declining global trade performance. Federal and state governments have sought to promote health exports, thereby creating confusion about a national brand and sometimes encouraging dysfunctional competition. Public funding for health export promotion has been modest and spasmodic. There is a pressing need for state and federal governments to work more cooperatively and in a coordinated way to foster greater export consciousness within the Australian health industry, and to identify and act upon export opportunities. The often competing interests of industry and governments are also explored by Smith (chapter 15). As Smith says, 'Food is a prerequisite for health and … is also a potential source of health problems.' So, food is always of interest to almost everyone.

Many of the chapters in the second edition of *Health Policy in Australia* emphasise the changes in values that have played such an important part in shaping and continuing to shape the health sector. Policy makers often adopt an internationally comparative approach, seeking to benchmark against world's best practice and explore performance indicators that might suggest reforms in Australia. These international values, however, do take on a particularly Australian flavour when implemented. It is a reciprocal process, whereby Australian health strategies and initiatives such as the tobacco campaign have been exported to many countries, and Australia has been a major contributor to disease studies worldwide.

PART 1

THE AUSTRALIAN HEALTH SYSTEM

1

Health Policy and Financing

Hal Swerissen and Stephen Duckett

Current arrangements

The past forty years of debate about the Australian health care system have been dominated by a debate about private versus universal insurance models to pay for health services, with the Liberal–National Coalition supporting the former, and the Australian Labor Party the latter. Following a long period of stabilisation through the reintroduction of a universal health insurance model by the Hawke government during the 1980s, the election of the Howard government in the mid 1990s saw a shift back to private insurance. International influences from Europe and the USA in the funding, planning, and management of the health system have been the subject of intense scrutiny in the recent past.

There is now a general recognition that significant improvements in the performance of the health system are possible, but to achieve them will require change in the relationships between the Commonwealth and state governments and in the way in which health services are planned, organised, and funded. The advocates for change range from the evolutionary to the revolutionary, but there are also significant interests in favour of the status quo.

In order to understand the pressures for change and their likely outcomes it is important to have first a reasonable understanding of the current features of the Australian system and how it has evolved. From there the discussion proceeds to current issues and the possible options for their resolution.

The Commonwealth derives its main powers for direct involvement in health policy through section 51(xxiiiA), section 51(ix), and section 96 of the Constitution. Section 51(xxiiiA) provides the Commonwealth's broad

Table 1.1 Total health service expenditure (current prices), by area of expenditure and source of funds, 1997-98 ($ million)

Area of expenditure	Government sector			Nongovernment sector				Total all sectors
	Commonwealth	State and local	Total	Health insurance funds	Individuals	Other	Total	
Total hospitals	6 343	6 437	12 780	2 607	418	1 095	4 120	16 900
recognised public hospitals	5 711	6 080	11 851	311	79	595	986	12 836
private hospitals	550	–	550	2 295	321	493	3 109	3 658
repatriation hospitals	15	–	15	–	–	–	–	15
public psychiatric hospitals	7	357	365	–	18	7	25	390
Nursing homes	2 575	137	2 712	–	608	–	608	3 320
Ambulance	90	281	370	106	129	38	273	643
Total institutional	9 007	6 855	15 862	2 712	1 155	1 133	5 000	20 863
Medical services	6 970	–	6 970	217	897	419	1 533	8 503
Other professional services	219	–	219	214	1 046	173	1 434	1 653
Total pharmaceuticals	2 785	16	2 801	34	2 463	37	2 534	5 335
benefit paid pharmaceuticals	2 783	–	2 783	–	593	–	593	3 377
all other pharmaceuticals	2	16	18	34	1 869	37	1 941	1 959
Aids and appliances	174	–	174	177	435	38	649	823
Other noninstitutional services	1 380	2 086	3 466	1 080	1 611	8	2 699	6 165
community and public health	775	1 357	2 132	1	–	–	1	2 133
dental services	76	328	404	568	1 611	8	2 187	2 591
administration	529	401	930	511	–	–	511	1 441
Research	427	96	523	–	–	129	129	652
Total noninstitutional	11 956	2 197	14 154	1 721	6 452	805	8 978	23 132
Total recurrent expenditure	**20 964**	**9 053**	**30 016**	**4 434**	**7 606**	**1 938**	**13 978**	**43 994**
Capital expenditure	70	1 400	1 470	n.a.	n.a.	n.a.	994	2 464
Capital consumption	34	538	572	–	–	–	–	572
Total health expenditure	**21 068**	**10 990**	**32 058**	**n.a.**	**n.a.**	**n.a.**	**14 972**	**47 030**

Figures in each cell have been rounded

Source: AIHW 2000, p. 404

power to provide health services and benefits directly to the Australian people through programs such as Medicare and the Pharmaceutical Benefits Scheme. Through section 51(ix) the Commonwealth has quarantine powers and section 96 gives the Commonwealth power to make grants to the states for specific purposes, such as health, as it sees fit. These tied grants, or Specific Purpose Payments (SPPs), are usually made as part of a Commonwealth–state agreement.

As table 1.1 indicates, total Australian expenditure on health in 1997–98 was $47 billion, of which the Commonwealth government provided $21 billion, the states and local government $10.9 billion, and the private sector $14.9 billion, made up of payments by health insurance funds and individuals. In 1997–98, 68.6 per cent of all health expenditure was provided by government (Australian Institute of Health and Welfare 2000).

In 1996–97 the Commonwealth government raised $3.6 billion through its 1.5 per cent Medicare levy on taxable income (Department of Health and Aged Care 1999a). The Medicare levy is not hypothecated for health expenditure but even if it were it would only have funded 18.5 per cent of 1996–97 Commonwealth health outlays. In reality, the Commonwealth's health expenditure is funded through its general revenue raising powers. The states fund their direct contributions to health outlays through their own, much more limited, revenue raising capacity.

That the states have insufficient revenue raising capacity to fund their outlays while the Commonwealth raises significantly more revenue than it needs for its own purpose expenditure is known as 'vertical fiscal imbalance'. To overcome vertical fiscal imbalance, the shortfall experienced by the states has traditionally been made up by the Commonwealth through Financial Assistance Grants (FAGs) and SPPs. Vertical fiscal imbalance gives the Commonwealth significant influence in state health policy, particularly through the use of SPPs.

Commencing on 1 July 2000, FAGs were replaced by funding provided to the states through revenue from a goods and services tax (GST). The Commonwealth, together with the states and territories, agreed on a range of matters related to the disbursement of the GST and related tax changes. In general, the replacement of FAGs by GST funding provides the states with access to a broadbased and growing revenue stream that they are able to use as they see fit. In principle this has the potential to reduce vertical fiscal imbalance.

However, the impact of these revised arrangements remains uncertain and a number of components of the new arrangements remain to be implemented. Additionally, it will be some time before the GST revenue stream is sufficient to reach the level of assistance that was provided through FAGs. In the interim, the Commonwealth continues to allocate additional funds to the states through Budget Balancing Assistance (BBA) grants to make up the shortfall.

Importantly, although the GST arrangements are intended as direct payments to the states, they remain the province of Commonwealth legislation, which can at any time be changed by the Commonwealth parliament. Similarly, although the Commonwealth has indicated that it does not propose to alter arrangements that apply to SPPs, there is no guarantee this will not occur when GST growth exceeds the FAGs payments that would otherwise have been made to the states.

Medical services, hospitals, pharmaceuticals, and nursing homes made up about 72 per cent of all expenditure in 1997–98 at a total cost of \$34 billion (see table 1.1). With the assistance of Commonwealth funds, the states are largely responsible for the direct funding and operation of public hospitals, psychiatric institutions, and nonmedical community and public health services. The Commonwealth directly funds medical and pharmaceutical rebates and residential aged care.

Primary care and medical services

Most Australians have their primary contact with the health system through consultations with general practitioners (GPs). The vast majority of GPs work privately in autonomous sole or small group practices earning income from fee-for-service consultations. Australian Institute of Health and Welfare (AIHW) data (1998) indicate that, in 1998–99, the majority of the population visited one of Australia's more than 44 156 GPs at least once. General practice provided around half of all Medicare rebated medical services—more than 102 million in that year (Health Insurance Commission 1999, table 6)—making it the main form of health care for the general community and the gateway to more intensive and specialised services such as hospital and institutional care.

Medicare is a national health insurance scheme, which ensures that Australians have universal access to affordable medical services. About 20 per cent of recurrent health expenditure goes to medical services. All Australians are able to claim a rebate for medical services through Medicare: 85 per cent of the Commonwealth Medical Benefits Schedule (MBS) is provided for services outside hospital and 75 per cent of the schedule fee for private patient services in public and private hospitals. A safety net limits the total yearly gap between the rebate and the schedule fee that families and individuals are required to pay.

Medical practitioners can send patient bills direct to the Health Insurance Commission (HIC), which administers Medicare, instead of billing their patients, provided they accept the 85 per cent rebate as full payment. What they lose in fees they avoid in bad debts and administrative costs. Many medical practitioners request direct payment from the HIC by submitting their patient bills as a bulk transaction on a regular periodic timetable. This practice is known as bulk billing. The proportion of bulk-billed services has risen steadily since the introduction of Medicare; 72 per cent of medical services were effectively free to patients through bulk billing in 1998–99. Consumer surveys conducted by the HIC indicate that 82 per cent of the community is highly satisfied with Medicare and 88 per cent supports the program (Health Insurance Commission 1999).

Of the $6.9 billion paid out in Medicare benefits for 1999/2000, $2.4 billion went to GPs, $1.1 billion to pathology, $1.1 billion to diagnostic imaging, and $1 billion to specialist consultations. A further $680 million went to operations, anaesthetics, and obstetrics (Health Insurance Commission 2000).

Since its introduction on 1 February 1984, Medicare expenditure has grown at an average yearly rate, adjusting for inflation, of about 5 per cent in real terms, although recently the real rate of increase has slowed sharply. Over the same period the average number of medical consultations per person in Australia has increased from 6.3 to 10.5. In 1998–99, Medicare provided 206 million services at a cost of about $351 per person (Health Insurance Commission 1999, table 16).

Over the past decade, the Commonwealth has moved to reform general practice. There are concerns about efficiency, effectiveness, quality, and access. Most importantly, Australia has too many GPs and they are too concentrated in urban areas, particularly in Sydney and Melbourne. As a result, while there is a significant oversupply in capital cities, some rural and remote areas struggle to attract a GP. Because Medicare tax funded rebates to GPs are delivered regardless of where they practice, it is difficult to create sufficient incentives to attract GPs to country areas.

Moreover, the oversupply of GPs has been one of the factors leading to unnecessary growth in Medicare costs. Few people who visit a medical practitioner are in a position to determine whether the services they receive are necessary or beneficial, particularly given that many of the conditions presented to GPs are self-limiting. As the supply of GPs has increased, the per capita consultation rate has gone up even though the average number of consultations per GP has remained relatively constant. Since the introduction of Medicare the proportion of services provided effectively without direct cost to the patients—that is, through bulk billing—has increased dramatically, reaching 80 per cent in 1997 with a slight decline to 79 per cent in 2000. This suggests that as the ratio of GPs per capita has grown, GPs have maintained their incomes by progressively increasing the number of consultations per patient. At the same time, competition between GPs has forced them to reduce out-of-pocket costs to patients through bulk billing. The net result is the unnecessary growth in the number of consultations and flow-on costs in diagnostics, pharmaceutical services, and referrals to specialists.

Despite its positive public image there are also significant concerns about the quality of general practice. Traditionally, general practice has been seen as a safety valve for those who were unable to gain entrance into specialist medical colleges. Specialist training and registration for general practice was not required, nor was continued practice conditional upon an ongoing commitment to further medical education and training.

Perhaps most importantly, because of its essentially isolated, small-business culture, accountability and coordination in general practice are poor. There are few requirements and incentives to act cooperatively with other health professionals and agencies. There are no requirements to participate in local health planning processes or to respond to community needs. Practices are not required to be accredited against accepted professional standards or criteria to safeguard treatment and patient rights.

During the period of the Whitlam Labor government (1972–75), attempts were made to reform primary care through the introduction of a community health program, which sought to establish community con-trolled health services to provide integrated primary health care, including medical and nursing care, particularly in areas with poor access to these ser-vices. Despite widespread opposition from the medical profession, resistance by some state governments and the curtailment and subsequent dissolution of the program by the Commonwealth, community health services devel-oped as an important focus for reform of the primary care system. In Victo-ria, for example, there are state-funded community health agencies in virtually all local government areas. In contrast to private general practice, these centres are community controlled and offer an integrated range of treatment, preventive, and advocacy services, in a number of cases including medical care. As well, the community health program led to a national (and international) focus on primary care through such developments as the establishment of the Australian Community Health Association.

Fundamentally, however, when the Commonwealth rolled community health funding into the Medicare grants and made community health a state responsibility during the 1980s it became difficult for community health ser-vices to be the main catalyst for change in primary medical care, given that the Commonwealth retained responsibility for these services through Medicare. By the early 1990s, a new approach, known as the general practice reform strategy, was developed.

The general practice reform strategy aims to improve access, quality, effectiveness, and efficiency.

First, general practice is being reorganised through the creation of Divisions of General Practice. Divisions provide the infrastructure to coordinate a range of activities relevant to general practice. Unlike the community health program, divisions are controlled by GPs and largely act as professional and administrative agencies. Typically, they coordinate project funds and other activities for between 100 and 300 GPs.

Second, the Practice Incentives Program has been introduced to provide incentives to improve the quality and accountability of GP services. Payments are made to practices for information management and technology, after-hours care, rurality, teaching medical students, and targeted programs such as immunisation and participation in prescribing reviews.

Third, incentives were provided to encourage GPs to practise in undersupplied rural areas through the Rural Incentives Program. This program provided payments to GPs for relocation to rural and remote areas, and for training expenses.

Fourth, the Commonwealth moved to improve GP training and reduce oversupply by requiring GPs to be vocationally registered in order to gain access to GP Medicare payments. Following an initial 'grandparenting' period, GPs were required to participate in a general practice training program run by the Royal Australian College of General Practice in order to become vocationally registered.

Most recently, with the stabilisation of the growth of Medicare expenditure on general practice, the emphasis of reform has shifted to the quality of general practice. The Commonwealth and the profession have established a Memorandum of Understanding that commits the profession and the Commonwealth to the development and implementation of a quality framework for general practice within agreed overall funding arrangements for GPs. The Commonwealth has also introduced changes to the fee schedule for GPs to encourage them to participate in care assessment, care planning, and case conferencing.

However, new pressures on general practice are emerging. Recently, there has been a significant trend towards the development of large general practice organisations through the corporatisation of existing practices. It is likely that general practice will progressively shift from a predominantly small-business, professional-ownership model to a mixed model that includes larger corporate business structures that employ GPs in vertically integrated organisations, including pathology and diagnostic services, private hospitals, and other health services.

It is also arguable that the Commonwealth's reform strategy is too narrowly focused on GPs. New information and care technologies, changes in consumer expectations, demand-pressures on acute and residential care, and increased demands associated with an ageing population are likely to see renewed interest in the development of a broader primary care and community services reform agenda.

Pharmaceuticals

Expenditure on pharmaceuticals makes up about 10 per cent of recurrent health outlays (see table 1.1). The Pharmaceutical Benefits Scheme (PBS) ensures that all Australians have access to affordable medicines as prescribed by medical practitioners. Those on low incomes who are eligible for health care cards have, for a relatively modest patient contribution per PBS item ($3.50 in 2001), access to drugs listed on the PBS. Prescriptions become free for concessional users for the remainder of a given year once they incur a cost of the equivalent of 52 patient contributions ($182 in 2001). Pensioners are provided with a yearly pharmaceuticals allowance equivalent to the cost of the safety net. General users, comprising the remainder of the population—that is, those without health care cards—are required to make a larger patient contribution per item ($21.90 in 2001), and the safety net ($669.70 in 2001) is less generous (Health Insurance Commission 2001).

In 1998–99 total expenditure on the PBS was $2.8 billion for 18.9 million scripts or an average of 6.6 prescriptions per person (Health Insurance Commission 1999, tables 14 and 15). The majority of this expenditure was made on concessional payments ($1.85 billion), with general payments making up the bulk of the remainder ($469 million). Expenditure on pharmaceuticals has increased as a proportion of recurrent health expenditure from 8.6 per cent in 1984–85 to 12.1 per cent in 1997–98 (Australian Institute of Health and Welfare 2000, p. 240). In the period 1982–83 to 1994–95 the average real annual cost increase for the PBS was 8.2 per cent—or, allowing for population growth, 6.8 per cent per person. Over this period the average yearly number of prescriptions per person fell by 0.3 per cent. The major reason that costs continued to increase while the number of prescriptions fell was the introduction of new, more costly pharmaceutical products, such as ACE inhibitors to treat hypertension (Sloan 1995).

Hospitals

The blend of public and private and Commonwealth and state that characterises the Australian health care system is nowhere more evident than in arrangements for provision and financing of hospitals. State governments establish, regulate, and fund public hospitals that provide both inpatient and ambulatory care. State governments also regulate private hospitals that have been established by private entrepreneurs and religious orders or bodies, as well as other not-for-profit organisations such as community hospitals.

Medicare ensures that all Australians can be treated, without charge, in public hospitals. This policy is effected through the Commonwealth–state Australian Health Care Agreements, which define the formulae by which Commonwealth funds flow to the states and territories for provision of care to public patients, and specify the obligations of the states in return for this funding. Under the Medicare agreements these Commonwealth funds account for about half the running costs of public hospitals. In 1997–98, the Commonwealth provided $12 852 million to the states and territories for public hospitals; the states provided $6437 million from their own sources (Australian Institute of Health and Welfare 2000). Over the period 1992–93 to 1997–98, in real terms and allowing for inflation, Commonwealth funding to the states and territories through the Medicare Agreements increased by 1.5 per cent, up to 45.2 per cent, while state and territory funding remained static at 23.4 per cent (Australian Institute of Health and Welfare 2000).

The current agreements run for five years from 1 July 1998. The Commonwealth provides its funding to the states from the Hospital Funding Grant (HFG). The HFG is distributed among the states by the Commonwealth on a needs basis, according to each state and territory's share of the total population, and weighted by age and sex to take account of different patterns of health service utilisation.

However, understanding funding for public hospitals is made substantially more complicated because the HFG is included in the calculation of FAGs' recommendations for the states and territories made by the Commonwealth Grants Commission (CGC). The allocation of FAGs is subject to a process known as fiscal equalisation. The aim of fiscal equalisation is to ensure that each state and territory has the capacity to provide an average level of services without being required to levy above average taxes and charges. The CGC makes recommendations to ensure that states and territories that face additional difficulties in providing public services as a result of remoteness, dispersion, climate, social composition, and other factors are compensated through FAGs.

The Commonwealth Grants Commission determines the relative funding allocations by calculating the average funding per person that would be required in each state and territory to achieve fiscal equalisation. These averages are known as per capita funding relativities. Among the factors that the CGC takes into consideration in determining relativities are the different shares of public and private provision of health services in different states. The logic is that if the private sector is providing more, then the state or territory has less need to provide public health services. Thus, states or territories with relatively high private provision, such as New South Wales and Victoria, have had funds redistributed away from them and towards states with lower private provision. Redistributions have also occurred in other functional areas and have generally disadvantaged New South Wales and Victoria.

In effect, the base HFG component—which makes up the bulk of the Australian Health Care Agreements—and FAGs are combined and allocated according to the CGC relativities. As a result the needs–based allocation of funds through the agreements is effectively overridden by the application of the CGC relativities. This has caused considerable irritation for successive Commonwealth health ministers and their state and territory counterparts.

In order to deal with these problems the most recent Australian Health Care Agreements have reduced the base HFG and redistributed these funds as bonus payments that are not subject to CGC adjustment. The agreements were designed to recognise the past efforts of states and territories in providing public access with bonus payments to reward future improvements in public access. These bonus payments replace the adjustments that the CGC has made to relativities based on their assessment of public and private shares in the health area.

Another feature of the latest agreements is to require states and territories to pay each other directly for services provided to their residents by other states and territories. This again replaces a function that has been covered by the CGC. In both cases, the adjustments in the Medicare arrangements were designed to be more timely, visible and understandable, and based on better and more up–to–date data than the adjustments made in the past by the CGC.

Public hospitals also admit private patients, who are required to pay an accommodation charge, which is about one-half of the cost of care; the balance is made up by a subsidy from the relevant state or territory government and the cost of medical care. A key distinction between public and private patients in public hospitals is that public patients are treated by the relevant specialist or, in smaller hospitals, by the general practitioner on duty for that type of condition or illness—under the terms of the Australian Health Care Agreement, the doctor nominated by the hospital—whereas private patients in public hospitals are able to nominate a specialist or general practitioner of their own choosing (who has an appointment at the hospital) to be responsible for their care.

Generally, public hospitals are accountable to a board of directors appointed by the state or territory minister for health. Boards employ a chief executive (who has day-to-day responsibility) and other clinical, support, and administrative staff. As a rule, boards have responsibility for a number of public hospitals and, in some states and territories, also have responsibility for nonhospital services (table 1.2).

Table 1.2 Hospital governance arrangements by state, January 1996

State*	Name of hospital governing entity	Scope	State funding basis
NSW	Area health service	Hospital and nonhospital health services	Population resource allocation formula
Vic.	Metropolitan health services	Hospital services in metropolitan area, usually including a teaching hospital, a smaller hospital, aged care, and mental health services	Predominantly casemix
	Hospital board	Normally responsible for multiple hospital complexes in rural areas, nursing homes, hostel and community health services	Predominantly casemix
SA	Hospital	Usually single campus	Casemix
WA	Rural health services board	Mixed; some boards responsible for single health service, other multiple services within a region	Casemix
	Metropolitan health services structure under review	All services in metropolitan area	
Qld	Zone (division of public services)	Hospital and nonhospital services	Transition to casemix
Tas.	Regional health authority (no board of directors)	Hospital and nonhospital services	Population resource allocation formula
ACT	Hospital (division of public service)	Hospital services only	Historic funding
NT	Hospital (division of public service)	Hospital services only	Historic funding

* In addition, religious hospitals function in most states and territories

Private hospitals have a variety of governance arrangements (for example, separate boards or part of a hospital chain). Patients in private hospitals are responsible for the full costs of accommodation and medical care. Medicare covers 75 per cent of the scheduled fee for medical services rendered to private patients in public hospitals and patients in private hospitals. Health insurance funds are able to cover the gap between the Medicare rebate and the doctor's charge when the doctor has negotiated a Medical Purchaser Provider Agreement with the fund, or only the gap up to the schedule fee in other cases. Health insurance funds also cover the accommodation charges.

Traditionally, the basis for public-hospitals funding from state and territory governments has been obscure: a hospital's budget reflects a combination of history, negotiating skill, political influence, and luck. Over the last few decades this has been changing. A number of states, including New South Wales, Queensland, and Tasmania, moved towards population resource allocation formulae as a way of funding regional health authorities. The formulae took account of population size, age distribution, and health need, the latter measured in a variety of ways. Funding arrangements between the regional authority and the hospitals for which it was responsible were on a mixture of methods, again involving history, luck, negotiating skill, and so on.

The major change in the way hospitals—rather than regions—are funded has occurred through the development of casemix or output-based funding using diagnosis related groups (DRGs). DRGs are a way of measuring the mix of inpatients ('cases', hence casemix) a hospital treats, distinguishing a patient who receives a heart transplant from one who has an appendix removed. Once patients have been classified into DRGs a standard price can be assigned to each DRG and hospitals paid on the basis of how many patients in each DRG the hospital treats. This method of paying for hospital care was first introduced in Victoria for the 1993–94 year and has since been introduced in South Australia to pay hospitals directly and to modify population formulae in a number of states (Duckett 1998). Noninpatient services of public hospitals (for example, ambulatory care, teaching, research) are also increasingly funded according to output-based formulae.

Using DRGs or other methods, private hospitals increasingly bill patients or health insurance funds on a casemix basis. Where casemix arrangements have not been negotiated between hospitals and funds, payment is usually on a per day of stay (*per diem*) basis.

In 1997–98 there were 5 563 074 separations from hospitals in Australia, with an average length of stay of 4.1 days. A total of almost 22 million days of care was provided (Australian Institute of Health and Welfare 1998, p. 198). Of all separations, 67 per cent were from public acute hospitals and 32 per cent from private hospitals (Australian Institute of Health and Welfare 2000, p. 270). Private patients are increasingly being treated in private hospitals rather than as private patients in public hospitals. About 40 per cent of private patients were treated in public hospitals in 1989/90, dropping to 31 per cent in 1994–95).

The overall capacity of the system measured in available beds has been roughly constant over the past few years (about 22 million bed days in 1997–98), but the mix of provision has changed slightly (67 per cent of bed days were in public acute hospitals in 1997–98 compared with 74 per cent in 1995–96), which in part reflects budget cuts in public hospitals. Despite the constant capacity, the number of patients treated is increasing overall (public patients up from just under 2 million in 1989–90 to 3.7 million in 1997–8; private patients are down slightly from 1.8 million to 1.7 million over the same period). The ability to cope with this increase is partly attributable to the increase in day surgery and day procedures (Australian Institute of Health and Welfare, 2000, p. 270).

Aged care

The Commonwealth has substantially taken control of care for elderly people. From 1971 to 1991 the number of people aged 65 years and over doubled, and it is estimated that this figure will grow by a further third by 2010 (Australian Bureau of Statistics 1994; Clare & Tulpule 1994). About four times more per person is spent on health services for those aged 65 years and over than on younger age groups. Expenditure is partly a function of the association of disease and disability with ageing, particularly for those aged 80 years and older, but it also varies depending on the appropriateness of services. In the past, services were overly focused on nursing home care.

Over the past decade the Commonwealth has embarked on a major aged care reform strategy. The aim has been to provide a needs-based continuum of community, hostel, and nursing home care to complement informal support provided by family, friends, and neighbours. As a result there has been a substantial effort to shift the balance of services from heavily medicalised residential care to greater support in community settings.

The Commonwealth has set a planning target of providing intensive residential and community support for the 10 per cent of those aged 70 years or over with the greatest need. Access to intensive (usually residential) support is determined by Aged Care Assessment Services. Different levels of funding are allocated, depending on the index of care an individual requires (Department of Human Services and Health 1995e).

State and territory governments, not-for-profit organisations, and for-profit providers provide residential care services, with the balance between provider types varying significantly between states and territories. High-intensity services (formerly nursing homes) and low-intensity services (formerly hostels) attract different levels of recurrent and capital subsidies. The Commonwealth funds residential aged care according to the dependency of the resident, measured using a Resident Classification System.

Residential care is complemented by community care provided through the Home and Community Care (HACC) program. The HACC program is jointly funded by the Commonwealth and the states and territories to provide a range of assistance for frail older people, people with disabilities, and their carers living in the community. Services are largely provided by local government and nongovernment agencies. These include nursing, home support, community support, and respite.

How does Australia compare?

In comparison to other member nations of the Organization for Economic Cooperation and Development (OECD), the 8.4 per cent of gross domestic product (GDP) Australians spend on health care is approximately as would be expected (table 1.3). In 1997, 17 of the 29 OECD member states spent between 7 and 9 per cent of GDP on health. Turkey at 4 per cent spent the least, the USA at 13.9 per cent the most. Average expenditure was about 7.8 per cent of GDP (OECD 1999).

Table 1.3   Total health expenditure as a percentage of GDP*

	1960	1965	1970	1975	1980	1985	1990	1995	1997
Australia	4.9	5.1	5.7	7.5	7.3	7.7	8.2	8.4	8.4
Austria	4.3	4.6	5.3	7.2	7.7	6.7	7.2	8.0	8.3
Belgium	3.4	3.9	4.1	5.9	6.5	7.3	7.5	7.9	7.6
Canada	5.4	5.9	7.0	7.2	7.2	8.3	9.2	9.4	9.2
Czech Republic					3.8	4.5	5.4	7.5	7.2
Denmark	3.6		5.9	6.3	9.3	8.7	8.3	8.1	8.0
Finland	3.9	4.9	5.7	6.4	6.5	7.3	8.0	7.7	7.4
France	4.2	5.2	5.8	7.0	7.6	8.5	8.9	9.8	9.6
Germany	4.8	5.1	6.3	8.8	8.8	9.3	8.7	10.4	10.7
Greece	3.1		5.7		6.6		7.6	8.4	8.6
Hungary							6.1	7.0	6.5
Iceland	3.3	3.9	5.0	5.8	6.2	7.3	7.9	8.2	7.9
Ireland	3.8	4.2	5.3	7.7	8.7	7.9	6.7	7.0	6.3
Italy	3.6	4.3	5.2	6.2	7.0	7.1	8.1	7.7	7.6
Japan	3.0	4.5	4.6	5.6	6.5	6.7	6.1	7.2	7.2
Korea			2.3	2.3	3.7	4.3	5.2	5.4	6.0
Luxembourg			3.7	5.1	6.2	6.1	6.6	6.7	7.0
Mexico							3.6	4.9	4.7
Netherlands	3.8	4.3	5.9	7.5	7.9	7.9	8.3	8.8	8.5
New Zealand	4.3		5.2	6.7	6.0	5.3	7.0	7.3	7.6
Norway	2.9	3.5	4.5	6.0	1.0	6.7	7.8	8.0	7.5
Poland							4.4	4.5	5.2
Portugal			2.8	5.6	5.8	6.3	6.4	7.8	7.9
Spain	1.5	2.6	3.7	4.9	5.6	5.7	6.9	7.3	7.4
Sweden	4.7	5.5	7.1	7.9	9.4	9.0	8.8	8.5	8.6
Switzerland	3.1	3.6	4.9	6.6	6.9	7.7	8.3	9.6	10.0
Turkey			2.4	2.7	3.3	2.2	3.6	3.3	4.0
United Kingdom	3.9	4.1	4.5	5.5	5.6	5.9	6.0	6.9	6.8
United States	5.2	5.9	7.3	8.2	9.1	10.6	12.6	14.1	13.9

* Gross domestic product

Source: OECD Health Data 1999

Health spending tends to grow as GDP grows, but when the rate of growth slows or GDP declines, it has proved difficult to rein in health expenditure. As with most other OECD members the proportion of GDP spent on health in Australia has almost doubled since 1960 (OECD 1999). Since the 1980s Australia has held its expenditure in check slightly better than average by holding down growth in real health expenditure per capita and medical-specific price increases.

There are clear differences across nations in their pattern of expenditure. Australia's pattern of health expenditure looks most like that of the USA and Canada. In 1997–98, 38 per cent of health expenditure in Australia was allocated to hospitals, 19 per cent to medical practitioners, 12 per cent to pharmaceuticals, 7.5 per cent to nursing homes, 5.9 per cent to dentists, and 3.8 per cent to other health services. By comparison in 1995 Germany allocated only 28 per cent to hospitals, while Japan spent 53 per cent on medical practitioners and only 1 per cent on nursing homes (OECD 1999).

Like other OECD nations, Australia had a relatively expansionary social policy in the three decades from World War II to 1975. Stable economic growth, low inflation, and low unemployment were accompanied by a perception—fuelled by Keynesian economics and postwar reconstruction—that governments were in the business of nation building. It was a time of comparative hope and optimism, when there was a desire to believe that the social democratic model of strong government could deliver a fair and just world that took care of everyone's needs.

The great insurance debate

Today's health policy had its genesis in the Curtin and Chifley Labour governments during and immediately after the war years. Chifley set the scene with his introduction of the 1946 amendment to the Constitution (section 51(23A)), which permitted the Commonwealth to legislate on—among other things—'pharmaceutical, sickness hospital benefits, medical and dental services (but not so as to authorise and any form of civil conscription)' Chifley's constitutional amendment, although limited by the civil conscription provision negotiated by Menzies at the urging of the British Medical Association in Australia (later to become the Australian Medical Association) forms the basis for the Commonwealth's subsequent development of the Australian welfare state, much of which, paradoxically, was put in place by the Menzies Liberal–National (then Country Party) Coalition government.

The ebb and flow of the health policy debate since Chifley has seen the central parameters remain relatively constant. The chief concerns have been about the mechanisms for financing health care, the extent to which government should direct and regulate hospitals, medical practitioners and other health care providers, and, insofar as these issues are resolved, the relative roles of Commonwealth and state and territory governments.

Chifley conceived a national, universal health care scheme, financed by noncontributory social insurance with government-run medical, hospital, nursing home, and pharmaceutical services as the central features. He envisaged equitable access at an affordable cost to hospital, medical, and pharmaceutical services. Although Menzies' civil conscription amendment largely scotched any notion of a dominant public, salaried medical service, Chifley's scheme nevertheless formed the basis for Labor's Medibank. But it was twenty-three years before the Whitlam Labor government was able to put it into place (see Sax 1984; Crichton 1990).

The Page plan

With the defeat of the Chifley government in 1949, Earle Page, who became Minister for Health during the early period of the Menzies government, modified Chifley's proposals to ensure consistency with Liberal (and Country) Party philosophy, which favoured greater reliance on individual rather than community responsibility. Although the Page plan introduced a framework for a national health system, it did so largely through subsidies and regulation of the private insurance funds for hospital, medical, pharmaceutical, and nursing home care.

In contrast to a universal tax funded scheme, the Page plan provided a safety net for the most disadvantaged while the majority of the population were required to make their own way, mainly through contributory (private) insurance funds. Little attempt was made to regulate or direct the relationship between service providers and the individuals who used them, or to give the states and territories incentives to manage their health care systems. Much to the delight of the AMA, the doctor–patient relationship and private practice were sacrosanct. Doctors charged patients, patients received rebates from insurance funds, and the Commonwealth provided a subsidy, either to the fund or directly to hospitals and nursing homes.

By the late 1960s, a number of inequities and failures had emerged to sow the seeds for the destruction of the Page plan. Seventeen per cent of the population had no insurance or access to public benefits. A further proportion was underinsured. In 1968, the Nimmo Committee, established to investigate widespread complaints about the health system, estimated that at least a million Australians suffered hardship because of the costs of insurance, because gaps between fees and rebates were variable and considerable, and because insurance cover discriminated against the chronically ill and those with pre-existing illnesses. The committee also found that the scheme was 'unnecessarily complex and beyond the comprehension of many'. There was also considerable evidence that the protection of the term 'doctor–patient relationship' was a euphemism for allowing the medical profession, private hospitals, and nursing home providers to capture the health system for their own interests. As a result, there was significant over-servicing, exorbitant and uncontrolled fee increases, and little in the way of sensible planning on the basis of need (Commonwealth Committee of Inquiry into Health Insurance 1969; Sax 1984).

At the time, the national debate split into three camps. The Left of the Australian Labor Party and sections of the union movement wanted to follow the United Kingdom and nationalise the health system. Others, mainly comprising the mainstream of the Australian Labor Party, wanted to introduce a universal social insurance model for health services. And there were those, including the Liberal and Country parties and the AMA, who wanted to retain the Page plan.

Medibank

The Whitlam Labor government's Medibank scheme, strongly influenced by Chifley's underpinning principles and the work of Scotton and Deeble (1968), finally became law in 1974 after a double dissolution and a joint sitting of parliament, which followed a two-year struggle with the Opposition, largely waged in the Opposition-controlled Senate, at the vigorous urging of the AMA, the private hospitals, and the insurance funds. Medibank was designed as a public, noncontributory, national health insurance model, which provided universal access to medical and hospital services, regardless of income. It established the HIC as the dominant insurer, set a schedule of medical rebates, and introduced a range of administrative reforms to improve the efficiency of insurance arrangements, including direct or bulk billing of the HIC by medical practitioners for their services at the level of the Commonwealth MBS rebate. The Commonwealth also used its power to make specific-purpose payments to the states and territories under section 96 of the Constitution, to fund them to provide free standard ward public hospital care (Scotton & MacDonald 1993).

The ink ratifying the Whitlam reforms was hardly dry before his government was defeated in 1975 and history set out on a repeat performance of the 1950s and 1960s. Although Fraser had committed a Coalition government to retaining Medibank, in fact the next seven years saw a faltering and confusing return to the basic Page plan. By 1981 universal, noncontributory insurance had been abandoned in favour of a safety net for the disadvantaged and contributory private insurance with tax rebate incentives for the rest of the population. Bulk billing was largely dropped and copayments became mandatory. Government subsidies were once again provided to private hospitals, nursing homes, and private insurance funds. Responsibility for hospital funding was handed back to the states and territories, which the Commonwealth attempted to force into introducing copayments for public hospital patients.

Fraser introduced these measures in part because the Coalition believed that in order to foster self-reliance and responsible use of services, individuals should provide for their own health care where they were able to do so. But

Fraser's primary problems were fiscal. After twenty-three years of relatively stable and steady economic growth, his government faced simultaneous double-digit inflation and unemployment, a phenomenon beyond the then dominant standard Keynesian economics. As well, in his desire to win the states and territories to his view, Whitlam had introduced extraordinarily generous—if unsustainable—cost-sharing arrangements for public hospital funding. In combination with the Commonwealth taking over responsibility for basic medical insurance, a very substantial increase in Commonwealth outlays was inevitable.

Consequently, much of Fraser's health agenda was driven by a desire to limit growth in Commonwealth health outlays, minimise the impact of health costs on inflation, and reduce overall expenditure on health. Unfortunately for Fraser, these aims were incompatible (Duckett 1984).

By the early 1980s, the same problems that had plagued the Page plan had re-emerged. Private insurance premiums were rising, aggregate costs were escalating, and many Australians were uninsured or underinsured because they were unable to afford the premium costs. People were confused about their responsibilities and entitlements; national health planning was paralysed while ad hoc expansion of hospitals, nursing homes, and other services proliferated, thanks to generous Commonwealth incentives (Sax 1984).

Medicare

Current arrangements (described above), including the Medicare scheme, the establishment of the Medicare Agreements for hospital funding, the continuing evolution of the PBS, and the reforms to aged care were largely put in place by Neal Blewett, Minister for Health in the first term of the Hawke Labor government, which was elected in 1983. More recently, during the period of the Howard government, strengthening private health insurance has again become a major policy objective.

The Howard government has raised concerns that decreasing participation in private health insurance will cause a crisis in public hospitals. From a preMedicare high of 68 per cent in 1982, the proportion of people with private health insurance had dropped to 30 per cent by 1998. People dropping health insurance have been principally the young and healthy, leaving health insurance funds with an older and sicker contributor base, which has been a contributing factor for health insurance premium cost increases. In part, this results from the Commonwealth's commitment to community rather than risk rating for insurance—that is, instead of allowing premiums to reflect the actual risk associated with various age groups, lifestyles, and other actuarial indicators of likely hospital use, which would inevitably result in older people paying higher premiums than younger people, health insurance premiums costs are equalised for all members. Premiums only vary as a function of the level of coverage provided. On average, younger, healthier people pay more than their risk warrants, while older people, as greater risks, pay less.

In early 1996 the annual cost for family health insurance to cover most accommodation costs in private hospitals ranged from about $1200–$2500, depending on the fund and the state or territory. As well, those using private hospitals often found themselves with multiple and substantial unanticipated out-of-pocket costs once they left hospital. These costs came about largely because specialist medical practitioners charged above the Medicare schedule fee. Individual patients had relatively little ability to negotiate fee levels with their medical practitioner and in many cases they received bills from practitioners, such as anaesthetists, whom they had never met.

Medical specialists have strongly favoured private hospitals and private health insurance because they have been able to charge substantially more than the remuneration received as visiting medical officers in the public hospitals, where they were largely paid on an hourly rate rather than by fee for service. It is worth noting that in 1993–94 the average fee income for the top 25 per cent income-earning cardiothoracic, plastic, urological, ophthalmic, and ear, nose and throat surgeons exceeded $500 000. The lowest average fee income for full-time surgeons in that year was $223 000 for paediatric surgery (Department of Human Services and Health 1995d).

By the mid 1990s consumers had, not surprisingly, identified that, compared to Medicare, private health insurance offered very poor value. In 1995, the Keating government introduced amendments to the *Health Insurance Act 1973* (Cwlth) and the *National Health Act 1953* (Cwlth) in order to improve the value of private health insurance to consumers. The amendments provided increased competition between insurance funds and gave them greater power to negotiate with private hospitals and medical practitioners on behalf of their members. For the first time the funds were able to offer 100 per cent coverage to members who agreed to use hospitals and medical practitioners under contract to the fund. As well, the amendments strengthened the rights of private patients to proper information on which they could make decisions; they also gave private patients access to complaints mechanisms if they felt aggrieved.

Predictably, medical specialists reacted badly to these proposals, claiming they would undermine the relationship between patients and their medical practitioners because insurance funds would force practitioners to make decisions on the basis of cost rather than quality. After a temporary aberration, when the AMA recommended briefly that medical fees should be capped (seemingly recognising that the unfettered ability of specialists to charge their patients whatever they liked might be driving proposals for change) the medical profession, including the AMA, reverted to its standard all-out opposition to any changes to fee-for-service arrangements.

Further changes to encourage private health insurance uptake were progressively introduced by the Howard government between 1996 and 2000. A 30 per cent rebate for private health insurance premiums, a surcharge on the Medicare levy payments for higher income earners who fail to take out health insurance, lower premium rates for those taking out private health insurance earlier in life, and hence penalties on those who defer taking out insurance until late in life when they are at higher risk (lifetime health cover) were introduced. By December 2000, as a result of these changes, private health insurance participation rates had risen to 45 per cent of the population (Willcox 2001).

However, private health insurance remains an inefficient and inequitable strategy for funding health services. Duckett and Jackson (2000) estimate that the cost of the private health subsidy is more than $2 billion. The available evidence suggests that private hospitals funded through insurance arrangements are less efficient than public hospitals. They argue that if the private insurance subsidy had been used to fund public hospital expenditure, around 60 per cent of private sector demand could have been accommodated.

The private health insurance rebate arrangements were also inequitable. The 30 per cent rebate was available regardless of income. Those with higher incomes have a greater capacity to pay and are more likely to take out private health insurance and therefore derive more benefit from the subsidy. It is interesting to note that in 1997 the Howard government abolished the publicly funded low-income dental scheme, which was targeted at health care cardholders, arguing it was a state government responsibility. Yet in 2000, the Commonwealth spent more on private health insurance subsidies for ancillary dental cover than it had on the low-cost dental scheme.

Current issues

By and large the reintroduction and consolidation of universal social insurance for medical and hospital services has been relatively successful, despite the consistent doomsaying of conservative critics. Concerns about equity of access to medical and hospital services have declined dramatically. Aided by a relative oversupply of medical practitioners, by 1995 nearly 70 per cent of all medical services were bulk billed and therefore effectively free for the patient. Some rural areas continued to have problems attracting medical practitioners, but this was a relatively minor problem compared to the distributional imbalance in services across affluent and disadvantaged areas of two decades earlier. By the early 1990s, survey results indicated consistently near-universal public support for the Medicare system for medical services (Health Insurance Commission 1995a).

However, because Medicare was introduced as an uncapped entitlement program based on fee for service payments to practitioners while remaining heavily subsidised or free to its users (patients) it inevitably suffered from the problem of 'moral hazard'; that is, with low or nonexistent copayments on the part of users, there were few financial penalties for using more services than necessary. The principal-agent relationship between medical practitioners and their patients is structured to provide incentives for both parties to seek more services: the patient to maximise health; the provider to maximise patient health and to increase income.

The logical response to the problem of moral hazard is either to constrain demand for services or their supply, most notably by either limiting the number of medical practitioners able to attract rebates or by the introduction of copayments (out-of-pocket patient contributions). The literature on copayments suggests that, all other things being equal, significant copayments have the ability to affect demand for services significantly, especially by the poor, but all other things are not usually equal. In the absence of changes to the supply of medical practitioners: they are likely to alter their behaviour in order to protect their level of income—for example, by seeing more concessional patients with health care cards when such patients are exempted from copayments (as they inevitably are). Moreover, patients decrease service use without discriminating between necessary and unnecessary services. Copayments also discriminate against the poor who have less money to spend on health and the sick who need more services (Richardson 1991).

On one hand, apart from one brief, highly contentious flirtation urged on by the Department of Finance in 1991, the Commonwealth has rejected compulsory copayments as a strategy for holding down medical expenditure. On the other hand, it did successfully introduce copayments for the PBS to reduce the use of over the counter items such as analgesics. Interestingly, the evidence for the PBS scheme is that following an initial decline in outlays, the growth curve re-established itself as practitioner and supplier behaviour adjusted to the new circumstances. It is also worth noting that for equity reasons, copayments for concessional users (health care cardholders) were kept to a minimum (Sloan 1995).

If copayments are not the answer then what of controlling supply? The Commonwealth did restrict supply of pharmacy services through an industry restructuring scheme introduced in 1990 despite a bitter campaign on the part of pharmacists. However, considering itself constrained by the problem of civil conscription the Commonwealth made only piecemeal and relatively unsuccessful attempts to limit the supply of medical services through restrictions for overseas-trained doctors, and changes to the requirements to access GP rebates.

Assisted by the oversupply of medical practitioners, the Commonwealth has used its monopsonist power to restrain growth in the unit cost of medical services (Medicare rebates) at or below inflation. Nevertheless, relatively rapid growth in Commonwealth medical benefit outlays occurred as the number of per capita medical services grew from 7.2 to 10.5 in the period from 1984–85 to 1994–95. As a result, expenditure grew from $2.3 billion to $5.6 billion—allowing for inflation, a real increase of 60.3 per cent.

But it is important to recognise that although unnecessary growth in Medicare outlays is a concern for the Commonwealth—particularly central agencies such as the Department of Finance—growth rates across areas of specialisation vary considerably. During the 1990s for example, despite concerns about general practice growth, the increase in Medicare services has been about 2.9 per cent per year compared with growth in pathology and radiology of 4.8 per cent and 5.1 per cent respectively. Solutions to unnecessary growth rates will vary with the nature of the services provided. Overall, the growth in primary care services is manageable and government has a range of options available for constraining those areas expanding at unsupportable rates.

Access to public hospital services also improved dramatically with the reintroduction of free public hospital care. However, in the course of re-negotiating funding for public hospitals through the Medicare and Australian Health Care Agreements, the Commonwealth effectively capped public hospital expenditure. Although this helped constrain overall spending on health, it led to ongoing disputes with the states and territories, which believed the Commonwealth's generous offer to provide free public hospital care was made at their expense. Faced with a narrow and fickle revenue base, a limited ability for deficit funding, and vertical fiscal imbalance, the states and territories set out to find ways to minimise public hospital outlays, which made up about 25 per cent of their spending. Most settled for some combination of shifting costs back to the Commonwealth by reducing their commitment to public hospital outpatients, pathology, and radiology, and increased productivity by reducing the length of patient stay in hospital, contracting services out and reducing staffing levels.

As cost control became an increasing feature of the public hospital system, medical specialists and hospital administrators responded by rationing services to elective surgery patients through the use of waiting lists. For members of the medical profession and for public hospitals, waiting lists became a useful tool in negotiating pay increases and hospital budgets. By the early 1990s, the lot of a health minister in a state or territory government was not a happy one.

In response the states have not been backward in blaming the Commonwealth for increased waiting lists. From their point of view the Commonwealth has underfunded public hospitals, particularly through reductions in the FAGs. Furthermore, they believe that Commonwealth policies have led to declining levels of private health insurance, thereby exacerbating their problems by shifting demand from the private to the public hospital system. Over the period of the 1993 Medicare agreements, Commonwealth Grants Commission data indicate that since 1989, while the Commonwealth increased its public hospital expenditure by about 26 per cent, the states and territories reduced theirs by around 10 per cent.

As public confidence in Medicare grew, health insurance became an increasingly uncompetitive product, particularly when patients discovered that despite their cover they were frequently victims of multiple, unexpected out-of-pocket expenses when they came out of hospital. Private insurance participation rates fell from 68 per cent in 1982 to a low of 30 per cent in 1998. The introduction of a lifetime community rating for private health insurance has seen rates reach 45 per cent again in 2000.

Those concerned to strengthen private insurance—the insurance funds, the medical specialists and the private hospitals—worried that at some point a threshold would be reached when older people and women in their childbearing years would drop out, resulting in serious decline in private insurance use and the private sector also suffering serious decline from commensurate transfer to the public sector. The private sector was happy to mount stiff campaigns in support of states and territories with the theme that a lack of Commonwealth incentives for private health insurance was causing waiting lists to blow out.

In fact, no hospital can use its resources sensibly without having some process for booking patients. The critical question is whether the time that patients wait is clinically appropriate. In 1993–94, there were 4.6 million hospital admissions to Australian hospitals, of which about 12 per cent were for elective surgery. The total waiting list was about 110 000, which would have taken about 2.3 months to clear. Although a small number of people waited longer than desirable for specific procedures in some locations, problems were within manageable proportions (Mays 1995).

However, given the incentives for the key stakeholders to highlight waiting list problems in the media, not surprisingly by the mid 1990s the public had significantly less confidence in the public hospital system than it did in Medicare and the PBS, leading to calls for tax breaks and other incentives for those who took out private health insurance, on the basis that this would cause a shift in demand from the public to the private sectors, thereby lessening the stress on the public hospital system.

By 1995 the Commonwealth, the states, and the territories had agreed to attempt to resolve their ongoing conflict about cost shifting, Budget reductions, declines in private insurance levels, and productivity gains. They agreed to renegotiate key sections of the Medicare and Australian Health Care Agreements to ensure that funding was increasingly tied to outcomes and performance on key indicators, such as elective surgery waiting times.

Where to from here?

In the almost two decades since the introduction of Medicare by the Hawke Labor government, Australian health policy makers have progressively shifted their concern from equity and social justice—first to cost containment, and now, to cost-effectiveness—a problem Duckett (1992) has referred to as the 'Goldilocks problem': are we spending too much, too little, or is our spending just right? These trends are neither unique to Australia nor to the management of the health system.

There is general concern among developed nations about the potential for increasing cost due to population ageing, changes in the technology of care, increased consumer expectations, and the ability of providers, such as medical practitioners and other health workers, to drive up the cost of health care in their own interests. As well, there has been significant criticism of the traditionally organised public sector bureaucracies for their unresponsiveness, inefficiency, and overproduction of services in relation to need. As a result a new paradigm of economic liberalism (or, in Australia, economic rationalism), for the management of health and welfare services has emerged, stressing the importance of efficiency and consumer responsiveness. Most important, the new approach shifts away from reliance on bureaucratic control of services, to decentralised management through new systems for measuring performance and the introduction of market mechanisms, such as contracts, to ensure control by government (Bellamy et al. 1992; Saltman & van Otter 1992; Taylor-Gooby & Lawson 1993).

The introduction of economic rationalism into the management of health services is not without controversy. As Culyer (1989) has argued, national expenditure patterns seem most related to per capita GDP, the extent to which health budgets are centrally controlled, and the extent to which health services are provided through the public sector. Countries with lower per capita GDP spend less of their national income on health. Health becomes relatively more important to wealthier nations.

Taking into account GDP, the fact that some health systems are relatively efficient compared to others seems to be most related to how planning, management and funding are organised. *Laissez-faire* health markets, such as those in the USA, have proved extremely inefficient. Consumers are poorly informed and organised, and have little purchasing power when it comes to health. As a result they are likely to seek private health insurance. In these circumstances the medical profession, hospitals, and other providers have a tendency to capture the market and design regulation and payment systems to suit themselves. In the USA this has led to widespread price fixing and overservicing, with no noticeable improvements in health outcomes (Saltman & van Otter 1992).

Where government plans, funds, and manages health services directly, as is the case in the United Kingdom, expenditures are more likely to be held down. However, central bureaucratic control and direction, rational planning, fixed or capped budgets, and the management of demand by rationing are all features of such systems. Planned public provision of health services through bureaucratically managed structures has been the dominant model for most OECD nations.

The fiscal crises during the economic downturn of the 1970s and 1980s produced a virulent critique of the so-called 'command and control' management of the welfare state, which had previously served government well. Governments forced to hold down expenditure growth in the face of simultaneous and incompatible demands for lower taxes and increased services began exploring alternatives. Neoclassical economic arguments for the revitalisation of the market experienced a renaissance, during which time the importance of competition, individual responsibility, deregulation, and private interest in the pursuit of efficiency and utility came to the fore. Changing community expectations, increased demand for services by the community, population ageing, and improved health treatment technologies were emphasised and placed pressure on government to provide greater flexibility and consumer choice.

Because resources are limited, expenditure on health services should attempt to optimise health outcomes and societal benefit. Ideally, the marginal cost of providing a health service should equal the marginal benefit it produces. Where the marginal cost of providing health services exceeds the health benefit produced, resources would be better allocated to other purposes, such as providing schools, childcare, or roads. Where the marginal benefits of health service provision exceed marginal costs there is an argument for allocating greater resources.

But the ideal is not easy to operationalise. It is not a simple matter to define, measure, and evaluate costs and benefits for even a single technology or treatment, let alone comparisons across technologies for the same outcome or comparisons of the costs for different outcomes. Even if there were general agreement about the costs and benefits of health care, there would be significant differences about the mechanisms by which resources should be allocated. Some would argue that utility to the individual is maximised by allowing the market to regulate the supply and demand for health services. Others believe cost benefit is maximised by rationally planned resource allocation.

By and large, even the most ideologically hidebound of politically conservative governments have recognised that health services represent particular problems for market solutions. Here, the classic arguments for market failure apply—the dismal failure of the USA, where deregulated market provisions have led to grossly inequitable health coverage at sky-rocketing costs, is a salutary lesson.

Most OECD governments, including that in the USA, are trying to find a middle road to planning, managing, and funding health and other services. This approach has variously been labelled 'managed competition', 'planned markets', 'the social market', or 'public competition'. Variants of these models are now being vigorously explored for potential application to health services by virtually all advanced economies (Appleby 1992; Saltman & van Otter 1992; Baldock 1993), the aim being to combine elements of market solutions (such as competition) with rational planning, public accountability, and democratic control. Information technology and accountability methodologies, which did not exist twenty years ago, now make it possible to consider alternatives that will reduce direct or bureaucratic management of health services while retaining planning, funding, and accountability within government control, thereby avoiding the folly of *laissez-faire* market solutions and the inflexibility of direct bureaucratic control.

It is these problems—how much to spend on health to optimise community benefit and the mechanisms to ensure that health services are efficiently produced—that fundamentally drive the microeconomic reform agenda of health. Australia is developing its own unique solutions to these issues.

The emerging Australian approach

As illustrated in the previous section, health policy is not determined in an ideological vacuum as a result of rational technocratic analysis. Rather, health policy is a result of the interplay of politics. Compromise through parliamentary, bureaucratic, and electoral processes is inevitable. The precise nature of the policy outcome in any period thus in part reflects which ideologies have political dominance and which bureaucratic or technical solutions are feasible.

The centralised solutions of the Chifley era are no longer in vogue, although many of the aims remain constant. Instead, the development of financing, planning, and evaluation technologies now make it possible to devolve operational responsibility to more localised control without direct involvement by state, territory, or Commonwealth governments. This is the rhetoric of governments 'steering not rowing' (Osborne & Gaebler 1992).

Accordingly, the next wave of policy should be about how to ensure that national social justice objectives can be achieved in an environment of decentralised decision making. The contemporary policy options will, in common with many other areas of public policy, focus on market or quasi-market solutions using economic incentives—for providers, not consumers—and will incorporate technocratic measurement solutions. There are three broad attributes that can be used to characterise future changes: the size or scope of the change, the role of government (Commonwealth, state, and territory), and the role of intermediaries (Duckett 1996).

Size and scope of change

The health sector represents a significant proportion of the Australian economy and, as a result, a significant number of Australians earn their income from the provision of health services or providing goods and services to the health sector. Any major change is likely to affect either the number of health providers or how much each one of them gets. It is thus not surprising that change in the health sector often involves vigorous debate from affected interests. Depending on the strength of the government and the popularity of proposed changes, health sector interests regularly defeat change proposals that they do not want to see implemented.

Change in any system occurs more easily when the system is unstable, so proponents of change often attempt to create a crisis or aura of instability in the health system. Malcolm Fraser, for example, almost created an expectation of regular changes to Medibank in the late 1970s. In the mid 1990s, supporters of tax concessions for health insurance created an imaginary threshold of 40 per cent of the population with insurance as indicative of a crisis and the unsustainability of Medicare, when there was no objective evidence to support this statistic and, logically, any fixed point on a continuous scale is no different in policy terms from adjacent points.

The role of government

Although Medicare has been part of the policy landscape for nearly two decades, the role of the Commonwealth, state, and territory governments is not settled. Medicare (MBS plus Australian Health Care Agreements) and

PBS consume about 10 per cent of total Commonwealth government out-lays and regularly attract attention as cost-saving targets, with the implicit assumption that private spending is somehow better for the economy than public spending.

There is also contention about the relative role of the Commonwealth versus the states and territories. Should the Commonwealth vacate health policy and leave it to states and territories, or should there be a single national approach to health policy? In theory, it makes more sense for one level of government to have primary responsibility for funding and direct-ing the whole of the Australian health system. In practice, for the states and territories to take over responsibility for medical and pharmaceutical expenditure or the Commonwealth to assume control of hospitals would require a very substantial reworking of the Australian federal system because of the expenditure transfers involved. Vertical fiscal imbalance makes it unrealistic for the states and territories to assume responsibility for Medicare and the PBS; for the Commonwealth to take over hospitals would mean a massive clawback of Australian Health Care Agreement and FAGs funding from the states and territories. Nevertheless, it is clear that the current arrangements led to cost shifting, duplication, inefficiency, and game playing, all of which distract attention from the objective of producing a better health system. Reforms to the current system are therefore inevitable.

The role of intermediaries

Health insurance funds have been a key part of the health sector since the early 1950s, mainly as conduits to transfer funds from consumers to providers without any management or planning intervention. The private health insurance reforms of 1995 marked a major change in role and fore-shadowed an important new function for the funds in negotiating with providers, both hospital and medical.

Many overseas health systems have identified an important new role in the health sector—that of purchaser (Saltman & van Otter 1992). The pur-chasing role is one that attempts to hold providers accountable for quality, efficacy, and cost of care, hopefully supplementing the accountability to the patient. In the USA, where health insurance is generally paid by employers rather than directly by consumers, this purchasing role is performed by managed care organisations such as health maintenance organisations (HMOs). Managed care is the fastest-growing sector of the health market-place in the USA. Other potential intermediaries who might purchase services on behalf of consumers—apart from insurance funds—include geographically based agencies such as area health authorities and case managers, or care coordinators such as GPs and Aged Care Assessment Teams.

Theoretically, by acting as purchasers for a product based on price, quality, and other important criteria, intermediaries create competition, thereby forcing providers to perform better on these factors. Whereas individuals who need health care often have very little ability to negotiate with medical practitioners and hospitals, by collectivising consumer interests, intermediaries create significant ability to force change and contract providers on terms more favourable to the consumer. Such a mechanism offsets the collective power of provider interests as exercised through organisations such as the AMA and the royal colleges. Early in the twentieth century the friendly societies were invented for a similar purpose.

In Australia, as elsewhere, health care has been captured partially by provider interests, to the detriment of consumers. There is little doubt that there is substantial room for improvement in performance. In combination with more juridical or rights-based strategies, funding, or purchasing mechanisms that create more powerful consumer agents could be an important mechanism for forcing a more responsive health care system.

However, there are risks with the introduction of intermediaries as purchasers. In the USA, for example, employers who purchase health insurance for their employees do not necessarily have the same interests as those employees. Much like in the example of workers' compensation in Australia (see Swerissen 1989, 1992), employers in the USA first try to minimise premium costs, while the quality and outcomes of care are likely to be secondary considerations, especially because of the difficulty of measuring these latter criteria. Employees in the USA have little choice about the cover purchased on their behalf. As a result there is now substantial concern about the quality of services provided through managed care in that country. While the medical profession in Australia has tried to defend its own interests by raising the spectre of USA-style managed care, in reality, while Australian health care consumers have a direct choice over their insurance cover and Medicare is available as a relatively inexpensive alternative, quality will remain a key criterion in purchasing decisions.

Restructuring proposals

Proposals to restructure the Australian health system and related community services are inevitably made within the context of Commonwealth–state–territory relationships. In April 1995, the Council of Australian Governments (COAG) established a wide-ranging reform agenda focused on improving the efficiency and effectiveness of service delivery by restructuring the planning, organisation, and funding relationships between Commonwealth, state, and territory governments for health and community services (COAG Task Force on Health and Community Services 1995; Duckett et al. 1995).

Initially, in the context of the forthcoming federal election in 1996, COAG avoided the vexed questions of funding and responsibility, and concentrated instead on the development of a relatively uncontroversial, idealised model for the structure and scope of the system as a whole. At the core of the debate about this model lay the question: What needs do people have and how can these needs best be met? In answer, COAG agreed that further policy development should occur within three streams of care: general, acute, and coordinated. These streams (see table 1.4) were intended as a heuristic policy development framework rather than a prescriptive formula for service organisation. Following the initial development of the care streams, for example, it became clear that the streams did not address population health issues sufficiently. Population health was therefore included as an overarching framework for conceptualising the system as a whole. It was also the case that not all aspects of the framework were equally well accepted and developed.

Table 1.4   Proposed care streams for health and community services

Care stream	Care needs	Service type	Referral and organisation	Payment model
General care	Uncomplicated care and support needs met by individual practitioners in community settings	Primary medical care, immunisation, community-allied health, child health	Self-referral and choice of provider	Fee for service and capitation
Acute care	Complex or intensive episodic needs met by specialist practitioners, multiple staff and/or specialised facilities	Inpatient stay and day procedures in hospital, crisis management in community settings for psychiatric and medical emergencies	General care or crisis referrals with care episode coordinated and managed through intake, treatment, and discharge procedures	Weighted episodic payment
Coordinated care	Ongoing complex and/or multiple care needs met by multiple generalist and specialist staff across general and acute care agencies	Individualised combinations of medical, pharmaceutical, allied health, community support, and personal care	General care or acute care referral leading to voluntary care planning and coordination by care coordinator with responsibility for organising an individualised program of services	Weighted case payment

In particular, while the concepts of general and acute care are relatively well understood as service delivery models—largely as primary and hospital care—this was not the case for coordinated care. Coordinated care represented a relatively new approach to the funding and organisation of services for those with ongoing needs for relatively complex or intensive services. It was intended to provide this group with ongoing care planned and organised with the assistance of a care coordinator in order to provide a more comprehensive, flexible, and efficient range of services across medical, hospital, pharmaceutical, and residential care, tailored to individual needs while maintaining freedom of choice and fiscal responsibility. At the core of this proposal was the identification of those needing coordinated care, the development of individualised care plans, and the purchase of the required services to implement the plan from a common pool of funds.

Not surprisingly, there were significant disputes between the Commonwealth, the states and territories, service providers, and consumers about the development of coordinated care. The states, territories, and the Commonwealth contested how the fund pool would be allocated, the scope of services to be included, the extent to which user and provider participation would be voluntary, whether compulsory copayments should be introduced, and which level of government should be responsible for startup costs. Providers such as the Royal Australian College of General Practitioners opposed any loss of their autonomy and control over service delivery. Consumers wanted assurances that participation would be voluntary, that Medicare would not be undermined, that quality and diversity would be protected, and that funding would not be reduced. As well, there were significant concerns that residential, community, and personal care would be overly dominated by the interests of medical practitioners.

In order to resolve these issues and allay the fears that had been expressed, the Commonwealth initiated a large-scale trial program to test the conceptual framework developed through the COAG process. These trials represent one of the largest health-systems research programs in Australian history. It is likely that further debate about the planning, organisation, and funding of health services within the structure created by COAG will require the Commonwealth, the states, and the territories (and consumers and providers) to determine the extent to which fundamental change is required to the principles that underpin the existing system. It is to these questions we now turn.

Possible policy options

There are three major policy options that might be pursued in the medium term, each of which places different emphases on the planning, organisation, and funding of health services. The Keating Labor government proposed an incrementalist restructuring of Medicare. This involved restructuring the existing hospital Medicare agreements—with their focus on outcome- and output-based funding organised in broad functional streams—with geographically based performance agreements. (The characteristics of outcome- or output-based funding of health services have been outlined by Duckett and Swerissen 1996.) This suggestion proposed a marginal increase in the role of the Commonwealth and no expansion in the role of intermediaries. Under the Commonwealth proposal, existing Commonwealth grants to states and territories would be restructured to involve regional allocations within broadbased streams (general care, coordinated care, public health, acute care), with funding tied to outcomes on a fixed price basis.

It would also be feasible to replace many of the individual, narrow-scoped, specific-purpose programs with a few broader programs incorporating agreed performance measures. For example, in the public health area, disparate programs across such areas as women's health, HIV/AIDS, immunisation, and drug addiction could be combined within one coherent public health strategy. Most likely, such a strategy would involve negotiation of a framework agreement between the Commonwealth and the states and territories that specified clear outcome requirements on important areas of performance, such as cervical and breast cancer screening, immunisation, and health education. Bilateral agreements with each state and territory would then tie funding to specific performance outcomes.

In the health sector, accountability on the hospital side has been facilitated by the development of DRGs and other casemix measures of hospital activity. Casemix has made it possible to measure state and territory hospital activity and thus hold states and territories accountable for hospital performance. The 1995 revisions to the Medicare agreement exemplify this trend: the amended agreements replaced a measure of activity based on proportionate change between states and territories in proportion to public bed-days by targets for each state and territory of DRG-weighted public separations, the latter being a direct measure of access by public patients in the state or territory. The amended agreements also include a measure for failed access, assessed in terms of the percentage of people in the state or territory who wait longer than is clinically desirable. The next stage of Commonwealth–state–territory negotiations will be to extend the measures of accountability, both in terms of range (for example, introducing quality measures) and specificity (for example, having measures at the regional or hospital level rather than at the state level).

An alternative policy direction, proposed by conservative analysts, is the *individual responsibility* option. This would involve the Commonwealth withdrawing from its major involvement in the sector, rolling the Australian Health Care Agreements into financial assistance grants, and devolving other responsibilities with broad framework agreements to the states and territories. This approach normally also supports incentives for private health insurance and a minimum safety net for the poor. While there is decreasing political support for this style of policy, given the strong popular support for Medicare, the Howard Coalition government took significant steps in this direction (that is, towards further withdrawal), despite its commitment to the maintenance of universal Medicare entitlements for both medical and hospital services. As with the Fraser Coalition government, which made similar promises, the Howard government has progressively sought to introduce greater individual responsibility for health care provision.

Similarly, the policies of conservative governments have led to an increase in the use of privately owned or managed facilities for the provision of care to public patients. Moves in this directions were taken by conservative Victorian, South Australian, Western Australian, New South Wales and Tasmanian state governments during the 1990s.

The most radical alternatives involve an emphasis on *managed care*, which involves a stronger role for intermediaries. There are a number of possible managed care options (Scotton 1995), but the most radical would see all health funding combined in a single pool for any one individual, regardless of whether that funding were provided by the Commonwealth, state, or territory governments or, for that matter, by private insurers. Individual entitlements to services would then be managed through brokers, who would negotiate service price, quantity, and quality with service providers such as hospitals, medical practitioners, and community agencies on behalf of consumers. Providers would, in effect, compete with one another for contracts or market share. Brokers might be areas or regions, or, in smaller jurisdictions, they could be the state or territory government.

Alternatively, brokers could be permitted to compete with one another by allowing consumers to choose between them. For example, private insurers or other agencies could be contracted to manage comprehensive health plans for their members on the basis of negotiated contracts with government based on their enrolments. Within this context it would be quite possible that private and public providers and brokers could compete with each other directly. As well, it would be possible to allow or force consumers to make copayments, depending on their ability to pay and the level of service desired.

Conclusion

After having been dominated by the question of equity and who should pay for health for three decades, the Australian health policy debate has moved on to questions about the overall cost of health care and its effectiveness.

The more radical solutions for dealings with these problems are relatively unlikely to be adopted in the short to medium term. There are significant interests that support some variant of the status quo, but there are also technical difficulties with these newer approaches: we do not know how to allocate on a per capita basis, and clear measurement of outcomes is a condition precedent for competition. Also, it is impossible to make meaningful comparisons of competing products. Ambitious privatisation, by removing protections developed over the last few decades (for example, Freedom of Information requirements, administrative law appeals, and so on) and, of course, reducing political accountability, also has consequences for answerability. Similarly, proposals based on introducing copayments need to acknowledge that if they are to have an impact on utilisation decisions they will discriminate against the poor.

Major structural change in the functional relationship between the Commonwealth and the states and territories also presents significant difficulties. It is unlikely that the states and territories would be willing to give up responsibility for hospitals and other health services to the Commonwealth, even if the Commonwealth was able to implement a system to manage them. The states and territories would not want responsibility for additional expenditure like Medicare and the PBS unless the problem of vertical fiscal imbalance were resolved.

This all suggests that the incrementalist approach—based on a move towards more emphasis on funding on the basis of outputs, and with incentives for improved outcomes—is the most likely direction in which the health system will evolve. This is not to say that this will eliminate political contests in the health sector as choices of goals, size of budget, and the relative role of Commonwealth, states and territories will still be present. It is likely that the politics of the health sector will be about which output and outcome measures are specified (for example, do HIV/AIDS policy or the National Drugs Strategy get a place in the sun?) and the sanctions or penalties associated with failure to achieve agreed outputs, their application, and so on. Debates on these issues will mean that health will remain high on the public agenda.

References

Appleby, J. 1992, *Financing Health Care in the 1990s*, Open University Press, Buckingham.

Australian Bureau of Statistics 1995, *Year Book Australia 1994*, AGPS, Canberra.

Australian Institute of Health and Welfare 2000, *Australia's Health 2000*, AIHW, Canberra.

—— 1998, *Australia's Health 1998*, AIHW, Canberra.

—— 1999, *Health Expenditure Bulletin No. 15: Australia's Health Services Expenditure to 1997–98*, AIHW, Canberra.

Baldock, J. 1993, 'Patterns of Change in the Delivery of Welfare in Europe', in P. Taylor-Gooby & R. Lawson (eds), *Market and Managers: New Issues in the Delivery of Welfare*, Open University Press, Milton Keynes.

Bellamy, P., Considine, M., & Watts, R. 1992, *Arguing About the Welfare State: The Australian Experience*, Allen & Unwin, Sydney.

Clare, R. & Tulpule, A. 1994, *Australia's Ageing Society*, AGPS, Canberra.

Commonwealth of Australia 1995, *Budget Paper* No. 1, AGPS, Sydney.

Commonwealth Committee of Inquiry into Health Insurance 1969, *Report*, AGPS, Canberra.

—— 1999b, *Annual Report 1998/99*, Commonwealth of Australia, Canberra.

Council of Australian Governments & Task Force on Health and Community Services 1995, *Health and Community Services: Meeting People's Needs Better*, a discussion paper, COAG, Canberra.

Crichton, A. 1990, *Slowly Taking Control*, Allen & Unwin, Sydney.

Culyer, A. J. 1989, 'Cost Containment in Europe', *Health Care Financing Review, Annual Supplement*, pp. 21–32.

Department of Health and Aged Care 1999a, *Reforming the Australian Health Care System: The Role of Government*, Occasional papers, New Series No. 1, Commonwealth of Australia, Canberra.

Department of Human Services and Health 1995a, 'Medicare Statistics', unpublished departmental paper.

—— 1995b, 'Hospital Funding Tables', unpublished departmental paper.

—— 1995c, 'Hospital Statistics', unpublished departmental paper.

—— 1995d, 'Medical Practitioner Incomes', unpublished departmental paper.

—— 1995e, *Annual Report 1994–95*, AGPS, Canberra.

Duckett, S. J. 1984, 'Structural Interests and Australian Health Policy', *Social Science and Medicine*, vol. 18, no. 11, pp. 959–66.

—— 1992, 'Financing of Health Care', in H. Gardner (ed.), *Health Policy: Development, Implementation and Evaluation in Australia*, Churchill Livingstone, Melbourne.

—— 1996, 'The New Market in Health Care: Prospects for Managed Care in Australia', *Australian Health Review*, vol. 19, no. 2, pp. 7–21.

——, Hogan, T. & Southgate, J. 1995, 'The COAG Reforms and Community Health Services', *Australian Journal of Primary Health-Interchange*, vol. 1, no. 1, pp. 4–10.

—— & Swerissen, H. 1996, 'Specific Purpose Programs in Human Services and Health: Moving from an Input to an Output and Outcome Focus', *Australian Journal of Public Administration*, vol. 55, no. 3, pp. 7–17.

—— & Jackson, T. 2000, 'The New Health Insurance Rebate: An Inefficient Way of Assisting Public Hospitals, *Medical Journal of Australia*, vol. 172, pp. 439–42.

Health Insurance Commission 1999, *Annual Report 1998–99*, Health Insurance Commission, Canberra.

—— 2000, *Medicare and PBS April Monthly Report*, unpublished HIC report.

Mays, L. 1995, *National Report on Elective Surgery Waiting Lists for Public Hospitals 1995*, AIHW, Canberra.

Organisation for Economic Cooperation and Development 1999, *OECD Health Data 99: A Comparative Analysis of 29 Countries*, OECD, Paris.

Osborne, D. & Gaebler, T. 1992, *Reinventing Government*, Addison Wesley, Reading, Massachusetts.

Richardson, J. 1991, *The Effects of Consumer Co-payments in Medical Care*, National Health Strategy Background Paper no. 5, Department of Health, Housing, Local Government and Community Services, Canberra.

Saltman, R. B. & van Otter, C. 1992, *Planned Markets and Public Competition*, Open University, Buckingham.

Sax, S. 1984, *A Strife of Interests*, Allen & Unwin, Sydney.

Scotton, R. B. 1995, 'Managed Competition for Australia', *Australian Health Review*, vol. 18, no. 1, pp. 82–104.

—— & Deeble, J. 1968, 'Compulsory Health Insurance for Australia', *Australian Economic Review*, fourth quarter, pp. 9–16.

—— & MacDonald, C. 1993, *The Making of Medibank*, Australian Studies in Health Service Administration, no. 76, School of Health Services Management, University of New South Wales, Sydney.

Sloan, C. 1995, *A History of the Pharmaceutical Benefits Scheme 1947–1992*, AGPS, Canberra.

Swerissen, H. 1989, 'Stress and Strain: The Role of Health Professionals in Workers' Compensation', in H. Gardner (ed.), *The Politics of Health: The Australian Experience*, Churchill Livingstone, Melbourne.

—— 1992, 'Workers' Compensation Under Pressure in Victoria', in H. Gardner (ed.), *Health Policy: Development, Implementation and Evaluation in Australia*, Churchill Livingstone, Melbourne.

Taylor-Gooby, P. & Lawson, R. 1993, (eds), *Market and Managers: New Issues in the Delivery of Welfare*, Open University Press, Milton Keynes.

Willcox, S. 2001, 'Promoting Private Health Insurance in Australia', *Health Affairs*, vol. 20, no. 3, pp. 1–10.

2

Australian Federalism, Politics, and Health

Linda Hancock

Federal–state relations remain a politically charged area of health policy in Australia. By far the most dominant recurring intergovernmental themes are concerns about funding, efficiency measures, jurisdictional issues, cost shifting between levels of government, and policy setting. There is an ongoing tension between the Commonwealth's desire for cohesive national policies on the one hand, and the states' and territories' desire for greater discretion, autonomy, and flexibility on the other. Added to these historically well-worn issues are new issues: the impact of the new goods and services tax (GST), implemented on 1 July 2000; on the future federal–state and territory tax and health funding mix; the re-emergence of the discussion of a centralised but more regionally devolved hospital system; and the implications of shifts in governance brought about by new public and private partnerships in health service provision.

Health policy and health services exist within an increasingly complex network of players comprising layers of partnerships between Commonwealth and state and territory governments, and between public agencies and public and private providers. The Australian health system is a complex mix of different levels of government and of public and private providers and funding. Insofar as government's role in health care funding is concerned (government pays for about two-thirds of total health services expenditure), unravelling the mix of Commonwealth, state and territory, and local government funding in health and the nature of public–private partnerships is a challenge for intergovernmental analysts. Understanding these shifting relationships is central to predictions about future directions of federal–state relations.

This chapter is divided into two main sections. First, it gives an overview of the basic characteristics of Australian constitutional federalism, intergovernmental relations, and their implications for health. The chapter sketches the constitutional foundations of federalism and notes the structural problems of funding that have dominated federal and state and territory relationships in health. Analysis of the intersection of federalism and the Australian health care system highlights the nature of federal practices, funding mechanisms, and institutional arrangements relevant to health, and focuses on how well they work in practice. The second section canvasses two issues, which highlight the complexity of federal and state and territory relations in health. These are:

- issues of cost shifting and state and territory differences in commitment to hospital and health spending, drawing on evidence from a study comparing Labor's and the Coalition's commitment to health spending, and highlighting the role of politics and ideology in health policy and the current weaknesses in terms of lack of state and territory accountability for state own-spending efforts under Australian Health Care Agreements
- shifts in the private and public mix of health care, in hospital and medical services, dental services, and private health insurance, and the implications of these for shifts in governance in health policy making and service delivery.

With regard to financing the health system, health is paid only partly (about 8 per cent of health expenditure) from a levy on income taxation (the Medicare levy), with the remainder of government contributions to health care costs paid from a mix of federal and state and territory government general revenues. Actual expenditure figures mask the source of funds, since the Commonwealth government is the major funder of Australian health care services, as would be expected on the basis of its monopoly on income tax collection. The states, territories, and local governments are the most important service providers, using Commonwealth funds directed to them for specific purposes, such as for hospitals, as well as from their own revenue sources. The Commonwealth government directly funds about 45 per cent of recurrent health expenditure; state, territory, and local governments fund about 24 per cent (some of this from Commonwealth funds paid through the states[1]); and the nongovernment sector, including voluntary private health insurance contributor schemes and individuals through service charges, fund about 31 per cent (see table 2.1) (Australian Institute of Health and Welfare 2000).

In the Australian context, 'health' includes medical and pharmaceutical services, institutions (including hospitals, nursing homes, ambulance), medical aids and appliances, noninstitutional services such as community

Table 2.1 Government and nongovernment sector expenditure (current prices) as a proportion of total health services expenditure, 1989–90 to 1997–98 (per cent)

Year	Government sector Commonwealth [a]	State and local	Total	Nongovernment sector [a]	Total health services expenditure
1989–90	42.2	26.1	68.3	31.7	100
1990–91	42.2	25.5	67.7	32.3	100
1991–92	42.8	24.6	67.4	32.6	100
1992–93	43.7	23.4	67.1	32.9	100
1993–94	45.3	21.4	66.7	33.3	100
1994–95	45.0	21.7	66.7	33.3	100
1995–96	45.6	22.2	67.7	32.3	100
1996–97	44.6	22.4	66.9	33.1	100
1997–98	45.2	23.4	68.6	31.4	100

(a) Expenditure by the Commonwealth government and the nongovernment sectors has been adjusted for tax expenditures.

Source: AIHW health expenditure database, AIHW 1999, p. 5; AIHW 2000, p. 235

services and public health, dental services, and health research (as defined by the Australian Institute of Health and Welfare 1998). However, three major items dominate health services expenditure and have, in turn, dominated policy reform debates. Expenditure in health is concentrated on institutions, including hospitals, nursing homes, and psychiatric care (about 46 per cent); medical services (20 per cent); and pharmaceuticals (12 per cent) (see tables 2.2 and 2.3, which show the dollar amount of current expenditure and the proportion of recurrent health services expenditure for different areas of expenditure).

Shorter hospital stays and capped hospital funding models have tended to ameliorate the influence of hospitals as drivers of increasing health care costs (Phillips Fox & Casemix Consulting 1999). Recent reform efforts have been directed at consumer- and provider-driven medical and pharmaceutical expenditures. At a more general level, however, many argue that more funds spent upstream on public health and disease prevention would reduce later downstream costs in terms of expensive hospital and medical services. While much of the debate on funding focuses on government expenditure, it should be acknowledged that a growing proportion of Australians seek out complementary health care, spending an estimated sum of over $1 billion per year on complementary medicines and therapists (Atkin & Kristoffersen 1997; Bisset 1996). A growing number of doctors are practising complementary medicine and some are charging upfront fees for these services.

The broader context of health care reforms and Australian health policy and practice reflects international trends similar to those in other Organization for Economic Cooperation and Development (OECD) countries, of government driving what may be identified as a neoliberal agenda in

Table 2.2   Total health services expenditure (current prices) by area of expenditure and source of funds, 1997–98 ($ million)

Area of expenditure	Commonwealth	Government sector State and local	Total
Total hospitals	6 343	6 437	12 780
recognised public hospitals	5 711	6 080	11 851
private hospitals	550	–	550
repatriation hospitals	15	–	15
public psychiatric hospitals	7	357	365
Nursing homes	2 575	137	2 712
Ambulance	90	281	370
Total institutional	9 007	6 855	15 862
Medical services	6 970	–	6 970
Other professional services	219	–	219
Total pharmaceuticals	2 785	16	2 801
benefit-paid pharmaceuticals	2 783	–	2 783
all other pharmaceutical services	2	16	16
Aids and appliances	174	–	174
Other noninstitutional services	1 380	2 086	3 466
community and public health	775	1 357	2 132
dental services	76	328	404
administration	529	401	930
Research	427	96	523
Total noninstitutional	11 956	2 197	14 154
Total recurrent expenditure	**20 964**	**9 053**	**30 016**
Capital expenditure	70	1 400	1 470
Capital consumption	34	538	572
Total health expenditure	**21 068**	**10 990**	**32 058**

Notes: Figures in each cell have been rounded.

Source: AIHW 2000, p. 404

relation to health and, more generally, social policy. These trends range from smaller government, a preference for market mechanisms in the provision of public services, and business-like management of public agencies, to devolution, shifts in risk management onto individuals, output-based funding and performance incentives, and a leaning towards private (for-profit) rather than public providers. In health, this is exemplified by recent policy trends that attempt to cut government expenditure on health through policies that transfer costs and risks onto the private sector and individuals, that withdraw government involvement from areas of previous government service provision, such as dental services, and the shift from public to private sector provision of services following privatisation and contracting out of services previously provided by government.

We now turn to an overview of Australian federalism, intergovernmental relations, and the implications for health.

Table 2.2 (cont'd)

	Nongovernment sector			
Health insurance funds	Individuals	Other	Total	Total expenditure
2 607	418	1 095	4 120	16 900
311	79	595	986	12 836
2 295	321	493	3 109	3 658
–	–	–	–	15
–	18	7	25	390
–	608	–	608	3 320
106	129	38	273	643
2 712	1 155	1 133	5 000	20 863
217	897	419	1 533	8 503
214	1 046	173	1 434	1 653
34	2 463	37	2 534	5 335
–	593	–	593	3 377
34	1 869	37	1 941	1 959
177	435	38	649	823
1 080	1 611	8	2 699	6 165
1	–	–	1	2 133
568	1 611	8	2 187	2 591
511	–	–	511	1 441
–	–	129	129	652
1 721	6 452	805	8 978	23 132
4 434	**7 606**	**1 938**	**13 978**	**43 994**
n.a.	n.a.	n.a.	994	2 464
–	–	–	–	572
n.a.	**n.a.**	**n.a.**	**14 972**	**47 030**

Australian federalism

The Constitution

Australian federalism (and the principle of power sharing between federal and state and territory governments) is written into the Australian Constitution of 1901. Federalism is based on a constitutional division of powers between two spheres of government: the Commonwealth, and the state and territory governments. A third sphere, local government, is set up under state constitutions and laws.[2] The founders of Australian federalism intended it to preserve a regional form of government in which states are free to pursue their own policies and the Commonwealth acts 'where national interest requires national uniformity' (Federal–State Relations Committee 1998, p. xvii).[3] Rather than separate and distinct governments

Table 2.3 Proportion of recurrent health services expenditure (current prices), by area of expenditure, 1989–90 to 1996–97 (per cent)

Area of expenditure	1989–90	1990–91	1991–92	1992–93	1993–94	1994–95	1995–96	1996–97
Total hospitals	40.6	40.1	39.7	38.6	37.7	37.6	37.4	38.1
public nonpsychiatric hospitals	32.3	31.3	30.7	29.8	28.8	28.5	28.2	28.8
recognised public hospitals	30.6	29.6	29.1	28.2	27.8	27.8	28.2	28.8
repatriation hospitals	1.7	1.7	1.7	1.5	1.0	0.6	–	–
private hospitals	6.3	6.9	7.2	7.3	7.5	7.8	8.0	8.4
private psychiatric hospitals	2.0	1.9	1.8	1.6	1.4	1.3	1.1	0.8
Nursing homes	8.3	8.6	8.4	8.1	7.8	7.5	7.5	7.6
Ambulance	1.5	1.4	1.4	1.4	1.4	1.2	1.3	1.2
Other institutional (nec)	0.2	0.2	0.2	0.2	0.3	0.3	0.4	–
Total institutional	*50.5*	*50.3*	*49.8*	*48.3*	*47.2*	*46.6*	*46.5*	*46.9*
Medical services	18.4	18.7	19.0	19.6	20.0	20.2	19.9	19.7
Other professional services	3.7	3.9	3.7	3.7	3.6	3.6	3.4	3.4
Total pharmaceuticals	9.3	9.5	9.9	10.4	11.0	11.6	11.8	12.2
benefit-paid pharmaceuticals	5.4	5.0	5.2	6.0	6.6	7.0	7.6	7.9
all other pharmaceutical services	3.9	4.5	4.7	4.5	4.4	4.6	4.2	4.3
Aids and appliances	2.1	2.2	2.2	2.2	2.2	2.1	2.0	2.0
Other noninstitutional services	14.4	13.8	13.8	14.4	14.4	14.3	14.7	14.2
community and public health	5.6	4.7	4.4	4.9	5.2	4.7	5.4	5.0
dental services	5.1	5.3	5.3	5.9	6.0	5.9	6.0	6.1
administration	3.7	3.8	4.1	3.6	3.2	3.6	3.3	3.1
Research	1.5	1.5	1.5	1.5	1.6	1.6	1.6	1.6
Total noninstitutional	*49.5*	*49.7*	*50.2*	*51.7*	*52.8*	*53.4*	*53.5*	*53.1*
Total recurrent expenditure	**100.0**	**100.0**	**100.0**	**100.0**	**100.0**	**100.0**	**100.0**	**100.0**

Source: AIHW health expenditure database, AIHW 1999, p. 16

with separate jurisdictions and policy responsibilities, Australian federalism is basically concurrent (Federal–State Relations Committee 1998; Galligan 1996). Thus, very few powers are held exclusively by the Commonwealth or state governments (section 90 defines the exclusive powers of the Commonwealth government over coining of money, initiation of referendums for constitutional change, and over customs and excise).[4] Section 51 of the Constitution of Australia sets out Commonwealth powers, the subjects on which the Commonwealth parliament may pass legislation, and forty heads of power. In these latter areas, the Commonwealth exercises power concurrently with the states, with Commonwealth law prevailing in instances of conflict.

One of the most remarkable features of Australian federalism is Commonwealth dominance over the area of personal income tax collection, a practice instituted during World War II. Hence, Australia is remarkable internationally for its extreme vertical fiscal imbalance, where Commonwealth revenue raising far exceeds its own expenditure needs.[5] The states, which are responsible for much of the service provision, have received grants from the Commonwealth under section 96, but historically these have not met their needs. Thus, funding transfers from the Commonwealth to the states are a central focus of much intergovernmental activity, conflict, and cooperation within Australian federalism. States have expressed difficulty with meeting their service obligations due to the Commonwealth's dominance over income tax, and due to recent High Court decisions that have prevented the states from imposing certain taxes on goods.

Amendments to the Constitution in 1946 gave the Commonwealth the power to make laws on pharmaceutical, sickness and hospital benefits, and on medical and dental services. The Commonwealth also operates the Medical Benefits Schedule (MBS) and Pharmaceutical Benefits Scheme (PBS) under the universal medical scheme, Medicare. Introduced in 1984, Medicare is a Commonwealth responsibility, providing universal access at little cost to medical, pharmaceutical, and public hospital care.

There are two main practice groups among Australian doctors: specialists and general practitioners (GPs), the latter being the first point of entry to medical treatment and those who are responsible for delivery of primary health care services. Under Medicare, GPs have the choice of bulk billing some or all patients, or none; the government automatically reimburses 85 per cent of the schedule fee for the consultation when it is bulk billed. As an equity measure, health care cardholders (qualifying Department of Social Security pension and benefit recipients) are bulk billed under Medicare. For nonhealth care cardholders, GPs may bill the patient for the full cost of a consultation, leaving it to the patient to recoup the 85 per cent reimbursement. Specialist fees, which are only partly reimbursed under

Medicare, involve a higher proportion of user contribution to the cost of consultations. Hill (1999) points out that specialist doctors' fees add significant amounts to health care consumers' out-of-pocket expenses.

The Commonwealth government provides for nursing homes, access to doctors, and pharmaceuticals under the MBS and PBS, which are administered by the Health Insurance Commission (HIC), a federal body. Universal access to free public hospital care is enabled through bilateral Commonwealth–State Health Care Agreements, negotiated every five years. The Health Care Agreements provide treatment beyond these public services, such as private hospital care and dental treatment. Treatment by other health care professionals is paid for by users, either directly or with the assistance of their optional private health insurance.

Commonwealth–state relations and health

Under a mix of Constitutional definitions and intergovernmental agreements, the Australian health system has a commitment to the following:
- the Medicare principles of universal coverage, bulk billing, free access to public hospital care, access to one's doctor of choice for out-of-hospital care, and the general freedom of doctors, within accepted clinical practices, to identify the appropriate treatment for their patients
- an overarching agreement between the Commonwealth and the states and territories on the principles and framework governing federal–state relations in the health and community services fields
- under the broad leadership of the Commonwealth, the joint setting of priorities, goals, and quality outcomes for both tiers of government, with the states and territories having increased responsibility for the delivery of services to meet agreed outcomes
- the negotiation and development of bilateral agreements between the Commonwealth and each state and territory, which canvass the incorporation of tied grants into a few broadbanded specific-purpose payments to the states and territories in agreed areas (Department of Health and Family Services 1996, p. 2).

These arrangements are mediated by two main agreements: the Public Health Outcome Funding Agreement 1997–98 and the Australian Health Care Agreements (replacing former Medicare Agreements), which cover public hospital funding grants to the states and territories. The current Agreement was renegotiated from 1998 and extends to 2003.

With shared or concurrent powers over health matters under the Constitution, attempts to divide responsibility for health care policy and service delivery between the Commonwealth and the states have been contested. Responsibilities for funding, service provision and dominance over policy direction are the main focus of intergovernmental tensions. There have been some attempts at division of responsibility with the Commonwealth over medical and pharmaceutical services, the states over public hospital and psychiatric services and public health, joint responsibility for Home and Community Care (HACC), and divided responsibility for disability services. As Duckett (1999) observes, responsibility is not shared in a coherent or consistent manner and comprehensive national policies are difficult to achieve.

The Commonwealth government, however, has played a central role in policy setting. In addition to Medicare, it has formed influential national policies. These include the National Health Strategy, National Mental Health Strategy, National Women's Health Strategy, Environmental Health Strategy, and the National Disability Strategy, along with national standards (such as those for regulating standards in nursing homes), and the hospital funding model (Casemix), which is now implemented in various forms by all states and territories.

The National Mental Health Policy illustrates state and Commonwealth governments' commitment to a national approach with an agreed policy framework, maintaining an agreed focus across Commonwealth and state jurisdictions. The second National Mental Health Plan (1998–2003) provides a national framework for mental health reform, with $300 million (indexed) for mental health services: $250 million allocated broadly on a per capita basis and $50 million for targeted reforms (Australian Health Ministers 1998). The plan identifies three broad themes: promotion and prevention, partnerships in service reform and delivery, and quality and effectiveness.

The Commonwealth sets national policy parameters such as medical fees, health insurance rebates, and fees for private patients in public hospitals (Duckett 1999). It has also been a driving force propelling the states into greater cooperation around nationally set agendas aimed at microeconomic reform, principally through the Council of Australian Governments (COAG) and National Competition Policy, both of which are discussed below. Health funding comes from a variety of sources. Central to government funding is a complex series of transfers from the Commonwealth to the states and territories, which is discussed below.

The mechanics of intergovernmental relations: Commonwealth–state transfers

Historically, the states have relied substantially on Commonwealth grants (for about 46 per cent of their revenue), but they raise the remainder of their own revenue mainly through property, gambling, and business taxes, since they are not permitted to levy income tax or, more recently, excise duties on the manufacture, distribution, and sale of goods.

Payments from the Commonwealth to the states and territories have historically been made principally as either General Revenue Assistance or Special Purpose Payments. Grants made under General Revenue Assistance were unconditional, constituting 51 per cent of total net Commonwealth transfers to the states (1999/2000) and comprising mainly Financial Assistance Grants (FAGs). In calculating these assessments, the Commonwealth Grants Commission uses a complex methodology, which takes into account differences in the per capita capacity of states to raise revenues and differences in per capita amounts that need to be spent to provide an average standard of government services (Commonwealth of Australia 1998, p. 17). FAGs were largely replaced in 2000/01 and will be further replaced in 2001/02 by revenue from the GST reforms which, the government states, 'provide the states with a secure, broad-based revenue source with which to fund community services such as schools, hospitals and the police' (Commonwealth of Australia 2001, p. 1).[6] However, the weightings in per capita relativities recommended by the Commonwealth Grants Commission are still an issue, with Victoria calling in late 2001 for an overhaul on equity grounds, given the different relativities applied to states such as Queensland.

General Purpose Payments (GPPs) and Specific Purpose Payments (SPPs) are mechanisms for overcoming both vertical fiscal imbalance and the horizontal fiscal imbalance that results from variations in revenue raising capacities of different states, and differences in the costs of providing goods and services across the country. With the open-ended nature of some of its programs, especially in the social policy area, the Commonwealth has increased its own outlays at a greater rate than its assistance to the states. The declining Commonwealth funding base paid to states is a source of persistent complaints from the states. Gross assistance to the states declined overall from 34 per cent of Commonwealth outlays in 1976–77 to 27 per cent in 1997–98 (James 1997, p. 1).

SPPs are subject to conditions reflecting Commonwealth policy objectives or national policy objectives agreed between the Commonwealth and the states. SPPs, of which there are over 100, must be spent by the states according to agreed conditions. These comprised 49 per cent of total net Commonwealth transfers to the states in 1999–2000 (Commonwealth of Australia 1999, *Budget Paper No. 3*), but declined to 40.2 per cent in the 2001/02 Budget.

Following the implementation of the new system, GST revenue collected by the Commonwealth on behalf of states and territories will largely replace FAGs. GST revenue comprises 53.6 per cent of total Commonwealth payments to the states, general revenue assistance comprises 6.2 per cent (the remainder of the old FAGs), and SPPs comprise 40.2 per cent (Commonwealth of Australia 2001).

Under the new tax system, SPPs will remain, although to what extent is uncertain. SPPs come in two forms. Payments from the Commonwealth through the states (about a quarter of SPPs or 12 per cent of total Commonwealth payments to the states) are payments not spent by the states but passed on to other bodies, such as tertiary institutions, nongovernment schools, and local government; there are no SPPs through the states for health. In cases where funding is passed on by the states and territories to other bodies, the states act as agents for the Commonwealth in what are essentially Commonwealth government programs, which for constitutional reasons the Commonwealth must fund via the states. In contrast, payments to the states (about three-quarters of SPPs or 29.5 per cent of total Commonwealth payments to the states) fund programs administered at the state level. These include hospitals, government schools, aged and disability services, housing, highways, and legal aid. Health Care Grants made under the Australian Health Care Agreements make up about half the payments to the states.

Most SPPs are tied grants, subject to conditions that reflect Commonwealth policy objectives or national policy objectives agreed to by the Commonwealth and the states. However, as discussed below, some of the mechanisms for states to account to the Commonwealth for their spending are weak and have been the subject of a Senate inquiry with potentially far-reaching effects. Although the conditions differ between programs, the provision of grants to the states in the form of SPPs is seen as a means for the Commonwealth to pursue national policy objectives in areas where the states are the primary service providers.

As noted previously, section 96 grants give the Commonwealth powers to make grants to the states on its own terms and conditions. Nevertheless, this is a controversial aspect of Commonwealth power from states' points of view. Conditions attached to SPPs can limit the ability of state governments to set their own spending priorities. Further, the ability of states to switch tied grants to other purposes is limited because a substantial proportion of SPP funding is for programs in which the Commonwealth exerts either direct control or imposes substantial conditions. Health grants are paid as Special Purpose Payments, although this has not always been the case.

Reflecting the role of the two main political parties that dominate Australian politics, SPP assistance has varied over time, with Labor governments generally favouring tied grants, and Liberal–National Party Coalitions reducing them.[7] The structuring of health grants as either part of general revenue to the states or as SPPs helps explain a large measure of variations in SPPs over the past twenty-five years as a percentage of Commonwealth grants to the states. Moves were made in the Council of Australian Governments in 1995 and 1996 to untie funds and to broadband previously separately funded programs into one payment, obliging states to meet Commonwealth objectives or outcomes but giving them discretion over the means to do so.

In recent years, states have put pressure on the Commonwealth to reduce the proportion of tied grants to enable states to determine better their own spending priorities. At the 1999 Premiers' Conference, the Commonwealth indicated that it had no intention of further reducing aggregate SPPs as part of the reform agenda outlined under the 1999 Intergovernmental Agreement on the Reform of Commonwealth–State Financial Relations. However, following implementation of the GST and the federal tax reform package, SPPs have decreased as a proportion of total government expenditure, to 40.1 per cent. In replacing a mixture of FAGs and state taxes, part of the selling point to enlist state support for tax reform was the promise of increased revenue and greater autonomy. However, the GST has also brought additional costs in the form of compliance costs and ongoing costs related to increased costs of supplies. Under the GST funding model, with projected increases of revenue flow to the states predicted after 2004, and for some states not until 2006, the longer-term impact of the new tax system for state revenue and for health funding will become clearer over time.

Institutional arrangements: the new federalism and the Council of Australian Governments

Historically, premiers' conferences have been the main vehicle for determining the amount and distribution of general revenue assistance to the states. Premiers' conferences have frequently highlighted states' claims about the negative impact of vertical fiscal imbalance and the need for more funds to flow in untied form to the states. Other mechanisms for intergovernmental cooperation include Commonwealth–State Ministerial Councils, the COAG, the Loans Council, and the Treaties Council, along with conferences in specific policy areas, officials' committees, and bilateral communications between Commonwealth, state and territory, and local government agencies. The Leaders' Forum, established in 1994, has been an important adjunct to states' and territories' involvement in COAG, allowing state and territory leaders to meet to develop a cooperative approach in their dealings with the Commonwealth. However, by far the most important driving force for national and intergovernmental reform has been COAG.[8] New federalism and the continuing role of COAG constituted the means of dealing with coordination of intergovernmental arrangements and, during the 1990s, new federalism set an agreed framework for improving Australian federalism.

COAG has played a central role in bringing about Commonwealth–state agreement on National Competition Policy, which in turn has profoundly shaped intergovernmental arrangements across a range of areas, including health. Building on the *Hilmer Report* (1993), in April 1995 the Common-wealth, state, and territory governments endorsed three intergovernmental agreements relating to National Competition Policy. Governments signed the Competition Code Agreement, the Competition Principles Agreement, and the Implementation and Funding Agreement, all of which commenced in 1997–98, and all of which committed governments to implementing significant reforms aimed at breaking down barriers to competition within and between public and private sectors, starting with electricity, gas, and road transport. For its part, the Commonwealth undertook to maintain the pool of FAGs (the main form of general revenue assistance to the states) in real terms per capita on a three-year rolling basis, and to make a series of payments to the states and territories. It is these grants that are replaced with the flowthrough to the states of Commonwealth-collected GST.

This national reform agenda has involved structural reform of public monopolies, competitive neutrality between public and private sectors, and oversight of prices charged by utilities with monopoly power. Reports congruent with its principles include those from the Industry Commission Inquiry (1996) into compulsory competitive tendering, which recommended greater use of contracting out and compulsory competitive tendering. The intention of national Competition Policy was to subject a range of sectors to international and domestic competition. This national agenda, which was strongly influenced by reforms urged by international bodies such as the OECD, has had important implications for federalism. State governments have been given some discretion as to how they implement National Competition Policy principles; some of them have taken a practical approach to implementation to minimise adverse community impacts and to implement sectoral reforms of perceived net benefit to business and the community. Examples of state government efforts to identify legislative restrictions on competition and a mixed market for health care include the Victorian Health Services Policy Review (Phillips Fox & Casemix Consulting 1999). National Competition Policy is clearly aimed at an integrated national economic policy and more consistent business regulation nationally, although it should be noted that critics warn of the tensions between its agenda, harmonisation, uniformity, and decreased regulation; and pressures for local diversity and increased regulation (Harman & Harman 1996). Others are critical of the impact of competition policy on areas such as employment, when outsourcing leads to changes in conditions and tenure of work, which may impact on quality. One example is the impact of agency nursing on work conditions and quality of care in hospitals, to the point that some hospitals have reverted to employing staff rather than contract nurses.

From a state's perspective, COAG has been seen as a potential circuit breaker on Commonwealth centralisation of government processes and an ongoing forum separate from traditional premiers' conferences, which dealt more with distribution of large FAGs from the Commonwealth to the states, whereas lower-priority tied grants were rarely dealt with (Hendy 1996). COAG's success might be perceived as uneven, emphasising micro-economic reform, but having less success in negotiations on reforming community services, childcare, public housing, the environment, and Native Title, and a lack of commitment to addressing the fundamental reform issue of Commonwealth–state financial arrangements (Hendy 1996). Although it is a significant milestone in intergovernmental relations, taking as it does a whole-of-government perspective on issues of national importance in recent years, it has been seen as a Labor invention, and meetings have been less frequent since the Howard government came to office in 1996. Nevertheless, in health, COAG reforms in program areas have emphasised the shift to output-based funding systems and broadbanded funding of related programs. This has given the states greater freedom in how they deploy funds but has tightened up constraints in terms of states having to demonstrate maintenance of their own contributions.

In 1995, COAG agreed on the need for major long-term reforms of health and community services. This approach represented a sharing rather than a separation of responsibilities. It sought to have joint setting of Commonwealth–state objectives, priorities, and performance standards; and joint funding. The Commonwealth would have a leadership role in public health standards and research, with the states having responsibility for managing and coordinating provision of services and for maintaining direct relationships with providers (COAG 1996). The boundaries of programs were redrawn and grouped into three streams:

- general care, including community and preventative health and welfare services
- acute care
- coordinated care, including a range of specialised services for the frail aged.

The reforms incorporated the assignment of programs to a care stream, output-based fundings, and a model of care where managers could purchase a mix of services within a set budget. In principle, the agreement marked an important shift of all health and related community services under a single multilateral agreement, with bilateral agreements covering funding and outcome measures.

Reforms aimed for improved outcomes for health care consumers, with better information, service coordination, and services, and increased efficiency through an outcome focus. In addition, there was investment in prevention and early intervention, planning, and managing services as close as possible to service delivery levels, as well as providing incentives for best practice (COAG meeting 1995). COAG has played an important role in the review of Commonwealth–state responsibilities and the devolution of much service delivery to the states, including the Aged and Community Care Program and broadbanding SPPs in the public-health and health-services areas. However, as illustrated by examples in 2000 and 2001 of substandard conditions in nursing homes in some states, a lack of proper regulatory inspection and proper reporting by states undermines achievement of national standards.

COAG has been a major driver of the implementation of National Competition Policy and the application of the Trade Practices Act to the health industry, both of which underlie the shift to managed competition in health— under policies such as Casemix—as a basis for capped hospital funding. Casemix funding is thus part of nationally initiated attempts at broader reform of hospital management and funding. With Casemix funding there are ongoing issues in relation to quality of care and the intensification of nursing work in hospitals. Length of hospital stay as a funding tool is problematic and, from the patient's perspective, concerns have been raised regarding quality of care, discharge planning, and significant increases in re-admissions following shorter hospital stays (Draper 1999). There are also arguments that early discharge has shifted costs that were formerly borne by hospitals onto community services and families. With shorter hospital stays, state governments have to confront issues of increased throughput of more acute-care patients. These are characterised by increased intensity of work for hospital health care workers, increased responsibility for hospitals in discharge planning and patient care in the community, and the need for a mix of high-tech, state-of-the-art, centralised hospitals and other hospitals capable of more routine day procedures.

Central to COAG's effectiveness—especially when it met more frequently under Labor—has been its location within the Department of the Prime Minister and Cabinet, the commitment to a national reform agenda, and its involvement of heads of government and senior ministers on agenda items in the national interest. In health, the redrawing of boundaries in acute care, coordinated care, and general (community and preventative) care has reset the basis for major funding agreements and outcome measures. Joint policy setting and an agreed division of responsibilities have attempted to address key issues of inefficiency and cost shifting. However, ongoing issues of quality care, nursing home provision, hospital waiting lists, community services for mental health, and home care services remain highly charged intergovernmental issues.

Attempts to rationalise programs involving multiple levels of government

The report of the National Commission of Audit (1996) to the Commonwealth government expressed its concerns about the involvement of multiple levels of government and called for a critical review of these arrangements. The report was critical of government management and reinforced the need for greater productivity, accountability, efficiency, and value for money. The Commission identified cost shifting as a major problem, conceding that this would remain even if problems of duplication and overlap were addressed. In the health area, the Commission identified a well-known cost-shifting issue. In response to capped funding and budget constraints in some areas, states have encouraged health services consumers to switch into uncapped, federally funded programs such as the Commonwealth funded Medical and Pharmaceutical Benefits Schemes, thereby shifting costs to the Commonwealth. The Commission acknowledged that it might be impractical to cede responsibility entirely to one level of government. It observed, however, that even with clear purchaser–provider delineation, with, say, Commonwealth programs run by the states, it would be difficult to avoid pressures for state involvement in standard setting or requests for additional funding, just as it would also be difficult to avoid Commonwealth involvement in program delivery as a way of verifying costs.

The Commission concluded that there is no easy solution to the problem but argued that, where practicable, it is best to avoid multiple levels of government involvement from the outset. It pressed for a review of all programs involving multiple levels of government, asking that the following questions be addressed:

- whether Commonwealth involvement is the only solution, even where national standards of service delivery are considered desirable
- whether uniform standards could be maintained as a result of state-level cooperation or competition
- whether the states, acting together as competitors, could deliver acceptable programs and standards, in which case the Commonwealth could vacate the field (National Commission of Audit 1996).

The Commission argued that the allocation of related programs over different levels of government is a design defect that not only facilitates cost shifting, but also creates incentives to engage in such practices. Accordingly, it put forth some program design principles for reducing cost shifting (National Commission of Audit 1996). The Commission laid down principles that should apply to Commonwealth–state funding arrangements.

- For programs entirely the responsibility of the states and territories, funding should be in the form of General Purpose Grants, allowing the states and territories allocative discretion between specific programs.
- For programs where there is joint Commonwealth–state responsibility, funding should go to pools that extend to all related programs, rather than being earmarked for specific programs. Again, this would allow the states some allocative discretion within funding pools.

• Where SPPs are considered necessary, the Commonwealth should focus on specifying policy objectives and establishing improved accountability frameworks and then give the states greater freedom in deciding program delivery. This would facilitate a reduction in the number of SPPs by grouping together or broadbanding SPPs that are directed at broad outcomes for particular groups, and would reduce administrative duplication, overlap, and inefficiency (National Commission of Audit 1996, p. 48).

The Commission further recommended that the administrative component of retained SPPs should be reduced and argued that any national policy bodies that are retained should be limited to national coordination, strategic directions, and the development of standards, benchmarks, and performance measurements. It took the strong view that the Commonwealth should not be involved in service delivery or approval of projects. These principles, delineated in the *National Commission of Audit Report* have influenced the more recent funding arrangements entered into by the Howard government, in particular the Australian Health Care Agreements and the Public Health Care Agreements. Even so, it should be borne in mind that not everyone agrees with these policy directions. Critics such as Painter regard 'neat and tidy' attempts to sort out clear and distinct roles and responsibilities, such as Commission audits, as misreading the constitutional logic of Australian federalism. 'It ignores the essential feature of concurrence in the division of powers in the Australian Constitution, and the adversarial and competitive dynamic of Australian federal politics' (Painter 1998, p. 8).

Issues in intergovernmental relations in health

Duckett (1999) encapsulates problems inherent in the intergovernmental system from the point of view of Commonwealth and state governments.

> The different responsibilities of the different players means that the players have different perceptions of the problems of Commonwealth–state relations. Reaching agreement on what the key problems are is thus difficult, making reaching agreement on solutions to those problems even more difficult (Duckett 1999, p. 73).

From the Commonwealth point of view, high on the list are growth rates of government expenditure on health care, wastage from service duplication, cost shifting between levels of government, and the difficulty of implementing national priorities. From the state point of view, high on the list of problems are vertical fiscal imbalance along with the states' poor revenue base. The latter drives dependence on the Commonwealth for funding, with costs resulting from duplication and waste due to Commonwealth–state program overlap and payment-related problems (such as the conditions of tied grants, which are perceived as undermining state autonomy and local diversity in implementation models).

Two issues, discussed next, highlight some of the ongoing debates around intergovernmental relations in health: cost shifting and state maintenance of effort, and shifts in the private–public mix of health care.

Cost shifting and state differences in funding commitment

It is now well recognised that health care costs, along with the quality of care, are major political and social as well as economic issues. Rising health care costs in Australia reflect a combination of factors. Some of the well-known drivers include growth in service intensity and demand pressures, an ageing population, growth in biotechnology, inefficient management, a provider-driven medical services system, and growth in pharmaceutical expenditure. Of further relevance to intergovernmental relations might be added system inefficiencies reflecting overlap and duplication of services, and cost shifting from the states to the Commonwealth in areas such as hospital outpatient, pathology and radiology services, emergency services, and mental health.

It is widely commented upon that, in comparison with other OECD countries, Australia has attained success in providing quality health care with reasonable public expenditure and that government has prioritised addressing issues of cost. Health expenditure in Australia as a proportion of gross domestic product (GDP) has risen from 7.5 per cent in 1989–90 to 8.3 in 1997–98 (Australian Institute of Health and Welfare 2000). This compares with lower expenditure on health in New Zealand (7.6 per cent) and the UK (6.8 per cent), and with higher expenditures in the USA (13.9 per cent) (Australian Institute of Health and Welfare 2000). However, growth in health care costs is occurring at a faster rate than general economic growth. The average annual real growth rate in health services expenditure is at a higher rate (4.1 per cent) than the average annual rate of real GDP growth (3.1 per cent) for the period 1989–90 to 1997–98, although the average rate of health services expenditure growth conceals an uneven distribution over this period. Compared with earlier lower rates, the real growth rate of spending on Australian health services had increased to 5.1 per cent for the year 1996–97 to 1998–99 (Australian Institute of Health and Welfare 1999).

Hence, rising health costs are becoming more of an issue. Notably, over the period 1989–90 to 1996–97, costs grew more slowly in areas of state service delivery responsibility.[9] Increases in medical and pharmaceutical services are in many respects provider- as well as consumer-driven, and constitute the two next largest areas of recurrent health services expenditure after hospitals.

Federal government Budget papers suggest that growth in Commonwealth outlays in health reflect higher utilisation of medical and pharmaceutical services with a 'drift towards more costly drugs and medical services' (Commonwealth of Australia 1997, pp. 4, 41–2). Medical services (33.2 per cent) and pharmaceutical benefits (13.2 per cent) constituted almost half of Commonwealth outlays on health for the year 1997–98 (Australian Institute of Health and Welfare 2000). They thus constitute an interrelated area where outlays are increasing and are difficult to cap, although the rate of growth in these two areas is expected to slow as a result of measures to constrain growth. These include both supply side measures such as caps on pathology spending, restrictions on the number of overseas-trained doctors entering the medical workforce, and reduced moonlighting by temporary resident doctors, as well as demand side measures such as revoking eligibility for Medicare for some classes of temporary residents.

Recognising that much of the problem of unconstrained expenditure centres on private medical practice, attempts have been made to reform primary care. These include General Practice Grants for activities that are not fee for service, such as research, evaluation, special training, and computer networking, the creation of Divisions of General Practice to work in cooperation with the staff of an area hospital, and piloting the concept of GPs as budget holders for patients, for example, in the Coordinated Care Trials.

Against this general backdrop of Commonwealth–state financial relations in health, system inefficiencies due to overlap and duplication have been perennial topics of discussion. Similarly, cost shifting post-Medicare in areas such as hospital emergency has been tightened up in subsequent agreements. However, responsibility for rising health care costs is consistently passed between Commonwealth and state governments. As Duckett (1999, p. 78) remarks:

> there are real problems of Commonwealth/state relations in terms of political process and accountability. The dissipation of responsibility in the health sector means that whenever state or Commonwealth politicians are under pressure they almost inevitably attempt to shift blame to politicians at the other level (the so-called 'blame game').

One area with scant discussion is that of the lack of enforcement of states' efforts in agreed areas of joint responsibility.

In a report on the first attempt to compile a state register of SPPs, significant discrepancies were found in the figures provided in the Commonwealth Budget and by the Victorian government. This has obvious relevance to assessments of both state and Commonwealth accountability under shared funding agreements and tied grants. The committee concluded that such discrepancies are obstacles to achieving a thorough understanding of the impact of SPPs on state government finances (Federal–state Committee 1999, p. 39). In an audit of SPPs in 1994, the Commonwealth Auditor-General questioned their program accountability and financial arrangements, and identified deficiencies in parliamentary reporting on SPPs. Trebeck and Cutbush (1996) pinpoint the main problem of SPPs, when duplication and overlap have 'no offsetting policy coordination or spillover internalising or uniformity of standard benefit for Australia'. They argue that vertical fiscal imbalance is only partly responsible, and emphasise 'deep seated confusion at both levels about the proper role of Government in society in the first place' (1996, p. 8).

It is significant that states effectively determine overall levels of service provided in the areas targeted by SPPs and that states have been known to substitute some of the Commonwealth SPP funds for their own contributions (Moore 1996, p. 7), thereby freeing their funds for other expenditures—such as deficit reduction in the case of Victoria during the 1990s—and contributing to significant per capita variations in spending between the states in areas of controversial social policy expenditure.

This is well illustrated in a study by Hancock and Cowling (1999) that analysed patterns of expenditure in Victoria during the Kennett Liberal government (1991–92 to 1998–99). It should be noted that political ideology is a strong driver of policy reform. The Kennett government has been widely identified with a neoliberal reform agenda, based on smaller government, outsourcing, privatisation, and the shift of government from service provider to regulator (Alford & O'Neill 1999; Hancock 1999). Spending on education, health, community services, and welfare in Victoria fell from 6.48 to 6.17 per cent of gross state product (GSP) over this time. Drawing on Commonwealth Grants Commission and ABS data, the study found that social spending in Victoria (on health, education, and welfare) had fallen 10.7 per cent, or $281 per head of population, over the 5 years from 1993–94 to 1997–98. By 1997–98, Victoria was behind the average of the other Australian states per capita by $138 in education, $174 in health and $8 in welfare (Hancock & Cowling 1999). Real per capita expenditure on health decreased 11.3 per cent ($797 to $707), with the greatest losses in nursing homes (−71 per cent, from $31 to $9) and hospitals (−11 per cent, from $574 to $511). Although spending on community health grew from $57 to $68 per head, that sector picked up load generated by cuts in other health areas, such as the effects of early hospital discharge and the deinstitutionalisation of the mentally ill.

Figure 2.1 compares shifts in Victorian per capita expenditure in health with that of New South Wales and the average of all states and territories excluding Victoria. Figure 2.2 shows the percentage shift in expenditure on health subgroups, showing the dramatic decreases in Victorian funding on nursing homes, hospitals, and public health (and lower growth rates in

Figure 2.1 Real per capita expenditure on health ($1997–98 = 100): Victoria and New South Wales compared with other states; 1993–94 to 1997–98

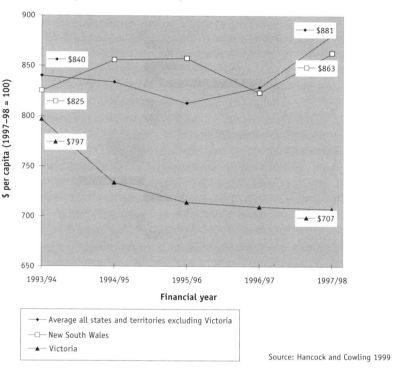

Source: Hancock and Cowling 1999

community health) compared with New South Wales and all states and territories, excluding Victoria.

These data illustrate how, from a starting point of roughly comparable per capita spending on health in 1993–94, Budget cuts up to 1997–98 resulted in a noticeable departure in Victorian funding. In the context of national goals and federal–state agreements on shared commitment to health care funding, Victorian citizens were not experiencing comparable levels of commitment.[10]

Arguments that lowered per capita expenditure was the outcome of improvements in efficiency need more complex examination. Analyses of contracting out in the hospital sector show that efficiencies from contracting out catering and cleaning to private sector operators, or moving from staffed to contracted agency nursing staff, have led to lower pay for workers, increased intensity of work, burnout, lowered quality, and, in some cases, increased hospital infection rates. Examples such as these show how weak the Commonwealth–state Funding Agreements really are and cast doubt on states' claims for more funding for the 'crisis in health', when they may in fact be prioritising their own funds for other expenditure.

Figure 2.2   Real per capita expenditure on health subgroups: Victoria compared with other states and New South Wales; five-year growth rate (per cent), 1993–94 to 1997–98

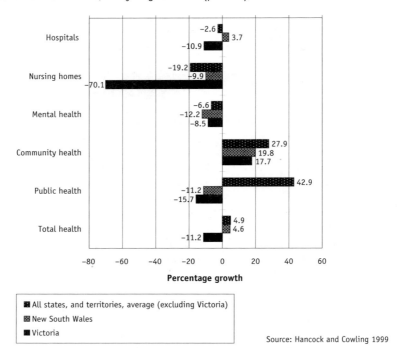

Source: Hancock and Cowling 1999

An alternative proposal, announced at the 2000 Labor Party National Conference (Macklin & Beazley 2000), was a Medicare Alliance model based on a nationally coordinated network of care across the health sector, including 24-hour clinics attached to hospitals. The model would combine agreed funds in state-based Medicare Joint Accounts from which health spending would be drawn initially for hospitals, aged care, medical benefits, and pharmaceuticals. Macklin and Beazley (2000) claimed that:

> Labor's Medicare Alliance will remove the artificial barriers that currently exist between Federal and state funded programs. It will bring an end to the era of cost shifting and Governments blaming each other. It will start a new era of cooperation and put the focus back on patient care.

Labor's proposal echoed the findings of a Senate report, *Healing Our Hospitals* (Crowley 2000), which concluded that the funding arrangement with the most support was a joint account, single fund model that would combine state and federal funds across a number of programs and that could be established in time for the 2003 Commonwealth–state Health Care Agreement:

The aim of the proposal is the creation of an environment in which the funding system facilitates, rather than obstructs, the provision of seamless, integrated health care. It would also give the community greater transparency to ensure that the funding commitments made by both levels of Government were kept. The lengthy debates over cost shifting will end when the facts are out in the open (p. xi).

Shifts in the private–public mix of health care funding and service provision

Shifts in the private–public mix of health funding have implications for different levels of government and nongovernment spending and thus for total health expenditure, as well as implications for equity and access to services. Two interrelated trends are discussed below: the higher rate of growth of the private hospital system, and recent government policy to grant income tax rebates for private health insurance payments in voluntary community-rated private health insurance schemes.

Shifts in public–private provision have effectively displaced formerly state-provided services onto the Commonwealth and onto individuals in the form of consumer copayments. One example is the closure of outpatient public hospital services resulting in a diversion of patients to private medical practitioners and the diversion of associated pharmaceutical costs onto the PBS. Similarly, privatisation of pathology and radiology services in public hospitals has shifted costs to the federal government and Medicare, and to patients when cases are not bulk billed (Kelly 1995).

Another subtle form of cost shifting occurs when private hospitals are colocated beside or as part of public hospitals. Kelly alludes to 'ambulance chasing' when patients covered by private insurance, transport accident insurance, WorkCover, or an expressed willingness to self-fund are 'diverted to the private hospital'.

> A symbiotic relationship is established between the public and the private hospital which allows the private hospital to skim off the cream of the private patients, with the public hospital providing back-up access to intensive care services … The result is that public hospitals' revenues from the treatment of private surgical patients decline, at the same time as they must pick up the cost of treating patients which the private sector is unwilling or unable to treat (p. 30).

Similarly, the private hospital share of total hospital admissions has been rising, while the number of beds in the public sector has been falling. The number of beds in the public system declined by 7375 between 1993–94 and 1998–99. The number of private patients being treated in public hospitals has declined, meaning a decline in patient revenue from 10.2 per cent of total recurrent expenditure to 8.6 per cent in 1998–9 (Crowley 2000, p. 9). This contributes to another subtle shift, that of surgeons moving from the public to the private sector, resulting in 'a gradual privatisation of acute care hospital treatment' (Kelly 1995, p. 31). The workload at private and public hospitals is also shifting, with higher cost, more intensive, longer-stay cases increasingly characterising public hospital casemix (Crowley 2000, p. 73).

Historically, in Australia, there has been a mix of private and public providers of hospital care, with private hospitals mainly run by the non-profit religious sector. Overall, about three-quarters of hospitals are funded from government sources and one-quarter from the private sector. That this mix is shifting is borne out by the figures. While funding to public nonpsychiatric hospitals as a whole fell from 31.5 per cent to 29.2 per cent of recurrent health expenditure between 1988–89 and 1997–98, expenditure on private hospitals rose from 5.6 per cent to 8.3 per cent. Recurrent expenditure on public nonpsychiatric hospitals grew at an average annual rate of 3.1 per cent between 1975–76 and 1997–98 compared with 6.8 per cent for private hospitals (Australian Institute of Health and Welfare 2000).

While a public health system dominates, government can, by various means, attain a degree of control over expenditure. It does this more successfully with public institutional care by capping public hospital funding and limiting the range of available services. In the area of medical services, government tries to do this by setting rebate levels for GP and specialist medical services—most providers being private practitioners—and through general practice reforms aimed at reducing medical expenses, as discussed previously. However, the mix of funding has been changing. Up to 1997–98 the proportion of total health expenditure funded by government fell from 71.9 per cent in 1984–85 to 69.1 per cent in 1997–98; nongovernment expenditure increased from 28.1 per cent to 30.9 per cent over the same period (Australian Institute of Health and Welfare 1999). Private hospitals represent an area of health expenditure where patients on average receive higher volumes of services and where higher charges are met by user payments and health insurance.

Looking to the future, in addition to cost shifting, in the case of growth in private hospitals, an increase in private provision can substantially increase overall health care costs as a proportion of GDP, even if costs to government remain unaffected. *Healing Our Hospitals* called for national investigation into the private management of public hospitals and for independent research on the strengths and weaknesses of colocation and cooperative sharing of resources between nearby public and private hospitals (Crowley 2000).

Before the introduction of Medicare in 1984, as high as 78 per cent of the population was enrolled in private health insurance (Owens 1998), which was in effect Australia's (inequitable) health insurance scheme. Since the introduction of Medicare, coverage declined to around 30 per cent by 1999,[11] although rates have risen following the health insurance rebate and a Medicare levy surcharge for higher income earners. Despite this decline, use of private hospitals has risen steadily since 1984 and the private hospital sector has grown faster than the public sector in terms of bed days and total admissions (Livingston 1997), with private health insurers contributing around 70 per cent of private hospital expenditure (Australian Institute of Health and Welfare 1998). According to Livingston's analysis, the cost of private health insurance premiums increased by 75 per cent from 1989–90 to 1995–96. By comparison, the Consumer Price Index (CPI) increased only 19 per cent over the same period. A 1997 Industry Commission inquiry into private health insurance attributed rising premiums to the rise in the proportion of fund members using private rather than public hospitals, rising average private hospital admission charges, increased admissions by private patients, and adverse selection; that is, entry of high-cost patients (Industry Commission 1997).

In 1996, the federal Labor government provided incentives for those privately insured to retain their membership and imposed a financial penalty on those high-income earners without private cover. Then in 1998, the Howard Coalition government's tax package promised a nonmeans-tested 30 per cent tax rebate to private health policy holders. In 1999, it announced the Lifetime Health Cover Scheme, which provides incentives for younger, lower-cost members to take up private health insurance, and penalties for older entrants. The combined effect of these reforms has been to increase coverage of private health insurance to 45.8 per cent of Australians by September 2000. Under the Australian Health Care Agreement, federal funding for public hospitals is to be decreased for every 1 per cent increase in private health fund membership above 32.2 per cent. Should private health insurance scheme membership increase too abruptly, there is concern that shifts to private hospital care could encourage overall health costs to become excessive. Added to moves by some states and territories to encourage the entry of for-profit providers in privatised public hospitals—which were previously more likely to be run by religious organisations—this could radically alter the private–public balance and eventually result in a two-tiered potentially inequitable system.

Inequity arises as a result of distributional factors (private hospitals tend to cluster closer to their wealthier clientele), differences in service mix (private hospitals offer a different range and quality of services), and cost barriers to private services for those reliant on a residual public system. Moreover, single-payer systems are found to be more efficient and more equitable than those with 'multi-payer, private insurance systems, where there are few controls on the activities of either doctors or hospitals' (Gray 2000, p. 8). It can thus be seen that this complicated mix of reforms is seen as having the potential to undermine the basic principles of universal access to quality hospital care, a foundation stone of national policy.

It could be argued that government subsidies on private health insurance play a role as subsidies to uncapped private hospital expenditure and to private hospital care for elites who can either afford to pay for care via personal funding or through insurance. Similarly, in the case of dental care, the Commonwealth Dental Scheme was scrapped in 1996, leaving responsibility for dental care to the states. This resulted in waiting lists of up to three years for low-income patients seeking state-subsidised dental care. However, reimbursement through health insurance funds has effectively cost-shifted Commonwealth funding via the health insurance subsidy paid to those able to afford private health insurance. In essence this also shifts cost from the now axed Commonwealth Dental Scheme, which used to service the disadvantaged, to a scheme accessible only to the well-off through subsidised private health funds. Moreover, profits from health care funds are disbursed to shareholders rather than being recycled into the health care system.

That private hospitals are increasingly run for profit is an important factor. A report on Victorian hospitals points out significant concentrations of ownership of private hospitals, which raises issues related to shareholder and owner interests (Phillips Fox & Casemix Consulting 1999). There is continuing controversy about the commitment of Commonwealth policy to propping up the private health insurance industry with tax-based measures for more privileged citizens. Critics argue that subsidies to the well-off in the form of tax rebates for private health insurance—costing approximately $2.8 billion per year—could be better used as direct funding to the public hospital and health system.[12] As Owens (1998) notes, tensions within the system between Medicare and community-rated private health insurance, between stakeholders (medical practitioners, insurers, and private and public hospitals), and between Commonwealth and state governments over cost shifting, really call for more fundamental review of the whole health system.

Conclusion

The Commonwealth's dominance over the financial operation of the federation in Australia has arisen largely because of the High Court's interpretation of the Constitution, which has allowed the Commonwealth government's wartime monopoly over income taxation to continue. In light of this, the most notable aspect of Australian Commonwealth–state relations is the extreme vertical fiscal imbalance, marked by the Common-wealth's control of major tax bases while the states bear most of the respon-sibility for expenditure and service provision. Tax reform is one attempt to address this issue, although, at the time of writing, it was too early to judge their effectiveness.

The provision of SPPs—tied grants—to the states under section 96 of the Constitution has enabled the Commonwealth to expand its role in the health system. Controversy surrounding tied grants is ongoing. From their own point of view, states would prefer fewer restrictions and view matched funding arrangements as restricting state budgetary flexibility, especially where such arrangements have not been agreed to on a cooperative basis. States perceive this to be the Commonwealth dictating the terms of service provision and advancing its own interests. States argue that SPPs result in unnecessary state–Commonwealth duplication and overlap, and reduce state government flexibility and responsiveness. From the Commonwealth perspective, SPPs are a means of satisfying Commonwealth demands for minimum national standards in areas such as health, with the Common-wealth setting strategic goals and fostering states' optional provision of ser-vices from available resources. States have been vocal in their continued complaints of funding shortfalls, which inhibit their capacity to deliver ser-vices to taxpayers. The Council of Australian Governments has been a cen-tral intergovernmental institution in terms of encouraging states to focus on national priorities and sorting out new demarcations in intergovernmental responsibilities in health.

Much of this chapter focuses on unravelling Commonwealth–state fund-ing of health and the role of institutions (such as the Council of Australian Governments) that are instrumental in forging a more effective and efficient national agenda in health. This agenda demands a national system with the capacity to generate comprehensive national policies related to health care and to implement national microeconomic reforms. These include the capacity of various components of the system to balance efficiency with equity and quality of care issues, the efficacy of intergovernmental institutions to facilitate better and more efficient Commonwealth–state cooperation, and the ability of a more efficient system to better address unmet needs (especially in aged and disability care).

Ongoing difficulties in policy implementation rely on negotiations between the Commonwealth and the states and give rise to distortions of priorities or goal shifting in the implementation phase. These issues really frame the challenge of effective intergovernmental relations. As Crowley (2000) comments: 'Systemic fragmentation, a lack of transparency of fund-ing arrangements, lack of knowledge about many key areas and differences between jurisdictions limit the extent to which Australia can claim to have a national health system' (p. 6). In responding to these problems, Australian Health Ministers agreed in July 2000 to a unified approach to strengthen primary health and community care. Other reforms are needed to properly address cost shifting and to recognise the broader impact on the public system of the shift to private hospital care.

References

Atkin, G. P. & Kristoffersen, S. 1997, 'Alternative Medicine: An Expanding Health Industry', *Medical Journal of Australia*, vol. 166, 19 May, p. 516.

Australian Capital Territory Government 1998, 'Intergovernmental Financial Relations', *Budget Paper No. 3*, Australian Capital Territory Government, Canberra.

Australian Health Ministers 1998, *Second National Mental Health Plan*, Commonwealth of Australia, Canberra.

Australian Institute of Health and Welfare 1998, *Australia's Health 1998*, AIHW, Canberra.

—— 1999, 'Australia's Health Services Expenditure to 1997–98', *Health Expenditure Bulletin No. 15*, Canberra, AIHW Health and Welfare Expenditure Series, AIHW Canberra.

—— 2000, *Australia's Health 2000*, AIHW, Canberra.

Beazley, K. & Macklin, J. 2000, 'Labor's Medicare Alliance', Media statement, 31 July, Australian Labor Party, Canberra.

Bisset, K. 1996, 'Alternative Medicine: Patients Spend $1bn', *Australian Doctor*, 8 March, p. 1.

COAG Task Force on Health and Community Services 1995, *Health and Community Services: Meeting People's Needs Better: A Discussion Paper*, AGPS, Canberra.

—— 1996, COAG Meeting Communique, 11 April.

Commonwealth of Australia 1997, *Budget Strategy and Outlook 1997–98*, Budget Paper no.1, AGPS, Canberra.

—— 1998, *Budget Paper Nos 1 and 3*, AGPS, Canberra.

—— 1999, *Budget Paper Nos 1 and 3*, AGPS, Canberra.

—— 2001, *Budget Paper Nos 1 and 3*, AGPS, Canberra.

Crowley, R. 2000, *Healing Our Hospitals: A Report into Public Hospital Funding*, Parliament of Australia, Senate, Community Affairs References Committee, Canberra.

Department of Health and Family Services 1996, 'A Healthy Future for Health and Community Services', Press release, Office of the Minister, Dr Wooldridge, Canberra.

Draper, M. 1999, 'Casemix: Financing Hospital Services', in L. Hancock (ed.), *Health Policy in the Market State*, Allen & Unwin, Sydney.

Duckett, S. 1999, 'Commonwealth/State Relations in Health', in L. Hancock (ed.), *Health Policy in the Market State*, Allen & Unwin, Sydney.

Federal–State Relations Committee 1998, *Australian Federalism: The Role of the States*, Second Report on the Inquiry into Overlap and Duplication, AGPS, Melbourne.

—— 1999, *Report on the Register of Specific Purpose Payments Received by Victoria*, Fourth Report on the Inquiry into Overlap and Duplication, vols 1 and 2, AGPS, Melbourne.

Fletcher, C. 1991, *Responsive Government: Duplication and Overlap in the Australian Federal System*, Discussion Paper No. 3, Federalism Research Centre, Canberra.

Galligan, B. 1996, 'What is the Future of the Federation?', *Journal of Public Administration*, vol. 55, no. 3, pp. 74–82.

Gray, G. 2000, 'Private Practice Publicly Supported: Equity in Hospital and Medical Financing', *Just Policy*, no. 18, pp. 4–14.

Hancock, L. 1999 (ed.), *Health Policy in the Market State*, Allen & Unwin, Sydney.

—— & Cowling, S. 1999, *Searching for Social Advantage: What Has Happened to the 'Social Dividend' for Victorians?*, Women's Audit Project, Stegley Foundation, Melbourne.

Harman, E. & Harman, F. 1996, 'The Potential for Local Diversity in Implementation of the National Competition Policy', *Australian Journal of Public Administration*, vol. 55, no. 2, pp. 12–25.

Hendy, P. 1996, 'Intergovernmental Relations', *Australian Journal of Public Administration*, vol. 55, no. 1, pp. 111–17.

Hill, S. 1999, 'Consumer Payments for Health Care', in L. Hancock (ed.), *Health Policy in the Market State*, Allen & Unwin, Sydney.

Hilmer, F. G. 1993, *National Competition Policy: Report of the Independent Committee of Inquiry*, AGPS, Canberra.

Industry Commission 1996, *Competitive Tendering and Contracting by Public Sector Agencies*, Industries Commission, AGPS, Melbourne.

—— 1997, *Private Health Insurance*, Report no. 57, AGPS, Canberra.

James, D. 1997, *Commonwealth Assistance to the States since 1976*, Background Paper no. 5, Parliamentary Library, Parliament of Australia, Canberra.

Kelly, R. 1995, 'Privatising Public Health: Private Profit at Public Expense', *Just Policy*, no. 3, June, pp. 26–32.

Livingston, C. 1997, 'Private Health Insurance: A Triumph for Market Ideology', *Health Issues*, vol. 51, pp. 27–9.

National Commission of Audit 1996, *Report to the Commonwealth/National Commission of Audit*, AGPS, Canberra.

Owens, H. 1998, 'Health Insurance', in G. Mooney & R. Scotton (eds), *Economics and Australian Health Policy*, Allen & Unwin, Sydney.

Painter, M. 1996, 'The Council of Australian Governments and Intergovernmental Relations: A Case of Cooperative Federalism', *Publius*, 26, pp. 101–20.

—— 1998, 'After Managerialism: Rediscoveries and Redirections: The Case of Intergovernmental Relations', *Public Policy and Private Management Conference*, February, University of Melbourne, Centre for Public Policy, Melbourne.

Phillips Fox & Casemix Consulting 1999, *Health Services Policy Review: Discussion Paper*, Department of Human Services, Victorian Government, Melbourne.

Summers, J. 1994, 'Federalism and Commonwealth–state relations', in A. Parkin, J. Summers, & D. Woodward (eds), *Government, Politics, Power and Policy in Australia*, 5th edn, Longman Cheshire, Melbourne.

Trebeck, D. & Cutbush, G. 1996, *Overlap and Duplication in Federal/State Relations*, Samuel Griffith Society, Sydney.

3

Moving Away from the Welfare State: The Privatisation of the Health System

Carol Grbich

Discussions on privatisation of the Australian health system have tended to take one of two broad positions. The first is that privatisation by stealth may be occurring; it has been suggested that such a covert approach is not in the best interests of Australian society (Costa 1999). The second position can be seen in statements, usually authored by governments or private corporations, which proclaim privatisation as the only logical solution to the problems of an overstressed health system. There is often an underlying sense of inevitability in both of these orientations, with the implication that somehow a combination of an ageing population, rapacious doctors rorting the system, the increasing costs of health care, and the globalisation imperative have all contributed to such a degree to problems in health funding that privatisation is the only solution. This chapter seeks to clarify moves towards privatisation of the health sector, to examine their efficiency, and to suggest how the interests of the general population might better be met.

The ideology of the welfare state

With the advent of Medicare in 1984, the values of the welfare state reached their greatest height. It was widely accepted that universal access, regardless of income, was essential and that health and health care were for the common good and should be provided through general taxation. The original welfare state principles sought economic security and wellbeing, human dignity and social solidarity, political participation, and empowerment, which, when implemented, should lead to community stability, a reduction in class difference, and a strong, cohesive national identity. With the radical restructuring of the Australian health care system over the past decade, these principles are under threat. Dharan Ghia, Director of the United Nations Research Institute for Social Development, views emerging ideologies and powerful interests as deliberately obscuring public vision by creating a focus on narrow structural issues such as age and technology, thus allowing the values of the welfare state to become sidelined (Esping-Andersen 1996).

In addition, the widely agreed on principles of primary health care from the *Alma Alta Declaration* (World Health Organization 1978), which highlighted the consumer health determinants and equity of access for all to basic health rights, also appear to have been compromised by a focus on economic factors and structural adjustment. These have led governments away from responsibility for individual health needs to an emphasis on user financing, diversity, competition, and cost recovery. This orientation has been facilitated by an increasingly global focus on economic rationalist theory implemented by managerialistic techniques.

Global capitalism

The global capitalist system, characterised by an emphasis on free trade and freely moving capital, has not allowed for integration with or the parallel development of the noneconomic needs of a global society (Soros 1998). The influence of global capitalism has seen the values of economic rationalism and managerialism dominate Australian public sector reform over the past twenty years. Simply translated, economic rationalism has been interpreted as a commitment to forms of self-regulating free market organisation that provide maximum space for the development of private markets. Deregulated markets are seen as the most efficient way to promote competition. Where competitive markets do not exist, the government's role is to create them by becoming a purchaser and administrator of contracts for service provision. Management of resources favours choice through user payments and the rejection of government provision of services.

Critiques of economic rationalism

Opposition to the economic rationalist perspective is provided by the social democratic critique (Pusey 1991; Stretton 1987), which postulates that limited debate about national purposes and values has affected the balance among three important entities: civil society, the political system providing needed goods and services equitably, and the preferred mixed economy consisting of the public, private, and domestic. Pusey indicates that one danger of economic rationalism is that it redefines the meaning and function of the 'system' from a tripartite entity to a narrowly based economic system with weak government control. Here, the needs of civil society are viewed as marketplace activities subject to corporate managerial practices and driven by profit. The public sphere (Habermas 1989), which is the conceptual arena for dialogue and ideas where societal consensus is sought, then becomes narrowly focused on the economy; the resources, particularly information, to enable wider debate are lacking.

Within the social democratic perspective, the pretence that questions of value and social purpose can be replaced by economic theory divorced from the real world is seen as problematic because economic rationalist principles are not value free. A refocus on civil society and the political system would emphasise issues of redistribution based on social need and highlight the interdependence of family, community, the economy, and government. The incorporation of the public sphere would further facilitate a movement away from solely market-driven decisions and would permit greater balance among the three entities.

The current emphasis on an economic orientation in the construction of a good health service by government has further led to the criticism that, in Weberian terms, technical (*zweckrational*—involving calculations for a desired end) rather than moral (*wertrational*—motivated by humanistic values) action is dominating (Hicks 1995). According to Hicks this emphasis, together with the increasing numbers of health managers in Australia in the late twentieth century, will have an impact on the health system for some time to come. Their growing presence and training will serve to reinforce the technical aspects of managerialism, which include economic efficiencies and measurable outputs, corporate management principles, privatisation of delivery of services, consumer cost sharing, and a shift away from the welfare state with its notions of social justice and equity.

The lack of debate within the public sphere, with its potential for identifying entrenched interests and its emancipatory capacity to transform these through the incorporation of other values, has allowed the government to 'legitimate' its actions (Habermas 1975) through the notion of 'economic crisis' (Deeble 1999).

Privatisation in Australia

The health care system currently comprises a complex mix of federal, state and territory, and private funding: two-thirds public and one-third private. Among the Organization for Economic Cooperation and Development

(OECD) countries, Australia is in a position second only to the USA in private sector health development. At the opposite extreme, the heavily government funded National Health Service (NHS) in the UK provides an opposing model for consideration by the Australian system.

Australia spends 8.5 per cent of the gross domestic profit (GDP) on health, in contrast to 15 per cent spent by the USA, and this figure has remained constant since 1992 when it was 8.1 per cent (Australian Institute of Health and Welfare 2000c). Government funding of health varied from 66.7 per cent to 70.0 per cent in the ten years between 1989 and 1999 (Australian Institute of Health and Welfare 2000c), and over the past decade-and-a-half was 'only a little more than average for the economy generally [but was] much less than consumer prices as measured by the CPI' (Deeble 1999, p. 2). Deeble is quite clear that Medicare has been destabilised by 'the unrealistically low rates of growth built into the Commonwealth's hospital contribution' (Deeble 1999, p. 10). Yet, quite remarkably, despite minimal increases since its inception in 1984, Medicare now supports 30 per cent more medical services and 87 per cent more public patient admissions per person (Deeble 1999, p. 11).

In 1999–2000, the 5.3 per cent upswing in health expenditure was largely due to the introduction of private health insurance rebate schemes and, to a lesser extent, to an increase in Commonwealth funding of the states' health services of public hospitals, medical services, pharmaceuticals, and veterans' affairs through the Health Care Agreements. The Australian government still controls the health system, maintaining the principle of universal access to acute hospital services. It provides input through Medicare, regulates private health insurance, provides patient rebates for medical consultations, procedures, and diagnostic techniques, and subsidises prescription drugs. But the question that has to be asked now is how much control does it actually have? For how long? And is what is happening in the best interests of the Australian people?

Hospitals

Since 1994, with the opening of the first privatised public hospital, Port Mac-quarie Base Hospital, there has been significant growth in the private hospital sector. Public capital has been shifted in the move to privatise public hospitals and to colocate private hospitals adjacent to public hospitals. This has resulted in a blurring of the boundaries between public and private. The privatisation model involves the private sector financing the construction of the hospital and the state government contracting with the private hospital operator to provide hospital services. State governments pay the capital costs of public patients per patient for up to twenty years or longer. In theory, financial risk is shifted from government to private operator. Payment for patients is by diagnosis-related groups (DRGs) and capped amounts. At the end of the contracted period the hospital may revert to public ownership under the build, own, operate, and transfer (BOOT) model.

As these shifts have occurred, large national and international private health care corporations have been positioning themselves closer to Australia, scenting profits to be made in both hospital management and the provision of diagnostic services. There has been a significant increase in partnerships between these corporations and the government.

The largest private corporation is Health Care of Australia (HCoA), owned by Mayne Nickless, with fifty hospitals (HCoA website, Mayne Health) and considerable pathology interests. Ramsey Health Care, Australian Hospital Care, Healthscope, and Alpha Healthcare—all with between twelve and seventeen hospitals each—follow this group. The two main not-for-profit companies are the Sisters of Charity Group and the St John of God Care Services, with nine hospitals each (Foley 2000). Some of these companies have been consolidating their positions by specialising: for example, Ramsey Health Care has a major focus on psychiatric and veterans' hospitals, and has purchased pathology and radiology services. HCoA has an annual turnover of around $300 million from diagnostic services alone (Mayne Nickless 2000). Given that Medicare rebates diagnostic services at 85 per cent, that makes diagnostic services a very lucrative area of investment.

Box 3.1
Case study 1—Port Macquarie Base Hospital

The first experiment in privatisation was not a success. The Port Macquarie Base Hospital in New South Wales needed rebuilding and refurbishing. HCoA was contracted in 1992 to construct a 161-bed public hospital. Privatisation was justified on the grounds of cost efficiency and the potential for upgrading public infrastructure through private sector input (Collyer 1996). The New South Wales Health Department was to be the purchaser and regulator, paying HCoA an annual service charge for public patients and an availability charge to ensure the hospital remained accessible to public patients. HCoA, as the provider, was to manage the hospital, deliver services, and employ staff. The New South Wales government's assessment in 1992 was that it would cost them $64 million to build the hospital and a further $417 million for running costs and wages over a period of twenty years if they did retain control. The private sector could build the hospital for

$49 million and the government would only need to pay $371 million on recurrent costs, providing the government with savings of $46 million (Collyer 1996). Further scrutiny of these figures by the Public Accounts Committee (1992, 1993) suggested that the government could match the private sector estimates. The committee also suggested that an underestimate of private sector costs may have occurred and that although the public option would be more expensive for the state government it would be cheaper for the Commonwealth. It recommended that privatisation should go ahead, but that the state should retain ownership and lease the services (Collyer 1996). A local referendum of the Port Macquarie community indicated that 61 per cent opposed privatisation (Dodd 1996). Residents protested that at the end of twenty years the hospital would belong to HCoA, who might then decide to close it down, which would leave the district without a hospital. These recommendations and concerns were ignored by the New South Wales government, which went on with its privatisation agenda and continued to sign contracts to the end of 1992.

In 1996 the Auditor-General of New South Wales independently examined the project. His report showed that over twenty years the government would not only reimburse HCoA an extra $143 million through annual availability and fee-for-service charges, but would also have given away ownership of both the hospital and the land. With these monies the government could have built the hospital three times over themselves. The Auditor-General seriously questioned the capacity of the government to negotiate balanced deals with the private sector and queried whether privatisation was in the state's best interest (New South Wales Office of the Auditor-General 1996).

Over time, further problems have appeared. Recurrent costs to the government have been between 20 and 30 per cent higher than for an equivalent hospital (Refshauge 1996) and, in addition, the hospital appeared to be operating less efficiently than comparable public hospitals in Dubbo, Albury, Lismore, and Orange (Refshauge 1997). Further hidden expenses have been exposed, including the drawing up and administering of a complex contract, the running of a community information program regarding the benefits of privatisation, the provision of separate delivery of health and preventative programs no longer provided by the hospital, and the amounts involved in shifting costs from the state to the federal sector through the higher Medicare payments associated with fee for service reimbursements in the privately owned hospital (Collyer 1997).

Community concern has further been registered regarding the lack of a requirement for public disclosure of financial information from HCoA, the inadequate level of service from the Accident and Emergency department, cutbacks in operating theatres from seven to five days, extensive waiting lists (including eighteen-month wait-ing lists for joint and ophthalmic surgery), the lack of delivery of the promised renal unit, the fact that an independent ombudsman had to be called in to monitor the hospital's lack of response to com-plaints about hospital service, and the increasing reliance on the employment of part-time and casual staff (Queensland Nurses' Union 1999). HCoA also is not pleased and threatened legal action against the New South Wales government over the funding short-falls encountered when elective surgery funding dried up four months before the end of the financial year (Watts 1999).

■

Box 3.2
Case study 2—Latrobe Regional Hospital

The Latrobe Regional Hospital in Victoria was the first of several pri-vate contracts to become operational during 1998. Australian Hospital Care (AHC), which was the private partner, agreed to provide services at 96 per cent of what the state would have paid had the hospital been constructed with public funds. The Latrobe Hospital contract involved a BOOT model in order to shift the risks of ownership to the private sector but avoid the ultimate transfer with the loss of the facility as in the Port Macquarie model. As part of the agreement, the Victorian government promised that no other hospital would be built in the Latrobe Valley for twenty years (Auditor-General of Victoria 1996–97). The Auditor-General's Report was critical of the fact that no cost-benefit analysis had occurred prior to the contract being undertaken and that there was no evidence that the private sector could deliver services any more cheaply than the government. Again, local residents were unconvinced regarding the advantages to them of privatisation. Death threats were made against a doctor hired from interstate, there were rowdy public meetings at which tomatoes were thrown at senior hospital executives (Walkom 2000), and meetings between the members of the public and the Liberal Minister for Health, John Hannaford, became abusive (Dodd 1996).

Once established, the hospital was accused of offering induce-
ments to rural doctors to send their patients to Latrobe rather than to
their local rural hospitals (Macklin 1999). In February 2000, after
enduring heavy losses at Latrobe, AHC sued the Victorian government for $10 million on the grounds that its contract was not being
interpreted properly (Gregory 2000; Quinlivan 2000). Late in 2000,
Premier Bracks settled the court action and bought the renamed
Latrobe Valley Hospital back into public hands at a cost of $6 million.

■

Continuing problems

Problems similar to those outlined in case studies 1 and 2 (see boxes 3.1 and
3.2) emerged in other states. The Western Australian Auditor-General's
Report (1997) of a performance examination on HCoA's Joondalup Health
Campus provides further documentation of costing problems. Based on the
assumption that the hospital would cost $51 million if it were to build it, the
Western Australian government originally estimated that it would save over
$20 million through this contract. A revision of costs in order to achieve the
standards required by government led to an increase from $27 million to $42
million between contract signing in April and project commencement in
June 1996. In addition, the benchmarking exercise on which cost savings had
been calculated apparently had neither taken into account a competitive public sector bid nor the value of the existing buildings, leading the Auditor-
General to conclude that there was 'no reliable estimate of the extent of any
savings' (Western Australia, Office of the Auditor-General 1997, p. 48). The
Auditor-General also suggested that the contract price had actually reduced
the competitiveness of facilities and that the contract had left the government
with limited capacity to control either quantity or quality of services. Further,
there was potential to provide 'financial incentives for the private operator to
influence admission, treatment and discharge patterns, and potential overpay-
ments because of incorrect coding of treatments' (1997, p. 4).

A *Follow on Report* by the Auditor-General in June 2000 provided a further examination and assessment of the Western Australian Health Department's management of the contract and of the performance of the Joondalup
Health Campus. In this document, problems identified included HCoA's
continuing claims on the government purse beyond agreed levels, their
inability to provide information when requested, and the existence of a
higher than average number of patient complaints. Other concerns lay in the
hospital's refusal to accept hospital transfers (only fifty-nine had been accepted

compared to the 1198 received by neighbouring benchmarked hospitals), some inaccuracies in medical recording and invoicing that favoured the hospital, and the provider's capacity to influence treatment, discharge, and transfer arrangements in order to enhance profitability (Western Australia, Office of the Auditor-General 2000). The report concluded that 'greater activity in setting activity profiles is required if the department is to have any real capacity to manage the types of services performed by JHC as is provided under the contract' (2000, p. 12).

It would appear that moves towards privatisation have largely occurred outside the public sphere (although local communities have attempted to clarify their concerns), and have been fraught by insufficient assessment, weak government contracts, and poor monitoring. The Auditors-General of each state and territory have been the major—often the sole—watchdogs. Some have expressed concern regarding lack of information and lack of public debate. Tony Harris, Auditor-General of New South Wales, noted that there was a 'growing trend' to secret government in Australia: 'It appears to me that governments just don't want to be accountable' (Morton 1998). The South Australian Auditor-General commented that the use of commercial confidentiality considerations by private sector operators to limit public disclosure with regard to privatisation was undermining the foundations of parliamentary democracy. Sir Anthony Mason, former Chief Justice of the High Court, stated that:

> It is unacceptable in a democratic society that there should be a restraint on the publication of information relating to government where the only vice of that information is that it enables the public to discuss, review and criticise government action (Morton 1998).

Does privatisation save money?

It would appear from the above case studies that savings to the public sector through the privatisation of hospitals are illusory. This is supported by United States research, which found that for-profit hospitals were 3–11 per cent more expensive to operate than not-for-profit hospitals, and in addition resulted in higher death rates (Ingelhart 1999). A British evaluation of a privatisation experiment found inequitable and inefficient allocation of scarce resources (Gaffney & Pollock 1997). Accumulated international evidence suggests that transferring ownership from the public to the private domain achieves limited positive results and may in fact be counterproductive in terms of the nation's health (Ernst 1997).

Another government claim is that privatisation will ease pressure on the public system and make waiting lists shorter. To date there is no evidence of this (Australian Institute of Health and Welfare 2000b; New South Wales, Office of the Auditor-General 2000). Perversely, government moves to increase the private health insurance sector may well result in waiting lists getting longer rather than shorter. Colocation of the latest technology, and new theatres and offices in the private part of the hospital, may act as enticements to surgeons (Walkom 2000). If specialists take up financial incentives to increase their contribution to the private sector, they will have less time to contribute to the public sector. This might also lead to spiralling costs as the public sector is forced to match incentive payments in order to maintain specialised staff.

Shifts in service focus have already occurred, with most colocated private hospitals concentrating on profitable same-day elective surgery. These are quick same-day or overnight investigations or minor procedures for which the facility is often the major provider, in particular for lens and procedures, dental extractions and restorations, and gastroscopy and colonoscopy (Department of Health and Family Services 1997). These day surgery procedures now account for close to 50 per cent of all hospital stays (Australian Institute of Health and Welfare 2000a). Although this shift has reduced hospital bed days, the cost remains the same. Any savings have been taken up by the increased use of expensive technology (Brown 1999). The logical extension of these changes will be public hospital purchasing of private hospital services (Lewis 1998), leaving the public sector with the less profitable, complex, and long-stay patients, all of which may result in the demise of the public sector as it becomes further run down and subject to takeover bids by its colocated, corporately managed neighbours.

These scenarios reinforce concerns that the Australian government is not using privatisation as a fiscal management technique but as a political strategy to serve special interests by creating distance from contentious administrative areas such as health (Browning 1999). These have not been cost-efficient exercises, as the state continues to pay premium costs for services. The strategy is facilitated by the use of legitimated means—using the language of economic rationalism—in order to transfer public monies to the private sector, thereby creating the illusion of good management while further increasing inequality, enhancing private wealth, and reinforcing class-based health access.

Privatisation or noncompetitive corporate oligopoly?

Concern for vanishing notions of access, equity, and primary health care have neither hindered transnational corporations from positioning themselves for takeover, nor much concerned Australian government regarding the extensive court records for poor service provision of some of these companies. For example, Kaiser, USA, with legal fines for poor managed care practices in the

USA (Kyle 2000) and a record of breaching patient confidentiality through its website (Brubaker 2000), has a contract in South Australia to help the Health Department reform its information systems. Sun Healthcare, USA, with major investments in Alpha Healthcare, has a record of fines for Medicare fraud in the USA and abuse of the elderly (Sikes 1999).

In 1994, Mayne Nickless (HCoA) was fined $7.7 million by the Australian courts for price fixing with regard to its trucking company. Mayne Nickless also has well-established links with the Health Corporation of America and Tenet Healthcare (National Medical Enterprises, USA), both of which are facing ongoing court action over major rorting of the United States health care system (Wynne 2000).

In 1994, the head of the FBI estimated that corporate fraud in health care was costing $100 billion annually (Wynne 2000). In 1997, HCoA developed close relations with AXA (France), which controls National Mutual Insurance Australia, and offered managed care contracts to doctors in HCoA hospitals in New South Wales and Victoria. The Australian Medical Association (AMA) resisted these arrangements (Wynne 2000). In March 2000, California-based Franklin Resources, the world's largest publicly trading mutual fund company, suddenly increased its interest in Mayne Nickless to more than 40 million ordinary shares (HCoA website). None of these moves bodes well for the stability of Australian health care.

The blurring of public and private was seen more clearly in 1998 when Dr Catchlove, senior executive of Mayne Nickless (HCoA), took the additional government position of head of the Health Insurance Commission. He was obliged to stand down from this position in October 1999 after the MRI imaging scam in which fifty-two scanners costing $3 million each to buy and house were ordered just prior to the May 1998 Budget. The Budget permitted a $475 Medicare rebate for this scanning service, enabling private operators to pay off their new equipment within two years. HCoA had, fortuitously for them, just purchased six of these scanners. The Medicare budget for radiology is now expected to exceed $1 billion (Wilkinson 2000). As well as standing down from his government position pending an inquiry, Catchlove also left his executive position in Mayne Nickless to become health and community services adviser at KPMG (Internet and Systems Integration Services, based in the USA). He remained a board member of Mayne Nickless (Mayne Nickless, news release, 9 February 2000) and retained his position as chairman of the board of the Institute for Magnetic Imaging Research (IMIR), the government-funded research institute attached to the University of Sydney (IMIR website).

Other national and transnational moves towards integration in the private sector can be seen in the 50:50 joint venture between Mayne Nickless and Ramsey Health Care to bid with the then Inner and Eastern Health Care

Network in Victoria for the highly controversial contract to build, own, and operate a teaching and research centre (Brooks 1999). This was to be the new Austin and Repatriation Medical Centre complex in Melbourne. The privatisation of the existing large teaching centre with a number of research institutes caused considerable public outcry (Birnbauer & Davies 1999; Brooks 1999) before Premier Bracks moved to retain this facility in public hands. From 2000, the Bracks government, which opposes privatisation, will spend $155 million to upgrade this facility and maintain its high teaching and learning reputation.

Despite moves by the private sector to consolidate its position, the process is not working as well as expected. Companies are not making the financial gains they had at first anticipated. Costs have grown, new technology, fewer than expected patients, and a minimal increase in rebates have forced profits down. In the twelve months to December 1999, share prices fell: Mayne Nickless by 39 per cent, Ramsey Health Care by 60 per cent, Healthscope by 59 per cent, Alpha Healthcare by 75 per cent, and Australian Hospital Care by 59 per cent (Ballard 1999). Profits have also dropped. HCoA's operating profit slipped from $13 million to $7.7 million between 1997 and 1999, Ramsey's net profit went from $14 to $10 million, Australian Hospital Care's profits went from $15 to $10 million, and all three showed further losses during the first half of the period 1999–2000 (Tolhurst 2000). The increase in private insurance following the July 2000 cutoff date improved share prices a little. For example, in 1998 Ramsey Health Care shares were worth $2.30, by April 2000 they had dropped to 76 cents, and they rose to $1.10 by August. Similarly, Mayne Nickless shares were worth $3.31 in February 2000, rising to $3.67 by August of that year. By 2002, however, their performance on the stock market was excellent (Greenblat 2002).

Colocation projects have also run into problems. North Shore Private in New South Wales and Flinders Private in South Australia continue to struggle for occupancy and viability. Ramsey Healthcare has already sold Flinders Private to a not-for-profit company, the Adelaide Community Healthcare Alliance, and has delayed the commencement of its successful tender to build and operate Princess Alexandra Private in Brisbane. HCoA withdrew from its bid to build the colocated Royal Brisbane Private and, together with AHC, appears to be reconsidering its Australian investments in the light of new (and more profitable) markets in Asia. Although there are clearly profits to be made, these might be less than previously anticipated. One unfortunate outcome of privatisation is that there are now too many private beds for the one-third of the population who are privately insured. Private beds have doubled from 2 per 1000 to 4 per 1000, which is twice the ratio of those available in the public sector (Kavanagh 1999).

The increasing control by insurers in the setting of prices for procedures has also put considerable pressures on the margins of for-profit private hospital firms (Tolhurst 2000). The uncertainty of demand, the potential for limited profitability against the lure of established and well-regarded teaching hospitals, and the lack of clarity regarding future health insurance arrangements have resulted in considerable uncertainty. More important, any public benefit from privatisation is a long way from being clarified.

Private health insurance

Inextricably linked with hospital privatisation is the issue of private health insurance. Private health insurance sits alongside the tax funded public Medicare system. Of the forty-eight health benefit organisations, the ten largest cover 85 per cent of the market (Standard & Poor's 2000). Since the early 1990s, all forms of health insurance coverage declined from 43.7 in 1991 to 30.6 in 1998. The main reason for the decline was the increasing cost of premiums, which were well above inflation rates. Consumers appeared to be viewing private insurance as an expensive luxury (Deeble 1999) and did not want to have to pay rising premiums, which would result in extra bills and out-of-pocket expenses. A CHOICE survey of 6000 members found that incentives for lower-income earners, or additional surcharges for higher-income earners, did not encourage many people to join. The Council on the Ageing (COTA) also saw tax penalties as further undermining the concept of universal health care (CHOICE and COTA 1998).

According to the Productivity Commission's *Report on the Private Health Insurance Industry* (1997), premiums increased because of two major factors. First, there was a shift by privately insured members in usage of private rather than public beds (patient numbers in private hospitals increased from 54 to 76 per cent in 1997–98), reducing revenue to public hospitals in terms of private hospital bed-days and increasing the costs for private health insurers. Deeble (1999) notes, however, that between 1985 and 1998 public hospital throughput was much greater. There was an increase of 87 per cent, as opposed to 15 per cent in the private sector.

Second, there was adverse selection, the growing concentration of high-risk members in the private insurance sector, with younger, fitter members dropping their cover because of increasing premiums, which offered no return because they were fit and healthy. Again, Deeble (1999) asserts that a close scrutiny of the figures shows no worsening of the risk profile of those privately insured. In any event, there has been a definite trend towards self-funding when those without private insurance pay for private care when they judge they need it (Australian Institute of Health and Welfare 1996–97). This has become more easily achievable with the lower costs associated with the increasing proportion of same-day surgery (Australian Institute of Health and

Welfare 2000a). All this suggests that the profit motive may have been an important factor in the increase of premiums by insurance companies.

Private health insurance: optional extra or widespread private coverage?

From 1998, the Commonwealth government provided up to $2.2 billion annually in tax rebates, equal to 30 per cent of any insurance premiums paid, in order to try to attract more members and to slow the persistent movement of the population away from private funds. It also placed increasing age-related penalties of 2 per cent per year on those older than 30 who entered after 15 July 2000. These moves might have increased the number of insured, but it seems likely that many who have taken out the lowest form of insurance to achieve the 30 per cent rebate and to avoid the additional Medicare levy, would still use the public system. As these manoeuvres do not address the inherent instability of the insurance system they are unlikely to have any long-term effect (Productivity Commission 1997).

Who exactly has benefited from these changes? The main beneficiaries appear to be those who were already insured and those who can afford to be insured, together with the insurance companies, which, in 1999, made a profit of $126 million after three consecutive years of losses (Standard & Poor's 2000). Beyond mid 2001, however, further losses are predicted as claims of new members escalate after the twelve-month curfew (Standard & Poor's 2000). In 2002, the government announced average premium rises of 6.9 per cent. The problem of gap funding still persists in a number of policies and if premiums continue to rise, as they inevitably will, individuals will again drop out of the system, negating recent gains and leading to cutbacks in services and further claims by private corporations on the public purse.

The average family paid around $1500 annually in premiums, putting the option of private health insurance out of the range of many. According to Schofield (1997), high-income families (the middle aged and couples without or with children) have the highest incidence of total cover. Those aged 15–30 and those aged 80 and over are the least likely to be covered, as are the poor, migrants, single parents, drinkers and smokers, and those in poor health. Given this profile, if the government continues to shore up the private health insurance system and to shift funding into the private sector, the likely outcome is the maintenance and extension of an increasingly divided two-tier system.

Private or public?

Private hospital funding is heavily reliant on private health insurance, with more than 70 per cent of revenue coming from this source. Dr Peter Davoren, president of the Doctors' Reform Society, asserts that the private health industry is 'more expensive, less efficient, less fair and has no better outcomes than the public system' (Davoren 1999, p. 9).

In a twelve-month review of patients attending the Department of Cardiology at Monash Medical Centre, a research team found that the average cost associated with 186 public and private patients treated for elective coronary angioplasty and stenting were similar—$5516 per public patient and $5844 per private patient. The average charges, however, differed with $13 347 being charged in the colocated private hospital and $14 978 in a standard private hospital. The revenue obtained from the government was $5664 in the colocated private setting, $5394 in the standard private hospital, and $6201 in the public hospital. The profit achieved by the private settings was thus in the order of $7500–8500 (Harper et al. 2000).

All of which begs the question of whether the extra monies involved could be more profitably spent in upgrading the public sector, given that the health outcomes for patients were found to be identical regardless of location. In addition, each patient tended to have the same doctor and health team and the same equipment. However, the availability of patients with private health insurance might lead to overservicing. The number of procedures performed on individual patients with acute myocardial infarction has been found to be greater when the patient is private (Robertson & Richardson 2000). On the basis of these findings, Harper et al. suggest that 'encouraging more people to take out private health insurance will paradoxically increase government costs as well as increasing overall health expenditure' (2000, p. 296).

The *Australian Health Insurers Report* (Standard & Poor's 2000) also predicted that, from 2001, increasing pressure on claims levels and the introduction of gap coverage, combined with fewer new clients, will create financial problems. As there are already too many players in the market, small companies will collapse and larger ones will pressure the government for further support.

Given the evidence presented here regarding private health insurance and hospital privatisation, it would be difficult to assert that Hsaio's (1992) three key criteria for evaluating a system's financial structure are being met in Australia. Universal coverage is teetering on the brink of inequality, equitable distribution of financial burden according to the individual's capacity to pay has not been satisfied, and the administrative efficiency of the financing scheme is highly problematic. It is difficult not to conclude that current reforms have been poorly researched and inappropriately assessed. In relation to privatisation, the principles earmarked for change—consumer choice, equitable allocation of services, and free market access—have not been well thought through.

Possible solutions

How, then, could the government maintain the principles of the welfare state and of primary health care while achieving administrative efficiency? There are a number of suggestions about possible solutions.

- *Place the whole matter in the public domain so that a properly informed debate can ensue.* As part of this process, the values of equity of access, quality, effective improvement in health status, and efficiency should be emphasised, and needs assessments and cost–benefit analyses of both public and private facilities and services should be undertaken.
- *Fund Medicare more appropriately.* Increase the Medicare levy by 1 per cent to put a further $2 billion into public health care in order to fund a universal health care system based on caring and best practice (Leeder 1999).
- *Accept that a health system with dependence on high-technology medicine is not cost-effective.* Changing personal behaviour with better public health and primary health care, and the delivery of health care in a more moderately technologised manner as the key to improving health.
- *Re-examine the medical system in terms of evidence-based medicine, best practice, and medical ethics, and use open debate to tackle the ethical issues around complex procedures.* These could include multiple bypasses that might give only limited years of life to an aged person, palliative chemotherapy and radiotherapy, fertility programs and in vitro fertilisation, sex change operations, the heavy use of diagnostic testing, and expensive drug alternatives.

People power

Apart from the absence of discussion about the public sphere, another aspect generally omitted from discussions regarding health delivery has been the role of health care workers and patients who are inheriting a privatised health system with all its limitations. The creation of new hospitals and the downsizing of others have already resulted in job losses and an emphasis on short-term and casual labour. The final product might well be a leaner and meaner workforce doing much more for less, but what will happen when, in an environment of reducing government support and in search of higher profits, private companies increase pressure for greater production and attempt further downsizing of their workforces? The general view has been that the combination of global companies, enterprise bargaining, and disparate and weakened unions will mean that strike action is likely—nationally and internationally—to be a rare and ineffectual event.

Two recent and successful strike actions have threatened this view. The first occurred in 1997 at United Parcel Service (UPS), a multinational company employing workers in the UK, the USA, Europe, Canada, and South America (among many other countries). Despite distance, the workers formed an international transport workers' union, which, through widespread strike action, was successful in preventing company moves to convert full-time jobs to part-time jobs. The workers also achieved pay increases and improved union control of wages and conditions (Mazur 2000).

The second action occurred in the USA at Boeing, which had announced it was going to eliminate 48 000 jobs over a two-year period because of competition from other aircraft makers. In early 2000, forty days of strike action were taken by the Association of Machinists (32 000) and by the Association of Professional Engineers (17 000). This action was successful in reversing the decision to sack people and, in addition, gained improved wages, improved medical insurance, and a stronger union voice. It is notable (and might provide a foretaste of the future in Australian health) that the engineers, like many professional groups, had no history of strike action and no strike fund to support such action. Both organisations insisted that the dominant issue was not so much jobs, wages, and benefits, but lack of respect. All believed the company had become too impersonal, focusing on profit rather than people and quality (Dube 2000).

Australian doctors on both sides of the political divide have reflected the concerns regarding privatisation of the health system. A submission to the Senate Inquiry into Public Hospital Funding chose to highlight patient care rather than efficiencies. It argued that in the public sector, where

> clinical staff provide a considerable amount of unpaid overtime for the benefit of their patients and the existing public hospital system, they could not be expected to provide 'honorary' services for a private for-profit operator, where resultant savings may simply be returned to shareholders (Australian Medical Association Victoria [AMA] 1999, Section 4).

The main resolution of this submission was 'that quality of care should be the cornerstone of the Victorian Public Hospital system and not just cost and throughput' (AMA 1999, Section 4).

In the final analysis, in the move away from the principles of the welfare state and of primary health care towards privatisation and private profit, an inequitable and unstable situation is being created. A weak political system, a lack of public debate, and poorly constructed agreements with companies without records of good care practice, make future health care delivery highly problematic.

References

Australian Institute of Health and Welfare 1996–97, *Australian Hospital Statistics*, AIHW, Canberra.

—— 1998, *Health Expenditure Bulletin*, no. 12, November, AIHW, Canberra.

—— 2000a, *Australian Hospital Statistics 1998–99*, AIHW, Canberra.

—— 2000b, *Waiting Times for Elective Surgery in Australia 1997/8*, AIHW, Canberra.

—— 2000c, 'Australia's Health Services Expenditure to 1998/99', *Health Expenditure Bulletin*, no. 16, AIHW, Canberra.

Australian Medical Association (AMA) Victoria 1999, *Trends in Hospital Funding*, submission to the Senate Community Affairs Committee Inquiry into Public Hospital Funding, October, AMA Victoria.

Ballard, J. 1999, 'Colocation: Opportunities and Threats for the Catholic Health System in Australia', address to the National Conference of the Little Company of Mary, 29 October, Hobart.

Birnbauer, B. & Davies, J. 1999, 'Critical Condition', *Age*, 31 May.

Brooks, P. 1999, 'Privatisation of Teaching Hospitals', *Medical Journal of Australia*, vol. 170, pp. 321–2.

Brown, D. 1999, Address by the Hon. Dean Brown, Minister for Human Services, South Australia, to the *Financial Review*'s Health Congress, February, Sydney.

Browning, B. 1999, 'Health, Values and Economic Rationalism', Paper presented at the Values Based Medicine Conference, Sydney.

Brubaker, B. 2000, ' "Sensitive" Kaiser e-mails Go Astray', *Washington Post*, 10 August, <http://www.washingtonpost.com/wp-dyn/articles/A64768-2000Aug9.html>.

CHOICE and Council on the Ageing 1998, *Private Health Insurance: A Policy Paper*, <http://www.choice.com.au/articles/a100221p3.htm>.

Collyer, F. 1996, 'Who Really Pays for The Provision of Private Hospital Services?: The Privatisation of the Port Macquarie Base Hospital', Paper presented at the Australian Sociological Association Conference, Tasmania, December.

—— 1997, 'To Market to Market: Corporatisation, Privatisation and Hospital Costs', *Australian Health Review*, vol. 20, no. 2, pp. 13–25.

Costa, C. 1999, 'Health Services in Transition: Privatisation by Stealth', Presentation by the past president of the Doctors' Reform Society to the National Conference, Sydney, August, <http://www.drs.org.au/conference/1999/Costa.html>.

Davoren, D. 1999, 'The Doctors' Reform Society on Public Funding', Submission to the Senate Community Affairs Committee Inquiry into Public Hospital Funding, October, *New Doctor*, vol. 72, Summer 1999/2000.

Deeble, J. 1999, 'Medicare: Where have We Been? Where are We Going?', Gordon Oration, available online at <www.pha.net.au/conferences/gordonoration.htm>; also in *Australian and New Zealand Journal of Public Health*, vol. 23, pp. 563–70.

Department of Health and Family Services 1997, *Australian Casemix Report on Hospital Activity 1995–96*, AGPS, Canberra.

Dodd, A. 1996, 'Public Patients, Private Profit', Australian Broadcasting Commission, Radio National, 20 October, <http://www.abc.net.au/in/talks/bbing/stories/s10626.htm>.

Dube, J. 2000, 'Back To Work?: Tentative Agreement in Boeing Strike' Australian Broadcasting Commission ABCNEWS.com, <http://www.abcnews.go.com.ns/business/Daily/News/boeing000317.html>.

Ernst, J. 1997, 'Public Utility Privatisation and Competition: Challenges to Equity and the Environment', *Just Policy*, no. 9, March.

Esping-Andersen, G. (ed.) 1996, *Welfare States in Transition: National Adaptations in Global Economies*, Sage International, London.

Foley, M. 2000, 'The Changing Public–Private Balance', in A. Bloom (ed.), *Health Reform in Australia and New Zealand*, Oxford University Press, Melbourne.

Gaffney, D. & Pollock, A., 1997, *Can the NHS Afford the Private Finance Initiative?* British Medical Association, Health Policy and Economic Research Unit, London.

Greenblat, E. 2002, 'Market Stars Perform in Sickness and Health', the *Age*, 1 January.

Gregory, P. 2000, 'Hospital Sues State for $10 Million', the *Age*, 23 February.

Habermas, J. 1975, *Legitimation Crisis*, trans. Thomas McCarthy, Beacon Press, Boston.

—— 1989, *The Structural Transformation of the Public Sphere: An Inquiry into a Category of Bourgeois Society*, MIT Press, Massachusetts.

Harper, R. et al. 2000, 'Costs, Charges and Revenues of Elective Coronary Angioplasty and Stenting: The Public Versus the Private System', *Medical Journal of Australia*, vol. 173, pp. 296–300.

Health Care of Australia, <http://www.hcoa.com.au>.

Hicks, N. 1995, 'Economism, Managerialism and Health Care', *Annual Review of Health and Social Sciences*, vol. 5, pp. 39–60.

Hsaio, W. 1992, 'Comparing Health Care Systems: What Nations Can Learn From One Another', *Journal of Health Politics, Policy and Law*, vol. 17, no. 4, pp. 613–36.

Ingelhart, J. 1999, 'The American Health Care System: Expenditures', *New England Journal of Medicine*, January, vol. 340, no. 1, pp. 70–6.

Institute for Magnetic Imaging Research, <http://www.imrr.org.au/aboutimrr.html>.

Kavanagh, J. 1999, 'Top 500 Companies, Health Funds on the Way to Recovery', *Business Review Weekly*, 6 August.

Leeder, S. 1999, 'How You Can Help Maintain the Health of Medicare', Keynote address to the Doctors' Reform Society National Conference, Sydney.

Lewis, G. 1998, 'Private Hospitals and the Private Health Insurance Conundrum', Research note 1, 1998–99, Social Policy Group, Parliament of Australia.

Macklin, J. 1999, 'How Shall We Judge the Success of the National Framework?', 5th National Rural Health Conference, 14–17 March, Adelaide.

Mayne Nickless 2000, *First Half Yearly Report 1999–2000*, 1 March, <http://www.maynick.com.au/investor/half_year_results.html>.

Mazur, J. 2000, 'Labour's New Internationalism: The Seattle Message', *Foreign Affairs (USA)*, January–February issue.

Morton, T. 1998, 'Shrinking Democracy', *Background Briefing*, Radio National, Australian Broadcasting Commission, <http://www.abc.net.au/m/talks/bbing/stories/s19075.html>, 1 November.

New South Wales Office of the Auditor-General 1996, *New South Wales Auditor-General's Report for 1996*, vol. 1, Audit Office of New South Wales, Sydney.

—— 2000, *Hospital Emergency Departments: Delivering Services to Patients*, Performance Audit Report, Audit Office of New South Wales, Sydney.

Productivity Commission 1997, *Inquiry into the Private Health Insurance Industry*, Report no. 57, February, AGPS, Canberra.

Public Accounts Select Committee of the New South Wales Parliament 1992, *Phase 1 Report of the Select Committee upon the Port Macquarie Base Hospital Project*, June, Phase 1, New South Wales Parliament.

—— 1993, *Report of the Select Committee Upon the Port Macquarie Base Hospital Project into the Funding of Health Infrastructure in New South Wales*, June, Phase 2, New South Wales Parliament.

Pusey, M. 1991, *Economic Rationalism in Canberra: A Nation Building State Changes its Mind*, Cambridge University Press, Cambridge.

Pyle, A. 2000, 'Woman Savors Victory in Long War with HMO', *Los Angeles Times*, 20 May, <http://www.latimes.com/news/nation/updates/lat_hmo000522.html>.

Queensland Nurses' Union 1999, *Submission to the Senate Community Affairs Reference Inquiry into Public Hospital Funding*, Queensland Nurses' Union, <http://www.qnu.org.au/htm>.

Quinlivan, B. 2000, 'Part Two: A Lingering Malaise', *Business Review Weekly*, vol. 22, no. 15.

Refshauge, A. 1996, 'Public Patients, Private Profit', *Background Briefing*, Radio National, Australian Broadcasting Corporation, 20 October.

—— 1997, Statement to Parliament, *Riverina Sun*, 26 March.

Robertson, I. & Richardson, J. 2000, 'Coronary Angioplasty and Coronary Artery Revascularisation Rates in Public and Private Hospital Patients After Acute Myocardial Infarction', *Medical Journal of Australia*, vol. 173, pp. 291–5.

Schofield, D. 1997, *The Distribution and Determinants of Private Health Insurance in Australia, 1990*, Discussion paper no. 17, National Centre for Social and Economic Modelling, Canberra.

Soros, G. 1998, *The Crisis of Global Capitalism: Open Society Endangered*, Perseus, New York.

Sikes, J. 1999, 'State Attorney Makes Deal with Nursing Home', *Gainsville Sun*, Florida, <http://www.sunone.com/news/articles/12-23-99f.shtml>, 23 December.

Standard & Poor's 2000, *Australian Health Insurers Report 2000*, Standard & Poor's Rating Agency, Sydney.

Stretton, H. 1987, 'The Corruption of the Intellectuals' and 'Tasks for Social Democratic Intellectuals', in *Political Essays*, Georgian House, Melbourne.

Tolhurst, C. 2000, 'Private Care Pinched to the Margins', *Australian Financial Review*, 29 May.

Victoria Office of the Auditor-General 1997, *Report of the Auditor-General on the Government's Annual Financial Statement 1996–97*, Audit Office of Victoria, Melbourne.

Walkom, T. 2000, 'Fixing Health Care: Hard Lessons Down Under, the Very Public Failure of a Private Hospital' and 'Condition Critical: Where Two-tier Hospitals are Failing', *Toronto Star*, <http://www.savemedicare.org/star.html>, 19 March.

Watts, A. 1999, 'Health Budget Crisis: HCoA says it will go to courts', *Port Macquarie News*, 24 February, p.1.

Western Australian Office of the Auditor-General 1997, *Performance Examination: Private Care for Public Patients: The Joondalup Health Campus*, Report no. 9, Audit Office of Western Australia, Perth.

—— 2000, *Private Care for Public Patients: The Joondalup Health Campus, A Follow-on Examination*, Report no. 4, Audit Office of Western Australia, Perth.

Wilkinson, M. 2000, ' "Scan Scam": A Mere Blip for Radiology's Rich List', *Sydney Morning Herald*, 13 March.

World Health Organization 1978, *The Declaration of Alma Alta*, Report of the International Conference of Primary Health Care, Alma Alta, USSR, WHO, Geneva.

Wynne, M. 2000, 'Health Care in Australia', <http://www.uow.edu./art/bmartin/dissent/documents/health/australia.html>, modified April 2000.

4

Health Information Policy

Rosemary Roberts, Kerin Robinson, and Dianne Williamson

Policies relating to health information management and health informatics have, until recently, been characterised by their ad hoc nature. National initiatives, such as the National Health Information Management Advisory Council (NHIMAC) and Health Online (NHIMAC 1999, 2001), have turned the spotlight onto the vital role that health information plays in improving Australia's health system. The need to agree upon national approaches for developments in electronic health records, record linkage, casemix, and population–based funding has forced an upsurge in health information policy statements at national and state levels. The policies have, in turn, been accompanied by planning statements dealing with resource and technology issues such as electronic systems, the health information and informatics workforce, and the role played by health professionals in creating and using health information.

This chapter focuses on recent developments in health information policy and their impact on managers and health service providers. It identifies the context in which these developments have occurred: the technological and cultural environment, the principal actors—governments, clinicians, health information professionals, and consumers—and the major issues of privacy, ownership and access, accountability, classification, casemix, quality, standardisation, and efficiency. Although the states and territories have their own jurisdictions, they are also involved in the creation of national policy through their participation in the National Health Information Agreement (NHIA).

The health information environment is reviewed and the boundaries of what constitutes 'health information' in the context of this chapter are defined. The chapter also covers the structures of data collections, national and state responsibilities, and policy background, especially in relation to electronic health records, and chronicles the major milestones in policy development to date.

The National Centre for Classification in Health (NCCH) is used as a case study to demonstrate the centrality of health information policy to the overall context of health services planning, research, quality of care measurement, consumer understanding of health, and efficiency of health service provision.

Health information defined

Health care *data* are the raw details such as facts, figures, ideas about, and observations collected on a patient or client, usually at the point of care. Health *information* comprises data that have been interpreted or manipulated into some meaningful form that is valuable to the user (Dombal 1996; Abedelhak et al. 2001). Health information is described by Waters and Murphy as 'pertaining to the physical, mental or social well-being of an individual or group of individuals' (1979, p. 33).

Three dimensions of health information derive from and support each episode of care (Southon & Holman 1996). These are

- *the patient dimension*—information gained from the patient and from the interactions of health care providers
- *the professional dimension*—information that supports evidence-based treatment and informs clinical knowledge
- *the management dimension*—information that meets administrative, financial, and evaluative needs of health services.

Clinical health data become health information when placed in a context, such as in comparison with similar cases, or matched with other, non-clinical, patient characteristics—for example, age, residential location, ethnicity, type of health provider, date of service provision, and occupation. Nonclinical data, for example, comparative length of stay or frequency of consultation, can also provide useful health information.

Health information can be collected and used at the level of the population, the service provider, or the patient (Smith 2000). At the level of the individual patient, health information derives from those items relating to the individual's physical and mental conditions and to the interventions of a health care provider to improve the individual's health status. This constitutes the medical or health record, created for the primary purpose of providing quality care to the individual patient.

At the aggregate level, data from the health records of many patients are combined to provide broader information, on a population basis, of health status and health interventions. Aggregate data do not identify the individual patient, although elements that allow separate records on the same patient to be linked may be included. Information from different providers or from the same provider at different times can be matched to provide information on a continuum of an individual's health or medical history and experience over several episodes of care. This continuum could extend from the birth to the death of the patient. Currently, this is not realistic because of the massive volume of lifetime health information that accrues in different places on any one person. There is, too, the involvement of many different providers and services across states and sectors, and the technical complexities of storing, linking, and retrieving relevant information for legitimate access while maintaining the security of the individual's health records.

Databases containing aggregate data tend to be established according to type of health service, such as the National Hospital Morbidity Database, which relates to the acute health sector; or to a specific condition, for example the National Diabetes Register. Death certification, the ultimate source of health information, records the cause of death and underlying conditions. These are aggregated in mortality databases.

The term 'health information' is something of a misnomer as most of the information collected relates to ill health or lack of optimum physical or mental wellbeing. From the patient's perspective, health information comprises clinical data on symptoms and disease, injury, congenital conditions, disability, and the pharmaceutical, surgical, and other interventions and measures undertaken to treat or prevent these conditions. An understanding of the health status of the population requires consideration of measures of ill health, including

- the number of patients to whom care is provided
- the incidence and prevalence of disease
- occupational injuries
- death rates and causes
- life expectancy
- the prevalence of disabilities.

Aggregate data may be based on the identification or treatment of health problems, for example, surgery for cholelithiasis or disease surveillance such as breast cancer screening. Much information in aggregate data collections derives from interactions between health care providers and patients where the contact is reported to a funding authority—for example, the Health Insurance Commission (HIC). There is, therefore, an incomplete picture of health problems for which patients self-medicate with over-the-counter remedies, do not seek treatment, or seek advice from health practitioners whose interventions are not recognised by governments and other agencies that collect intervention data. For example, episodes of care provided by a physiotherapist in private practice, a naturopathy practitioner, or a psychologist, are not registered on these databases.

The context of databases containing aggregate data is determined by the stated purpose of the collection, which might be funding and payment, public health research, disease surveillance, service evaluation, or service planning. Users of health information are frequently frustrated by the limitations of databases when the content of the collection does not match the desired potential use—for example, data collected for financial purposes might not be useful to epidemiologists.

Data elements—that is, specific items of data—need to be defined carefully to ensure the quality and the usefulness of the data. For example, the data element 'age' could be measured in days or years at the time of the episode of care, or derived from the date of birth. Although the element 'country of birth' may be collected, some data users may be more interested in ethnicity or language. Other issues surround the method of recording the patient's residential location because of variability in postcode, municipal boundaries, or the catchment area of a regional health service or health network.

Most data collections are episode-based and do not match individual patient interactions with health services over time, making it difficult for users to monitor the quality of health services. We may know about the length and nature of the consultation, but not the outcome in terms of long-term improvement in health status; an exception to this is the relatively blunt measure of mortality data. This deficiency has major implications for policy on linking records and patient identifiers at local, state and territory, and national levels.

Hargreaves (1999) describes difficulties with Australian health information caused by gaps within and between the classification systems used to record health data. These have occurred because of historically fragmented approach to the development of health information databases. The work being undertaken by the National Centre for Classification in Health both to improve classifications and the quality of data is described below.

Health information as a strategic resource

The fact that health information is integral to all aspects of health care and health care delivery, evaluation, service planning, and funding, places it in a special position with respect to policy negotiation and development. Its universality, especially in terms of the number and breadth of categories of stakeholders, ensures that the processes and plays in policy change and development are highly contested and often protracted. This is exemplified in the conflict surrounding the policy on health consumers' access to their personal health records.

At times, efforts to frame health information policy are fragmented and appear to be poorly organised. These characteristics are in common with other shifts in the negotiated order of the health care system as identified by Degeling and Anderson (1992). The complexity of health information and the fact that it is so fundamental to the health system and to its stakeholders inevitably ensures a weaving and shifting of coalitions of interests. In policy development in health care, the dominant structural interests were described by Alford (1972) (and later applied to the Australian health care system by Duckett (1984)), who identified the 'professional monopolists' as the medical profession (represented by the Australian Medical Association) and medical researchers, and the 'corporate rationalists' as health bureaucrats and large health facility managers. The contemporary Australian equivalent of Alford's third group, the 'community population', comprises the health consumer representatives. Each of these interests, working in various coalitions, has influenced health information policy in Australia in the past decade.

During the 1990s, there was a shift towards increased use by the corporate rationalists of high-quality, timely health information. Evidence of this trend was the introduction of casemix-based funding systems. However, the trend to evidence-based medicine and the incorporation of quality management in health care have led to an increasing emphasis by clinicians on the wider uses of health information. Consumer groups have led the push for improved rights of access by patients to their medical records.

National health information structures

Although many health care providers collect and use health information for effective management of individual patients and health services, there is a multiplicity of reporting requirements at local, state and territory, and national levels. These can be a burden for providers when collection agencies require different data items, definitions of data elements, and reporting time frames. A single episode of care relating to a single patient might need to be reported, in different formats and combinations, to several data collection agencies.

According to Armstrong (1995), it is not necessary for national health information to be collected or stored as a nationally based collection, but it is important that information is both relevant and comparable at a national level. Eagar and Innes (1992) highlighted the problems with state and territory approaches to health information. They reported a lack of standardisation of data items and definitions resulting in difficulties in identifying the health service needs of the population and the health services provided to the Australian community. For example, there was no national agreement on the terms 'hospital', 'inpatient', or 'length of stay'. Eagar and Innes recommended a national approach to health information to enable the Commonwealth government to monitor expenditure, to enable comparison of service provision, and to support casemix-based funding.

In 1987, the Commonwealth government established the Australian Institute of Health and Welfare (AIHW) as a statutory authority with a mission to improve the health and wellbeing of Australians through informing community decision making, collecting, analysing, and publishing health information, and developing methods to ensure information quality (Australian Institute of Health and Welfare 1999). The AIHW Knowledge-base, a key source of metadata on health information collected in Australia, is accessible from the AIHW website, <http://www.aihw.gov.au>.

In the early 1990s, a series of national forums furthered the development of priorities for a national health information development plan for Australia (Armstrong 1995). The plan is embodied in the National Health Information Agreement (NHIA), which brings together state, territory, and Commonwealth agencies, the AIHW, the Australian Bureau of Statistics (ABS), and the HIC for the purpose of improving and sharing health information at a national level. The NHIA was signed in 1993 and renewed in 1998 for a further five years. The National Health Information Management Group (NHIMG), which is chaired by an appointee of the Australian Health Ministers' Advisory Council (AHMAC), and whose membership includes the signatories to the NHIA, coordinates the work program of projects targeted to meet the agreed national priorities of the NHIA.

The NHIMG works at a practical level, identifying the data that should be collected and developing strategies for transferring these from the states and territories to the AIHW. A subcommittee of NHIMG, the National Health Data Committee (NHDC), advises on the detail of data items and how they are defined. These data items are then included in the *National Health Data Dictionary (NHDD)*, which is managed by the AIHW. The *NHDD*, in turn, defines the data items and classification systems for the elements of the National Health Information Model (NHIM), providing a common language to standardise the collection of data and to facilitate useability (Australian Institute of Health and Welfare 2001).

The NHIM was developed in 1994 by the AIHW to provide a shared vocabulary and framework, identify areas for improvement, and coordinate development of national health information (Mercer & Moss 1995). The NHIM defines information needs, the data items required to meet those needs, and the organisational structure of the information including definitions, classifications, and interrelationships. It provides a conceptual basis for viewing the components of the health system as the underlying structure of the *NHDD*.

The National Health Information Management Advisory Council (NHIMAC) met first in 1999, having been established to provide expert advice to health ministers on efficient and effective utilisation of information technologies in health care. Later that year, following collaboration with the states and territories, NHIMAC released *Health Online: A Health Information Action Plan for Australia* (NHIMAC 1999). The plan describes priority activities aimed at increasing the use and quality of health information.

> Policy makers and planners, faced with limited resources and the need to maximise efficiency at the same time as maximising quality of care, are seeking greater amounts of comprehensible data to determine where and to whom the public dollar should be directed and to measure how well services are being delivered (NHIMAC 1999, p. 8).

Health Online is discussed below under policy development for electronic health records. The second edition describes progress on initial action plans as well as new strategies and projects for future implementation (NHIMAC 2001).

McGlynn et al. (1998) emphasise the problems faced by decision makers in the health system where there is a lack of data uniformity and completeness. Health policy makers need timely access to quality data to formulate policy and to monitor subsequent changes to the health system. The American Health Information Management Association (AHIMA) data quality model describes ten characteristics of data quality, which are equally applicable in Australia:

- accessibility
- consistency
- currency (immediacy)
- granularity (level of detail)
- precision
- accuracy
- comprehensiveness
- definition
- relevance
- timeliness (available when required) (AHIMA 1998).

Indeed, in Australia in the past decade there have been concerted efforts to expand and improve health information to meet the requirements of data users.

Key issues in health information policy

The somewhat inconsistent approach to Australia's health information policy development and implementation can be observed, in varying degrees, in health information and health planning, accountability, quality health information, privacy, access and ownership, and policy development for electronic health records. Policy in these areas is evolving. A recent example of a focused approach to informed policy development has occurred in electronic health records.

Health information and health planning

The comprehensiveness of Australia's health data collection must be improved to increase its utility for health planning. While Australia has a number of high-quality, key health data sets, deficiencies remain in some areas of health information. These include chronic diseases in people who are not hospitalised, disability in the community, and morbidity diagnosed in the primary care environment.

Various health surveys go some way to identifying illness and the prevalence of disability, and provide a picture of the nation's health status (Britt et al. 2000). The paucity of structured health data collections that enable regional, national, and international comparison creates an unnecessary obstacle for health planners wanting to identify and forecast needs for health services, facilities, and promotional programs, and for determining the appropriate mix of the health workforce.

Accountability, quality, and health information

In any discussion of health information within the context of accountability in health care, there needs to be acknowledgment of the multiple players and the varying degrees and levels of accountability. All health care workers, health bureaucrats, health educators, and patients themselves, ultimately have a responsibility, directly or indirectly, for the quality of health care. The common objective should be provision of the highest possible quality care at the lowest possible cost. Wilson and Goldschmidt (1995) believe that the key factors propelling hospitals towards quality management are medical technology, changes in the hospital environment, and general expectations about quality and accountability. They observe that the health record is 'the core of the totality of information relevant to patient care, quality management, and healthcare administration and policy' (Wilson & Goldschmidt 1995, p. 509).

Health information underpins the measurement of the quality of care or service provided throughout the health industry, and accountability for high-quality health information rests with the professionals who care for patients and with the health information managers who code, manage, and analyse health information. The accurate coding—classification—of health information requires a skilled workforce. Considerable effort has been expended in the past decade to assess the workforce characteristics of health information managers and clinical coders. Continuing education has been provided through NCCH publications, conferences and seminars, and the Health Information Management Association of Australia (HIMAA) distance education program. Clinical coders are encouraged to monitor coding quality using Performance Indicators of Coding Quality (NCCH 2000) and the Australian Coding Benchmark Audit (NCCH 2000), and several states conduct regular recoding audits to ensure the accuracy of coded data. The HIMAA has developed a set of competency statements for clinical coders in conjunction with a national coder accreditation process to establish benchmarks for individual coders (HIMAA 1995, 1996; Groom et al. 1998; McLachlan 1999; NCCH 2001a, b).

In the late 1990s, dedicated efforts were made to introduce policy for a culture of quality in Australian health care. The National Expert Advisory Group on Safety and Quality in Australian Health Care reported to the Minister for Health and Community Services in July 1999 and recommended priority actions to improve the safety and quality of health care in Australia. Earlier work—for example, that of the Victorian Quality Assurance Task Force (1987)—demonstrated vigorous negotiation by the key professional and other health industry stakeholders for a say in how and by whom quality assurance is conducted, and how and to whom results are disseminated. These efforts have resulted in diverse national and state and territory legislation for statutory immunity for quality assurance information. The statutes generally have not achieved wider objectives, such as the education of health industry personnel in quality assurance techniques. The Australian Council for Safety and Quality in Healthcare (ACSQHC) was formed in January 2000. It identified, as one of three priority areas, the better use of data to identify, learn from, and prevent error and system failure. ACSQHC has established a data-and-information working group subcommittee to refine data on adverse events in health services (ACSQHC 2000).

Privacy, access, and ownership

It is widely accepted that people have a right to privacy regarding information contained in their health records. Most health consumers expect that their health information will be protected from unauthorised or inappropriate release to, or access by, any other person or body for subsequent use without their consent.

The Office of the Federal Privacy Commissioner has played an active role in the development of legislation, standards, and guidelines concerning privacy of personal information (Office of the Federal Privacy Commissioner 1999). The Information Privacy Principles adopted by the Commonwealth in the *Privacy Act 1988* (Cwlth) and the *Privacy Amendment (Private Sector) Act 2000* (Cwlth), and by a number of states, originated in nonhealth settings. Consequently, there are practical difficulties in applying some of the principles to health information systems. The application of others requires some creative problem solving by health information managers because existing or emerging networked electronic health record systems produce their own special difficulties, especially in relation to developing and managing systems to control unauthorised access by multiple users (Mulligan 1999). The principles derive from international law and provide guidelines for clinicians, researchers, health information managers, and others who create, design, or manage health records and related systems (Mulligan 1999). The version of principles formulated by the Office of the Commonwealth Privacy Commissioner (the National Principles for the Fair Handling of Personal Information) includes guarantees concerning the collection, handling, and disclosure of information. In 2001 the Office of the Federal Privacy Commissioner developed health privacy guidelines. The extent of the work undertaken in this area can be observed on the website of the Office of the Federal Privacy Commissioner at <http://www.privacy.gov.au>.

The consequence of the privacy principles extends beyond personal health information to large holdings of aggregated data. For example, consumer advocacy groups, some health care researchers, and custodians of large epidemiological and health databases hold differing views about which data should be held, who should be entitled to access these data, and for what purposes they may be used. Researchers and database custodians believe that care can be improved by data sharing. Consumer advocacy groups believe that stricter controls should apply to the exchange of data or information without the consent of the subject, regardless of its de-identified status (Mulligan 1999).

There has been a gradual shift in the perceived nature of health records. The old view was that they were an *aide memoire* for doctors and other health professionals. The contemporary concept is of health records being information held in trust by medical practitioners for patients as part of a fiduciary relationship (Breen et al. 1997). Consumer representatives and the medical profession have contributed actively to the public debate on the rights of patients in the private sector to access their own health information. The existence of enabling legislation in some other countries has provided the impetus for Australian jurisdictions to move towards the development of policy favouring consumers' rights to access their health records.

Freedom of Information statutes in the Commonwealth, states, and territories have provided people with the right of access to their health records created and held in the public sector, with provision for constraints and prohibitions. An example of such limitation occurs where the subject of the record is likely to suffer harm as a result of access to the information.

Box 4.1
Summary of key points of the Information Privacy Principles

- Personal information will be collected only when necessary, and in a fair manner.
- The subject of the information collected will be informed of who is collecting what information, and what they intend to do with it.
- Wherever practicable, information will be collected directly from the subject.
- Wherever possible, where information is collected about an individual from somebody else, the subject will be advised to this effect.
- Personal information will be protected by the record-keeper via security safeguards against loss, unauthorised access, or misuse.
- Information collected will only be used or disclosed in ways that are consistent with the subject's expectations, or as required in the public interest.

Source: Adapted from the 'Information Privacy Principles', in
Privacy Amendment (Private Sector) Act 2000 (Cwlth);
see also, website, Office of the Federal Privacy Commissioner,
<http://www.privacy.gov.au>

The right of ownership of medical records in the private sector rests with the individual or the organisation that creates the record as part of a contractual relationship between patient and provider or provider organisation. Exceptions to this occur in situations where a patient requests the preparation of a medical report for a third party, such as a life insurance company. A corollary to ownership has been the right of the owner of the record to regulate access by the subject. This was confirmed in the *Breen versus Williams* (1996) decision, in which the High Court of Australia concluded that medical practitioners hold all rights of ownership of the health records that they create about their patients. The exception is investigative reports such as pathology and radiology results.

In *Breen versus Williams* the plaintiff, Mrs Breen, was denied access to her medical records held by her plastic surgeon, Dr Williams. The records were being sought for a separate legal action being brought by Mrs Breen against the manufacturer of her silicone breast implants. Following the High Court decision, consumer advocacy groups increased pressure on various governments to legislate for consumers' rights to gain access to their own health information. The Australian Law Reform Commission had an active interest, and the Senate Community Affairs References Committee held a wide-ranging inquiry (1997), resulting in recommendations for legislated access which, in turn, have preceded federal and other legislation (see box 4.1 for the key points in information privacy principles).

The issue of ownership of electronic records is less clear than is the case for hard copy records because of the potential for multiple owners across several practices and facilities. The concept of custodianship and the rights to exercise control over the content and use of data held electronically have been suggested as a more appropriate approach to dealing with ownership of electronic health records (National Electronic Health Records Taskforce 2000).

Policy development for electronic health records

In 1998 the Commonwealth government set the national strategic direction for Australia's information economy by identifying key issues and priorities for action in ten areas, including health (National Office for Information Economy 1998, p. 8). *Health Online: A Health Information Action Plan for Australia* is a blueprint for national progression of the health information management and information technology agenda (NHIMAC 1999, 2001). The plan, whose development and implementation involves participation by the Commonwealth and all states and territories, identifies the three key structural interests, namely consumers, providers, and policy makers and managers. The plan is framed in a broad interpretation of health information, which includes

- personal and aggregated health information and issues associated with collection and access
- information transfer in interactive services and situations, such as online access to medical consultations, online claims, and electronic prescribing.

The pressures surrounding policy development concerning national electronic health records have meant that a wide range of organisations and individuals have been taking an active interest in developments. For example, at the National Health Online Summit in 2000, there was productive exchange of ideas among key interests and subgroups, including the Australian government (through the NHIMG), NHIMAC, health care consumer representatives, the medical profession, the health information management profession, informatics and information technology specialists, epidemiologists and researchers, and commercial software industry representatives.

The National Electronic Health Records Taskforce (NEHRT) was established to develop a coordinated approach to electronic health records in Australia, to avoid the potential for system incompatibility and duplication, and to allow the electronic exchange of clinical information between providers and across regional and state and territory boundaries. The taskforce reported to the Australian Health Ministers' Conference in July 2000, in *A Health Information Network for Australia*, on the possibilities, benefits, and potential difficulties of a national approach based on the application of new technologies (Briggs 2000; NEHRT 2000). The project's working title was changed subsequently to HealthConnect in order to promote the notion of an improved partnership between consumers and providers, on the basis that electronic health records would be available to all providers, with patient consent, to facilitate clinical decision making. NEHRT states that Australians will enjoy substantial benefits from a national electronic health records system, These benefits include

- empowerment of consumers
- improved health outcomes for all Australians, for example through reductions in the number of medical misadventures and dangerous drug interactions
- reduction of unnecessary repetition of tests
- enhanced privacy and confidentiality of health information
- a flexible, seamless, and integrated process of care
- better access to care, especially in rural and remote areas
- confidence that important medical details will be available when most needed (Briggs 2000; NEHRT 2000; <http:www.health.gov.au/healthonline/nehrt.htm>).

Many contentious or logistically problematic aspects of electronic health records are in the slow process of technical development or political negotiation for longer-term resolution. These include

- national coordination mechanisms and partnerships
- policy and legal issues governing electronic exchange of health information
- common standards for information collection and its electronic storage, transfer, and handling, and for international compatibility
- infrastructure issues
- standardised clinical terminologies
- logistics of data entry by providers
- difficulties of integration of electronic health records with other forms of information (Briggs 2000; Heard et al. 2000).

Serious concerns about the maintenance of confidentiality and privacy of personal health information held electronically, including in large databases, have been raised by the medical and the health information management professions, health consumer representatives, the federal Privacy Commissioner, and a legislator (Carter 2000; Crompton 2000; Phelps 2000; Macklin 2001). Practical difficulties remain to develop tamper-free systems that will ensure patient confidence in a high degree of health information security (Frawley 1999).

Another issue is legitimate access to health information. Consumer representatives have long advocated a balance between what might be considered private information and what is a necessary sharing of information at a multidisciplinary level (Draper 1992). The need for this balance will not change with the advent of electronic health records. The electronic transfer of clinical information between health care providers has the potential to increase the standard of care through enhanced communication; however, patients may not wish to make available all of their health information to all of their health care providers. NEHRT recommends the provision of opt-in and opt-out facilities, in which patients can elect to have all, or some, components of their record accessed by other health care providers (opt in), but have the option of withdrawing their permission for access (opt out) at any time. Yet to be resolved are the technical challenges, which include enabling individual patients to provide signed consent for release of all or nominated components of their electronic health record, to have such consent stored against the respective individual episodes of care, and to manage the system to prevent any breach of confidentiality. Another issue concerns the development of digital signatures and the registration of users to enable electronic authentication and encryption of messages containing sensitive health data exchanged between health care professionals. This is being addressed by the Health e-Signature Authority (for information on further developments, see <http://www.hesa.com.au>).

The aim for national compatibility of health information systems and for extensive intraprovider networking of these, is very ambitious. Indeed, the rejection in late July 2001 of the proposed Better Medication Management Scheme, a planned integrated information system for prescribing and dispensing medication, is indicative of the rocky road along which funding, developing, and implementing networked health information systems travel. The development cost for electronic patient record systems is potentially prohibitive, and large-scale information technology projects have a high record of failure. In spite of this, key stakeholders generally have greeted enthusiastically the policy process associated with HealthConnect. A reason for this might be that HealthConnect is being developed and implemented incrementally through a structured process of negotiation by the various stakeholders to achieve balanced health information systems that are technically feasible, affordable, secure, and manageable. These four characteristics offer significant challenges to all involved in health information policy development and implementation. Underpinning information about health and provision of health services is the language we use to communicate health concepts, so these concepts need to be ordered and classified to ensure a common understanding of the meaning of health data. The Australian experience in turning health data into health information through development of standards for health classification is described in the following case study.

Box 4.2
Case study—National Centre for Classification in Health

The National Centre for Classification in Health (NCCH) was established in 1997 as a joint venture between the University of Sydney's National Coding Centre (NCC) and the Queensland University of Technology's National Reference Centre for Classification in Health (NRCCH). The NRCCH was created in 1992 with funding from the AIHW and, more recently, from the Australian Bureau of Statistics. The NCC was established in 1994 and funded through the Casemix Program of the Commonwealth Department of Health and Aged Care. Although health classifications of one kind or another had been in use in Australia for many decades, the will to promote national standards in the application of classifications did not materialise until data about diagnoses and procedures were required for casemix classification and hospital funding. Policies regarding use of international classifications had existed by default, but there was no clear statement about national application of particular classifications for hospital morbidity statistical collections. In espousing the World Health Organization (WHO) International Classification of Diseases (ICD) for cause-of-death coding, Australia had a foundation on which to build a national policy for morbidity coding.

The issue of responsibility for data collections is an important one. In this case, the ABS oversees the cause-of-death reporting and coding, the Australian Institute of Health and Welfare collects data on mortality and morbidity statistics, and the Commonwealth Department of Health and Ageing sets standards for the national implementation of casemix classifications. Other federal government departments, such as Veterans' Affairs and Defence, are also involved, as are state and territory governments whose health departments are charged with delivering care and maintaining morbidity collections. But being responsible for data collections does not necessarily bring with it responsibility for classifications that allow meaning to be derived from the data. It was only when that meaning was attached to dollars that the need for a policy initiative relating to health classifications became apparent. In the case of NCCH, the introduction of casemix funding was the trigger for a national policy on coding and classification.

The immediate catalyst to NCCH (then NCC) being formed were the recommendations of the National Patient Abstracting and Coding Project carried out by Eagar and Innes (1992). One of their recommendations was to establish a national coding authority to oversee the development and implementation of national coding standards.

Another event that fostered policy development and implementation was the development of an *Australian* casemix classification with the Australian national and now the Australian refined diagnosis related groups (AN- and AR-DRGs). Until this occurred, Australia had inherited international (usually WHO) disease and procedure classifications or United States modifications. Australia did not have a centre of expertise in health classifications and there were many perceived advantages in adopting an existing international system. This approach allowed comparison of statistics on mortality and morbidity and on the use of health services nationally and internationally. There was little questioning of the appropriateness of classification structure or terminology for Australian health services. AN-DRGs changed all that. And so did the involvement of clinicians in the development and refining of the Australian casemix system. Together, these factors involving the use of classified or coded material have led to questioning the disease and procedure classifications that form the foundation of casemix groupings. They highlight the need for flexibility in an Australian modification of the classification, which allows the introduction of new Australian codes to give specificity or reflect new technology, especially for procedures. Although a mechanism for updating ICD-9-CM existed in the USA, Australia had no official say in what was approved, and the process was long and cumbersome. There was a need to develop Australian expertise in coding and classification in order to be able to respond to the need for a dynamic disease and procedure classification while maintaining some stability for comparison over time. The Australian Casemix Clinical Committee was established in 1988 to provide clinical input into the casemix system. This process has been instrumental in establishing clinical credibility for the Australian DRGs. There was also the need for standards for application of the classification and for standard definitions of terms and code sequence. When the NCC was established in 1994, there were still differences between Australian jurisdictions in interpretation of the principal diagnosis definition. This had major implications for casemix grouping, the principal diagnosis being critical in the logic of grouping to major diagnostic category.

NCC's early activity reflected its origins in casemix, in that most energy was applied to updating the classification for clinical currency and for practical and credible casemix application. The need for coder education and validation of coding quality was also established in these early years, although coding quality activities have still not received the attention they deserve at the national level. It has been at the state and hospital levels that audit action has been most intense, predominantly to ensure that hospitals accurately reflect their casemix and throughput for funding purposes. Australia's decision to implement ICD-10 and to create an Australian modification, including an Australian procedure classification, was a landmark in the progression to a major centre of expertise in classification issues that we now see in the NCCH. Experience acquired during the creation of that classification has formed a solid base on which NCCH can build its future and on which policy on health classifications can be developed without being merely responsive to crises. There is the opportunity for this to become a reality with the incentives to use clinical vocabularies to support the introduction of electronic health records. It is of prime importance that the bridge between classifications and vocabularies is recognised and maintained. Classifications usually have an index of terms, which allows the user to relate a specific disease or procedure to a class. The terms, which appear in ICD-10-AM, provide a comprehensive list of words used in the language of health communication for the acute care sector. Conventions governing the structure of terms in this index need to be understood to use the classification as it is, but also to create from this index a useful list of the vocabulary used by all clinicians. Only when this is done will it be possible to tap the electronic health record using terms that can be converted to a classification so that they can be recognisable and commonly understood by users. The National Health Information Standards Plan recognises the need for a standard clinical vocabulary.

Such policies on health classification must be developed in parallel with policies and practice relating to health records, in particular electronic health records. The technological environment of information creation, storage, exchange, and analysis is such that it is impossible to separate out any one of these elements. With the development of an electronic version of the ICD-10-AM classification, NCCH has placed itself in a position whereby this classification instrument can be used in health system applications to guide data users. The ability to incorporate ICD-10-AM into software applications supports current initiatives to widen the scope of NCCH activities beyond acute hospital inpatients to ambulatory services. The exchange of electronic health records between health facilities and individuals means that there must be a common language of health, with terms included in the classification for clinicians in all specialties, disciplines and settings. There is also an argument for gearing the terms to relate to the health literature, so that terms used at the bedside are the same as those used to access medical knowledge.

All these approaches bring together the use of information for public health and health services research, funding, and monitoring the utilisation of health services. Decisions on what terms and classes to include or make prominent in the classification are based on the clinical importance of diseases and procedures, evidence of efficacy, and the need to establish outcomes of treatments for similar conditions. The use of codes in quality monitoring is a study in itself. One could use a similar parallel to that of casemix in following current moves to use codes for adverse events to help monitor interventions and improve patient safety in hospitals.

The Australian experience in creating a national version of an international classification has allowed it to participate in the international arena of classification and vocabulary development through the WHO and the International Organization for Standardization (IOS) Health Informatics Technical Committee. Australia now chairs the Update Reference Committee for ICD-10 for WHO because of the expertise acquired in working with clinicians to build an Australian classification. This will provide a strong foundation for use of clinical terminologies to make possible the creation and use of electronic health records.

■

This case study demonstrates the expedient nature of policy that led to the formation of NCCH. Its existence has brought to the forefront the need for Australian standards for health classifications and brings together responsibility for morbidity and mortality classifications in one organisation. The case study also addresses the efficiency and quality of the coding process. This is especially important with electronic systems becoming more pervasive, so that the classification acts as a catalyst for realisation of electronic health records. In regard to scope and interface between classifications, the AIHW has formed an Expert Group on Health Classifications to be responsible to NHIMG for recommending classifications for specific settings and creating of terminology so that the languages can be used and understood by all health professionals.

Conclusion

The introduction of casemix funding and pressure to implement the electronic health record provide a basis for policy in the development of Australian health information and health informatics. The nature of these changes and the issues of privacy and access ensure that providers, consumers, and health informatics professionals will be involved in driving health information policies to match cultural and technological environments.

Legislators and other decision makers in Australia cannot afford to neglect their responsibility to create policies that guide the use of technologies to give access and utility to clinical data while providing a secure environment for sensitive health information. Structures and procedures must be established, resources allocated, and the workforce educated. These are the foundations upon which data can be organised and classified to enable users to understand and interpret its meaning in a consistent way. The many users of health information must be recognised and their energies harnessed to improve data quality, as well as efficiency of data collection, analysis, and application.

References

Abdelhak, M. et al. 2001, *Health Information: Management of a Strategic Resource*, 2nd edn, W B Saunders, Philadelphia.

Alford, R. R. 1972, 'The Political Economy of Healthcare: Dynamics Without Change', *Politics and Society*, winter, pp. 127–64.

American Health Information Management Association, Data Quality Management Taskforce 1998, 'Practice Brief: Data Quality Management Model', *Journal of the American Health Information Management Association*, vol. 69, no. 6, insert.

Armstrong, B. 1995, 'National Health Information: Directions and Management', *Proceedings of 16th Conference of the Health Information Management Association of Australia*, HIMAA, Sydney.

Australian Council for Safety and Quality in Healthcare 2000, *Safety First: Report to the Australian Health Ministers' Conference*, Commonwealth Department of Health and Aged Care, Canberra.

Australian Institute of Health and Welfare 1995, *National Health Information Development Plan*, AIHW cat. no. AIHW 407, AIHW, Canberra.

—— 1999, *Australian Institute of Health and Welfare Corporate Plan 1999–2000*, cat. no. AUS 18, AIHW, Canberra.

—— 2001, *National Health Data Dictionary*, Version 10, AIHW cat. no. HWI 30, AIHW, Canberra; online version available at Australian Institute of Health and Welfare website, <http://www.aihw.gov.au>.

Breen, K. J., Plueckhahn, V. D., & Cordner, S. M. 1997, *Ethics, Law and Medical Practice*, Allen & Unwin, Sydney.

Breen versus Williams, 1996, 186 CLR 71.

Briggs, L. 2000, 'A National Approach to Electronic Health Records', *Proceedings of the National Health Online Summit*, Adelaide, 3–4 August, Department of Health and Aged Care, Canberra.

Britt, H. et al. 2000, *General Practice Activity in Australia 1999–2000*, AIHW cat. no. GEP 5, Australian Institute of Health and Welfare, Canberra.

Carter, M. 2000, untitled paper presented to 'Laying Sound Foundations: Enhancing Privacy and Confidentiality in the World of e-health: Keeping Personal Health Information Safe', *Proceedings from the National Health Online Summit*, Adelaide, 3–4 August, Department of Health and Aged Care, Canberra.

Crompton, M. 2000, untitled paper presented to 'Laying Sound Foundations: Enhancing Privacy and Confidentiality in the World of e-health: Keeping Personal Health Information Safe', *Proceedings from the National Health Online Summit*, Adelaide, 3-4 August, Department of Health and Aged Care, Canberra.

Degeling, P. J. & Anderson, J. M. 1992, 'Organisational and Administrative Dimensions', in H. Gardner (ed.), *Health Policy: Development, Implementation, and Evaluation in Australia*, Churchill Livingstone, Melbourne.

Dombal, F. 1996, *Medical Informatics: The Essentials*, Butterworth Heinemann, Oxford.

Draper, M. 1992, 'For Whose Eyes Only? Health Records, Access and Privacy', *Australian Medical Record Journal*, vol. 22, no. 1, pp. 7–9.

Duckett, S. J. 1984, 'Structural Interests and Australian Health Policy', *Social Science and Medicine*, vol. 18, no. 11, pp. 959–66.

Eagar, K. & Innes, K. 1992, *Creating a Common Language: The Production and Use of Patient Data in Australia*; Report of Patient Abstracting and Coding Project for Department of Health, Housing and Community Services, Canberra.

Frawley, K. A. 1999, 'Case Study: Confidentiality and Security of Health Information', in G. F. Murphy, M. A. Hanken & K. A. Waters (eds), *Electronic Health Records: Changing the Vision*, W B Saunders, Philadelphia.

Groom, A. et al. 1998, 'Developments in Coding Quality Measures', *Proceedings of the Tenth Casemix Conference in Australia*, 6–9 September, Department of Health and Family Services, Canberra.

Hargreaves, J. 1999, 'Gaps in Classifications', Paper presented at the Australian Institute of Health and Welfare Conference on ICD-IDH, 3 May.

Health Information Management Association of Australia 1995, *The Australian Coder Workforce*, National Coder Workforce Issues Project, HIMAA, Brisbane.

—— 1996, National Coder Workforce Issues Project, *Coder National Competency Standards and Assessment Guide*, HIMAA, Brisbane.

Heard, S. et al. 2000, 'The Benefits and Difficulties of Introducing a National Approach to Electronic Health Records in Australia', in *A Health Information Network for Australia: Report to Health Ministers by the National Electronic Health Records Taskforce*, Department of Health and Aged Care, Canberra.

McGlynn, E. A. et al. 1998, *Health Information Systems: Design Issues and Analytic Applications*, Rand, Santa Monica, California.

McLachlan, J. 1999, 'Report on the Audit of 1998–99 Victorian Public Hospital Data Coded in ICD-10-AM', *Proceedings of the 20th Conference of the Health Information Management Association of Australia*, HIMAA, Sydney.

Macklin, J. 2001, 'Health Information Database Created by Private Company', Media release from the Office of the Shadow Minister for Health, 19 February.

Mercer, N. A. & Moss, E. 1995, 'The National Health Information Model', *Proceedings of the 16th Conference of the Health Information Management Association of Australia*, HIMAA, Sydney.

Mulligan, E. 1999, 'Information Privacy Principles: Are They Just Too Difficult to Apply in Networked Health Information Systems?', *Proceedings of the 20th Conference of the Health Information Management Association of Australia*, 27–9 October, HIMAA, Sydney.

National Centre for Classification in Health 2000, *International Statistical Classification of Diseases and Related Health Problems, Tenth Revision, Australian Modification—ICD-10-AM*, 2nd edn, National Centre for Classification in Health, Sydney.

—— 2001a, *Australian Coding Benchmark Audit* (computer program), National Centre for Classification in Health, Sydney.

—— 2001b, *Performance Indicators for Coding Quality* (computer program), National Centre for Classification in Health, Sydney.

National Electronic Health Records Taskforce 2000, *A Health Information Network for Australia: Report to the Health Ministers*, Department of Health and Aged Care, Canberra; online version available at <http://www.health.gov.au/healthonline/nehrt.htm>.

National Expert Advisory Group on Safety and Quality in Australian Health Care 1999, *Implementing Safety and Quality Enhancement in Healthcare: Final Report to Health Ministers*, Department of Health and Aged Care, Canberra.

National Health Information Management Advisory Council 1999, *Health Online: A Health Information Action Plan for Australia*, Commonwealth of Australia, Canberra; online version available at <http:www.health.gov.au/healthonline/nehrt/htm>.

National Office for Information Economy 1998, *A Strategic Framework for the Information Economy: Identifying Priorities for Action*, Commonwealth of Australia, Canberra.

Office of the Federal Privacy Commissioner 1999, *Privacy Commissioner's Report on the Application of the National Principles for the Fair Handling of Personal Information to Personal Health Information*, Office of the Federal Privacy Commissioner, Canberra; online version available at <http://www.privacy.gov.au>.

Phelps, K. 2000, 'Enhancing Privacy and Confidentiality in the World of e-health: Keeping Personal Health Information Safe', *Proceedings from the National Health Online Summit*, Adelaide, 3–4 August, Department of Health and Aged Care, Canberra.

Quality Assurance Task Force 1987, *Quality Assurance in Health Care in Victoria*, Department of Health, Melbourne.

Senate Community Affairs References Committee 1997, *Report on Access to Medical Records*, Senate Printing Unit, Parliament House, Canberra.

Smith, J. 2000, *Health Management Information Systems: A Handbook for Decision Makers*, Open University Press, Buckingham.

Southon, G. & Holman, J. 1996. 'Information, Management and the Organisation: The Role of IT', *Proceedings of the 18th National Conference of the Health Information Management Association of Australia*, HIMAA, Sydney.

Waters, K. & Murphy, G. 1979, *Medical Records in Health Information*, Aspen, Germantown, Maryland.

Wilson, L. & Goldschmidt, P. 1995, *Quality Management in Health Care*, McGraw-Hill, Sydney.

5

Structural Reform and Cultural Transition: Reflections on the National Public Health Partnership

Vivian Lin

In 1996 Australian health ministers agreed to embark upon a two-pronged approach to national reforms in public health: a multilateral policy forum, the National Public Health Partnership, and the broadbanding of program dollars, the Public Health Outcome Funding Agreements. This chapter focuses on one aspect of these reforms, the National Public Health Partnership (NPHP). There is a great deal of information in the public domain about the background, objectives, and activities of the NPHP,[1] and the intention here is not to dwell on these details. Rather, this chapter reflects on what has occurred and what that might mean for the field of public health. A brief review of the original context and intent provides a basis for assessing the processes involved and the progress to date. The early experience of the NPHP provides a number of lessons for other policy arenas and processes. The NPHP breaks new ground in a number of respects, including, inter alia, intergovernmental relations, public administration, and a whole-of-system approach. Other issues raised by the NPHP experience include forming and sustaining collaborative arrangements, government and external stakeholder relations, the importance of implementation research, and the contemporary history of public health as a field of professional practice. More importantly, the intersection of this intergovernmental mechanism and its activities allows for some observations about the state of the public health industry in Australia. Some suggestions about the remaining agenda and direction will, it is hoped, serve as the basis for discussion and debate.[2] A conclusion is that structural reform of institutions of governance is a necessary, but not sufficient, condition of cultural transformation.

Development and intent

The NPHP was developed between 1995 and 1997 in response to a range of issues. At the most practical level, Australia had seen myriad single-issue vertical programs that were increasingly rigid in their boundaries. The 1980s was an expansionary era for the health system in general, and a renaissance period for public health in particular (NPHP 1997; Lewis and Leeder 1998). Through the late 1980s, a number of Commonwealth–state cost-shared programs were funded, including HIV, drugs, women's health, cancer screening, and services for homeless youth. While some were well resourced, others were less so. Over time these programs became tightly targeted and increasingly locked into historical patterns of allocation. Yet people's lives did not necessarily respect the program boundaries created by governments and bureaucrats. People often had multiple needs, which fell in between the boundaries of the programs, creating the need to think about how programs could be better coordinated to address the real needs of people.

Public health funding at the Commonwealth level, unlike funding for personal health care—that is, Medicare and pharmaceutical benefits—was capped and time-limited. Every three years, it was necessary to go through the Budget process for re-authorisation. This naturally limited the types of programs and projects that could be pursued. From the early 1990s, all jurisdictions began to move into a more restrictive fiscal climate. At the state and territory level, it was easier to reduce budgets in areas not locked into cost-shared agreements with the Commonwealth and to reduce budgets in areas that were less immediate or visible in the public eye. As a consequence, public health funding began to decline.

The combined dynamic of fiscal restraint and tighter targeting called into question the underlying paradigm for public health programs. At one level, there were targeted programs, with strong constituencies, able to articulate specific short-term objectives. On the other hand, questions were raised about whether these programs were sustainable and if they increased the capacity of organisations, communities, and citizens to tackle proactively new health challenges.

Within this broad context arose an interesting configuration of individuals who were able to develop and drive the NPHP. At the senior levels of the Commonwealth Department of Health were several key people. These included a secretary who had long been identified as a health economist with public health understanding and commitment, a chief medical adviser who was a founder of the Public Health Association in Australia, and a first assistant secretary long identified as a champion of system change through public health and primary care approaches.

In addition, the chief health officers in the relevant jurisdictions had long-established relationships and were voicing common concerns about the quixotic nature of resource allocation and the desirability of change.

This confluence of personalities occurred during a window of opportunity in Commonwealth–state relations: specifically, at the very time of debates about structural reform of the health and community services system. The notion of a partnership approach signalled an avenue of reform that a new minister for health, in a newly elected government, and one who had a predisposition towards public health, could adopt.

Key features of the National Public Health Partnership

Australian health ministers endorsed the establishment of the NPHP in late 1996.[3] During the course of 1997 all ministers signed a five-year intergovernmental memorandum of understanding (MoU). The MoU (NPHP, n.d.) dictated the objectives as a concern with

- improving collaboration across the national public health effort
- enhancing coordination and sustainability of national public health strategies
- strengthening public health infrastructure and capacity.

The priority work program areas identified in the MoU were information, legislation, workforce development, research and development, planning and practice improvement, and national strategies coordination.

Health ministers had determined that the partnership would be limited to an intergovernmental mechanism, although public health efforts required the mobilisation and participation of multiple interests in and out of government, as well as inside and outside the health sector. The NPHP Group determined to set up a nongovernment advisory group comprising organisations interested in the broad public health effort and system (see figure 5.1 for the structure of the NPHP).

So, what is new?

There are a number of features in the NPHP arrangements that represent significant developments—if not departure points—for public health governance and intergovernmental relations in Australia. In that sense, it represented a major step in structural reform.

From the public health viewpoint, rather than focusing on specific health issues, the NPHP has a whole-of-system focus. In addition, the NPHP is concerned with the infrastructure of and capacity required in the system in order to achieve the desired health outcomes.

From the viewpoint of intergovernmental relations, the NPHP represents a radical step forwards. Instead of a mechanism that is constituted to negotiate around dollars—and therefore the policies associated with the dollars—the NPHP provides a separation of policy debates from mechanisms to debate funding arrangements. Finally, the establishment of the advisory group was the first time that a forum had been created to bring nongovernment organisations together to address public health system issues. Members included the Australian Health Promotion Association, the Australian Institute of Environmental Health, the Australian Nursing Federation, the Consumers' Health Forum, the National Aboriginal Community Controlled Health Organisations, the Public Health Association, the Public Health Education and Research Program, the Royal Australian College of General Practitioners, and the Royal Australasian College of Physicians.

Figure 5.1   The NPHP structure

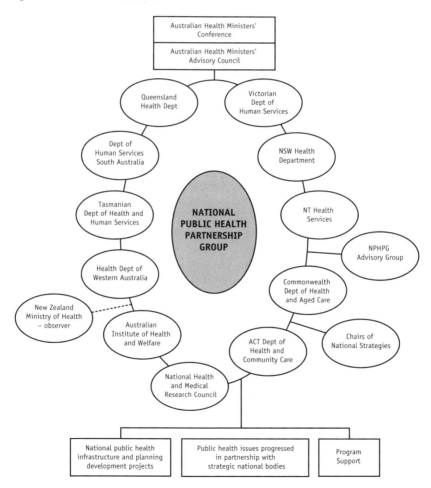

From a public administration viewpoint the NPHP secretariat arrangement contributed to innovation. First, it was policy driven. This meant it was an intelligent secretariat rather than one solely concerned with administration matters. Second, it was located in a state jurisdiction, Victoria. This was to signal clearly that it was not operating a Commonwealth agenda. Additionally, the commissioning of an evaluation at the outset, concurrent with implementation, was what could be termed a 'courageous' decision. To commission a significant piece of action research where the explicit aim was to improve performance by identifying and overcoming weaknesses is virtually unheard of in public sector management.

The first three years

The achievements

From the group formation perspective, the NPHP's first three years are not distinctive, in that they could be characterised as a period of 'forming, storming, and norming'. Any newly established group will take some time to determine the manner in which it operates and the nature of its internal group dynamics before it settles into a mode of operation.

A range of operational and developmental issues had been worked on during this time. The NPHP's annual report, *Progress Through Partnerships* (NPHP 1999a), provides a detailed account of the public health effort, which includes, *inter alia*,

- a national public health information development plan (NPHP 1999b)
- a program of legislation review on issues including passive smoking, immunisation, and notifiable diseases
- the identification of priorities for workforce development, such as environmental health, health promotion, and public health leadership
- the development of position papers on public health research and development to feed into the National Strategic Review of Health and Medical Research
- submissions to other national reviews—on food regulation and on blood supply and blood products
- guidelines for partnership with private industry (NPHP 1998)
- best-practice guidelines for development and coordination of public health strategies (NPHP 1999c)
- the development of a schema to evaluate evidence for public health interventions (Rychetnik & Frommer 2000)
- a Delphi study on core public health functions (NPHP 2000a)
- a framework for planning public health practice (NPHP 2000b).

More importantly, these activities have seeded debates, linked people and groups, and provided a stronger public health voice within governments. Chairs of national strategies met for the first time and began to share information about their activities and to identify areas of common interest in, for example, youth health, Indigenous health, and working with general practitioners (GPs). Public health professionals from different disciplines, and working in different settings, were put together in workshops to debate issues, such as what constitutes evidence for public health and what are appropriate methods for resource allocation and quality management. The Chief Health Officers offered comparable policy advice within their jurisdictions. While a new consensus was forged between the professions and within governments on some matters, there were tensions about other issues. There was a range of underlying conflicts over issues such as priority setting for the group and whether to pursue the concurrent evaluation.

The NPHP implemented a communication strategy, which included a widely distributed newsletter, a booklet about how public health in Australia is organised, and an annual report on the national public health effort. This program has led to a higher degree of visibility for all public health activities. Evaluation and anecdotal feedback suggest that government activities in public health became more transparent as a result and that practitioners began to forge more links across jurisdictions.

From the perspective of intergovernmental relations, the NPHP was definitely a good news story, with items consistently appearing on the Australian Health Ministers' Advisory Council agenda and being endorsed. Those working on public hospital funding issues began to consider whether Australia's health financing debates might be better served by separating the policy mechanism from the forums where funding battles were fought.

The creative tensions

There was a degree of confusion, disagreement, and tension, both within the NPHP and between the NPHP and external public health interests. This occurred for a range of reasons, but was generally a product of the diversity of the field in terms of disciplinary background, practice settings, understanding of public health, and ideology. It also reflected a field that lacked coherence and a common voice.

In light of the existence of over twenty national public health strategies, each with its own machinery to progress matters, the NPHP had clearly determined that it would not duplicate the efforts of individual strategies. Instead, efforts would be directed at value adding and improving coordination across strategies. For some, this was problematic. Given the contemporary tradition of targeted funding programs and the established history of public health as a social movement advocating specific change, the fact that the NPHP was not focused on particular health issues posed difficulties for a number of people in the field. Many working outside government looked for specific health objectives and outcomes. They expected to see advocacy for issues through Budget initiatives or other forms of government statements. That the NPHP would be concerned with system development seemed to be a diffuse and unfocused venture. The notion of improved public health governance was foreign, if not undesirable, probably because it used language comparable to that of the hospital sector.

It is a fundamental tenet of public health science and practice that much of the historical improvement in the health of the population relates to improvements in economic, environmental, and social conditions, rather than to health services delivery. Thus, the notion of intersectoral collaboration is central to contemporary public health strategies. For the NPHP to be concerned about ensuring that the public health house was in order through better means of planning and financing as well as through quality assurance mechanisms for public health practice was again anathema to many advocates and practitioners.

With epidemiology as a core scientific base for public health knowledge and, more recently, the rise of health, social, and behavioural sciences to complement epidemiology, much of the academic public health leadership has been concerned with a better understanding of the nature of the problem. In other words, the concerns have centred on public health discovery. In contrast, the practitioners, administrators, and government officials are focused on public health delivery. At the same time, while the administrators are necessarily concerned about investments and trade-offs, the practitioners are championing local community issues. The consequence is a tension between the researchers and teachers, the community-based practitioners, and those in decision-making positions.

Within the group of government officials that constituted the NPHP Group, there were differences and tensions. The states and territories shared many common concerns, such as having to cover the full spectrum of issues, be ever prepared for unexpected priorities, and ensure that the management of statutory obligations did not falter. However, there were also differences. The smaller jurisdictions had fewer expert resources, but were closer to operational concerns in the community. The larger states had to contend—on a daily basis—with medical and other interest group politics, from the industries that were being regulated through public health legislation. The Commonwealth had responsibilities distinct from the states and territories, in part because of broader constitutional arrangements. The delicate balance for the NPHP Group between their role in serving the Commonwealth government and their leadership role in addressing the national interest, which transcended jurisdictional boundaries, was a constant challenge. In terms of public service culture, to shift from controlling and enticing the states and territories with funding proposals to working in partnership with them was another challenge. An additional challenge in change management at the Commonwealth level related to human resources. Whereas the public service in the states and territories often drew from professionals working in the field, the Commonwealth public service culture was geared towards promoting generalist public administrators. Frequent personnel shifts and a lack of professional training in public health constituted another complicating facet of partnership building.

The challenges ahead

In reflecting on the tensions that surfaced in the NPHP's first three years, it is possible to be either dismissive about the possibility of change or to accept tensions as challenges that need to be addressed. If we accept that, given the diversity of the field, those tensions will always exist in some form, then the question becomes how tensions can be seen in a creative light and how they might be managed.

From the viewpoint of the NPHP, the most immediate challenges rest with how to build a broader partnership within the terms prescribed by governments. The need to involve local government is paramount, given its general and historical contribution to public health, although it is constitutionally a creature of the state and its specific roles vary considerably across Australia. There is also the need to build stronger links with the medical profession, particularly the primary care sector, given the prevalence of primary care practitioners and their role as frontline observers of health problems among individuals. Beyond these are the questions of how to form strategic and meaningful partnerships with the community sector and with other sectors. Although the NPHP Group represents a starting point, informational asymmetry makes it difficult for those outside government to appreciate the bureaucratic imperatives and therefore to make a substantial contribution. Similarly, while the actions of other sectors may be critical for the health of the public, the values and imperatives that drive their decision making might be quite different. Thus, effective points of engagement might differ from issue to issue.

As the peak governance body for public sector policy and investment in public health, the NPHP Group also faces the challenge of developing and effecting new paradigms for funding and programming. Accepting that political interests will continue to drive the definition of vertical programs, the managerial challenge is to ensure that these programs are translated into a horizontal delivery framework that can meet the health needs of the community and of people's lives. Additionally, there remains the challenge of how to reorient health service delivery towards prevention and cost-effective care.

Those with a public health understanding necessarily champion a health investment framework for the whole of the health system. The NPHP has a role as an internal advocate to advance such an agenda.

For the wider community of public health academics and practitioners, the challenges are also substantial. The field of public health is steeped in a tradition of critical analysis and social activism. The skills of advocacy, however, need to be honed through experience, backed by sound political analyses, and modified in accordance with circumstances. The combination of post-Cold War era politics and the new economy call for the development of more sophisticated approaches to advocacy.

A more fundamental challenge for the field of public health is a cultural transformation—to move from tribalism to integrative practice. Public health practice for much of the twentieth century was dominated by a command-and-control model, led by a chief medical or health officer. With the social movements of the 1960s and 1970s came pluralism and competing schools of thought, each often contending for a new hegemony. The dichotomisation of old versus new, social marketing versus media advocacy, behaviour change versus community development, and risk factors versus structural determinants, has supported the development of diverse practice but has failed to recognise the complementarity of these practices. An integrative practice would recognise the value and need for multiple strategies to be practised simultaneously. It would also support the development of a multiskilled workforce.

Public health may have an image problem. Because of the diversity of the field there is not a public health voice that is able to communicate clearly with the public. A survey of the American public in 1996 found that while people supported public health initiatives—for example, 90 per cent supported communicable disease control and 80 per cent supported toxic waste control and the provision of safe drinking water—only 3 per cent answered correctly when asked what public health was (Levy 1998).

Public health is about preparedness and vigilance as much as it is about a specific issue or set of issues that are easy to express. This makes it difficult to engage with the community. There has been significant erosion of the infrastructure in public health. This is not visible until a major issue, such as the problems with Legionnaire's disease in Melbourne in 2001, arises. The NPHP, because of its whole-of-system approach, has been able to identify the infrastructural weaknesses, but effective communication of the systemic issues to the wider community remains a challenge.

Culture: critiques and transformational possibilities

During the 1990s the field of epidemiology underwent a period of criticism and self-criticism. In a critique, McKinley and Marceau (2000) argue that the thinking and practice of epidemiology and public health have been absorbed by biomedicine and hence are based on biophysiological reductionism. Like Krieger (1994), they see the discipline as lacking in theoretical sophistication and overly reliant on methodological development. As such, the field is limited by its dichotomous thinking, fixated as it is on risk factors, and confuses observational associations with causation. These problems lead to dogmatism shaped by study designs. If epidemiology has been the core science for public health, it is possible to extend the critique to public health practice.

Coye (1994), a public health leader in the USA, suggests that the culture of public health is perhaps its own worst enemy. According to her critique, the culture of public health reflects two related dimensions: the corporate culture of public health and the corporate culture of government. Coye identifies a number of key features in the corporate culture of public health:

- a belief and reliance on entitlement
- antipathy to organisational discipline
- resistance to accountability
- scorn for cost-effective considerations
- suspicion of the private sector
- ignorance plus disdain for the medical care sector.

Key features of the corporate culture of government, which overlays public health practice, include

- an inability and slow response to environmental change
- a categorical approach to program design and implementation
- an inability to work across programs
- an inability to focus and prioritise efforts.

The combination of these factors has led to the erosion of public confidence in the public sector, resulting in declining investment in infrastructures and systems. The combined cultures work against the bureaucracy's capacity to reinvent itself. While government has outsourced to nongovernment organisations, many of these organisations mirror the public sector in suffering the same corporate culture. A downward spiral is thus set in motion.

In Australia these problems are not as stark as they appear to be in the USA. The ossification of the United States system that Coye finds so frustrating has been avoided here. In part, this is because of the very significant changes experienced by the government sector in general and the health sector in particular in Australia during the 1980s and 1990s. However, some of the problems Coye identifies are still observable.

Turnock (1997) also argues for a more effective public health system, but less so from the perspective of the underlying culture. For Turnock, the lack of current effectiveness can perhaps be attributed to the fact that all the easy problems have been solved. The remaining intractable problems require different tools. He suggests that when only one set of tools has been in use, they tend to be applied to problems that actually require different solutions—or, in other words, when you are a hammer, the whole world looks like nails. Further, given limited-term funding, low rewards, and lack of incentives, the public health workforce is unlikely to be highly entrepreneurial or risk taking. When challenges emerge or when they fail to be addressed, a response of 'nobody told me it was my job', although not surprising, is inadequate for the future of the public health system.

Coye suggests that transformational tools are needed at the conceptual, structural, and system design levels, and that these are available. At the conceptual—organisational and cultural—level, she proposes the necessary developmental directions as transformational leadership, learning organisations, and a culture of quality management. At the structural level, she proposes the need to integrate across programs, to have performance incentives that support initiative and risk taking, and to have systems of coaching and teaching. At the system level, she argues for connections across the whole of health. Here, the necessary tool would build data linkages that could track investments, interventions, and outcomes. Such a tool would underpin the development of accountability systems for access, quality, and productivity.

Turnock's solutions are not dissimilar, albeit less prescriptive. Given that a friend in need is a friend indeed, he argues for the need to develop partnerships, particularly beyond traditional alliances. In doing so, public health professionals would acquire new skills for collaborative action and adopt a range of professional tools that promote more integrative public health practice. At the organisational and system levels, new strategic investments would be required and possible, and clearer expectations for outcomes and evidence-based practice could be set and supported.

A medium-term vision for a national public health system

The period of reflection and rebuilding of public health in the USA was given impetus by the 1988 Institute of Medicine Report, *The Future of Public Health*. These deliberations occurred during a period of significant infrastructure decline, as the Reagan brand of neoliberal policy reform swept through the USA. Although Australia has not encountered the same degree of difficulty, trends in public sector management have been in the same direction. The advent of the NPHP offers the possibility of setting a new direction without having to rebuild from a purely defensive position.

Prior to the establishment of the NPHP, public health governance in Australia could be seen as a rather messy set of nonintersecting Commonwealth–state committees with occasional, issue-specific participation by community and professional groups. Separate from these links, each jurisdiction went its own way in terms of issues such as investments, approaches to addressing health issues, and system architecture. The NPHP did not seek to impose a national superstructure but to facilitate better coordination, with a focus on infrastructure development. Through the NPHP processes, further commonalities emerged in thinking about public health investments, how systems might be designed, and ways to tackle health issues.

Given the federal system of government, a medium-term vision for a national public health system in Australia necessarily has to recognise the continued centrality of intergovernmental relations. An intergovernmental focal point, inclusive of local government, is needed and should have as its focus policy and investment issues. Such governance needs effective support from the three arms that interact with each other, and may be illustrated as follows.

Figure 5.2 The future of public health governance

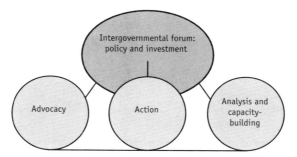

A broad public health coalition, bringing together a range of organisations, is needed as the advocacy arm. Such a group should engage with change from within as well as act as a ginger group from the outside. It has a role to 'keep the bastards honest', but should also be negotiating the broad public health agenda with governments and helping to build broader community support for the public health approach.

The imperatives of government do not necessarily support the analytical and capacity-building work that is necessary to construct a sound public health evidence base and ensure a strong multiskilled workforce. A virtual public health institute, drawing from organisations across Australia, could help overcome the 'tyranny of distance' and build the critical mass of resources needed. The virtual institute would need to have strong links to government and be part of building and implementing a national public health agenda.

Policies need effector arms and each jurisdiction implements public health action through its own workforce and through funding a range of health service and community organisations. Much public health action is local and requires only technical guidance from state and national levels. Some public health needs, however, are complex, extend across boundaries, or are of national significance. A national action arm, such as a virtual national centre for disease control, could be a rapid-action coordination mechanism that would deploy resources and expertise as the need arose. Such a networked mechanism could also serve as a quality assurance and practice-improvement mechanism, using methods such as Breakthrough developed by Berwick and the Institute for Healthcare Improvement (Voelker 1997). It could also support the improved documentation and promulgation of best practice.

The most critical features of a national public health system are effective leadership, strong delivery system infrastructure, and a workforce with adaptive skills. The system must achieve dynamic efficiency; that is, have the capacity to anticipate issues, respond to them, and evolve with them. The e-revolution may be a new tool to support national public health system development.

How to get there: some immediate agendas

A number of agendas need to be fulfilled to reach the medium-term vision. Some of these require leadership from governments while others rest with public health academics and practitioners. All of them will require the cooperation of these different groups.

From the system design perspective, more empirical information is required about current public health infrastructure and capacity. This will help define current optimal practice and the efforts required to ensure that all communities have infrastructure and practice that meet contemporary standards. Mechanisms for continuous transfer of research-and-development evidence into practice in a way that meets the needs of practitioners, are necessary to support the improvement of local practice. This may require further investments in translational or implementation research into how to effect a better takeup rate of research evidence, particularly around the more intractable areas of public health, such as health inequalities, and evidence-based health policy.

In the USA, a list of ten basic public health practices was developed for the Centers for Disease Control and Prevention (CDCPs) (Roper et al. 1992). More recently, the Pan American Health Organization (PAHO) has been working on measures to improve public health through the definition and measurement of the essential public health functions (PAHO 2000).

Public health practice needs supportive policy and managerial framework and investments. The NPHP has only begun to point to the agenda in resource allocation (Deeble 1999; NPHP 2000c), quality management (NPHP 2000d), and performance measurement (NPHP 2000c). Better policy and management tools, such as resource allocation methods, public health laws, advocacy approaches, and quality assurance mechanisms, need to be developed and taught to, or appreciated by, the workforce. Public health leadership networks spanning governments, health service providers, and community organisations, also need to be fostered to promote dialogue from perspectives driven by different constituencies. The identification and development of common agendas and directions will help secure a more coherent voice for public health interests.

In the USA, following publication of the *Institute of Medicine Report* (IOM 1988), the W K Kellog and the Robert Wood Johnson Foundations seeded the Turning Point Program[4] to assist local public health authorities to improve their planning and management capacity, including working with community organisations. It is interesting to note that, arising from these experiences, collaboration is being established on public health law reform, performance management, social marketing for public health, and information technology.

The investment in public health workforce development is ultimately crucial to a vibrant and effective public health system. The Public Health Leadership Institute (PHLI) in the USA is a collaboration between the CDCPs and partners including the University of California. The PHLI offers a year-long program with the aim of strengthening 'the public health system by enhancing the leadership capabilities of senior health officials' (Center for Health Leadership 1998, p. 13). It notes that 'over 97 per cent of graduates report direct contributions to their leadership skills and over 80 per cent report enhanced communication, motivation and conflict resolution skills' (Center for Health Leadership 1998, p. 13). The Australian public health workforce has demonstrated its effectiveness in health analysis in epidemiology and the health, social, and behavioural sciences (Nolan et al. 1999) and, to some extent, in the implementation of local public health interventions (National Health and Medical Research Council 1997). In the most immediate term, there is an urgent need to develop the workforce capacity for public health policy analysis and development. In most health authorities, strategic analysis and thinking has been focused on the development and management of the hospital sector. Increasing attention is being paid to the community care sector. Public health planners need to be engaged in these debates.

In the longer term, there is a need to ensure the public health workforce has the right balance of critical analytical skills and practical skills. Public health action relies on good problem identification as well as problem solving. It also requires an understanding between the different forms of public health as social enterprise, a knowledge base and a set of techniques, a delivery system, and a profession, in order to strengthen the connectivity between the different elements.

At the triennial conference of the World Federation of Public Health Associations (WFPHA) in Beijing in September 2000, George Alleyne,

Director of PAHO, suggested that it was time for a change in the culture of the public health movement. He urged those involved to

- celebrate the achievements
- create and support political will and move away from factionalism and blame shifting
- adopt a systems approach rather than a dichotomised and reductionist approach
- partner other sectors (especially economists)
- focus on operationalising the issues (rather than simply being rhetorical).

It would appear that there is convergence on many of the problems that afflict the public health movement as well as on the potential solutions.

Some questions about deep structures

Public health decision making is fundamentally concerned with the interplay between science and society. Public health science has been uncovering not only the causes and distributional patterns of health and disease, but also the social institutions shaping people's views and choices about health practices. The establishment of the NPHP is a significant attempt at structural reform in terms of reshaping the institutional arrangements for public health governance. As such, it signals some new parameters in how business will be done and creates conditions for the development of new business rules.

What is less considered seems to be the deep structures that underpin the institutional arrangements shaping the delivery of public health activities. To transform the culture of public health practice will require a better understanding of the interface of the cultures of the various professions that make up the field of public health. These include the cultures of specific programs and organisations, the gender and ethnic dimensions within organisations, and the jurisdictional cultural differences. These cultural issues are shaped by history and, in turn, shape the labour process. While what public health people do can be described, what motivates what they do, how their activities are changing, and what is driving those changes are less well understood. The 1980s and 1990s saw an increasing rate of public sector management reforms and health reforms. But to what extent did public health practices change?

Public health professionals, in their initial meetings, seldom seem to be able to advance beyond a discussion about the definition of public health. This may be an inevitability resulting from the diversity of the workforce and the issues being addressed. It may also reflect some underlying preoccupation with professional identity and a collective uncertainty about power and marginality.

In the struggle by public health professionals to define boundaries and preserve their special identity—in part through self-differentiation from medical care—there appear to be considerable tensions about whether it is better to be championing the underdogs from the margins or seizing control and being at centre stage. This may be the most fundamental challenge for a cultural transformation of the public health field.

Acknowledgment

The assistance of Prue Bagley is gratefully acknowledged.

References

Centre for Health Leadership 1998, *Development of the Public Health Workforce: A Preliminary Compendium of National Resources*, Public Health Leadership Society and the Centre for Health Leadership, <http://www.cfhl.org/phli/compend.pdf>.

Coye, M. 1994, *Our Own Worst Enemy: Obstacles to Improving the Health of the Public*, Milbank Memorial Fund, <http://www.milbank.org/mrlead.html>.

Deeble, J. 1999, *Resource Allocation in Public Health: An Economic Approach*, National Public Health Partnership, Melbourne; online version available at <http://www.nphp.gov.au/ppc/resalloc/deeble/index.htm>.

Institute of Medicine 1988, *The Future of Public Health*, National Academy Press, Washington, DC.

Krieger, N. 1994, 'Epidemiology and the Web of Causation: Has Anyone Seen the Spider?', *Social Science and Medicine*, vol. 39, pp. 887–903.

Levy, B. 1998, 'Creating the Future of Public Health', *American Journal of Public Health*, vol. 88, no. 2, pp. 188–92.

Lewis, M. & Leeder, S. 1998, 'History of Public Health in Australia since 1945', in B. Furnass (ed.), *Infectious Disease in Humans*, Howard Florey Centenary Symposium, Canberra.

Lin, V. & King, C. 2000, 'Intergovernmental Reforms in Public Health', in A. Bloom (ed.), *Health Reform in Australia and New Zealand*, Oxford University Press, Melbourne.

McKinlay, J. & Marceau, L. 2000, 'To Boldly Go …', *American Journal of Public Health*, vol. 90, no. 1, January, pp. 25–33.

National Health and Medical Research Council 1997, *Promoting the Health of Australians: A Review of Infrastructure Support for National Health Advancement*, AGPS, Canberra.

National Public Health Partnership n.d., *Memorandum of Understanding to Establish a National Public Health Partnership for Australia*, National Public Health Partnership, Melbourne; online version available at <http://www.gov.au/mou.htm>.

—— 1997, *Public Health in Australia*, National Public Health Partnership, Melbourne; online version available at <http://www.gov.au/broch/contents.htm>.

—— 1998, *Issues for Consideration in Industry Partnerships for Public Health Initiatives*, National Public Health Partnership, Melbourne; online version available at <http://www.nphp.gov.au/indust/index.htm>.

—— 1999a, *Progress Through Partnerships: Annual Report*, National Public Health Partnership, Melbourne; online version available at <http://www.nphp.gov.au/ar99/index.htm>.

—— 1999b, *National Public Health Information Development Plan*, National Public Health Partnership, Melbourne; online version available at <http://www.nphp.gov.au/nphidp/index.htm>.

—— 1999c, *Guidelines for Improving National Public Health Strategies Development and Coordination*, National Public Health Partnership, Melbourne; online version available at <http://www.nphp.gov.au/natstrat/index.htm>.

—— 2000a, *National Delphi Study on Public Health Functions in Australia: Report on the Findings*, National Public Health Partnership, Melbourne; online version available at <http://www.nphp.gov.au/ppi/corefunc/delphi/index.htm>.

—— 2000b, *A Planning Framework for Public Health Practice: a Systems Perspective*, National Public Health Partnership, Melbourne; online version available at <http://www.nphp.gov.au/ppi/planning/planfrwwk/index.htm>.

—— 2000c, *Performance Indicator Frameworks for Population Health: Report of the Workshop held on 16 March 2000*, National Public Health Partnership, Melbourne; online version available at <http://www.nphp.gov.au/perfinds/ index.htm>.

—— 2000d, 'Promoting Quality in Public Health', *National Public Health Partnership News*, no. 11, March; online version available at <http://www.nphp.gov.au/mar00/quality.htm>.

Nolan, T., Bryson, L., & Lashof, J. 1999, *Independent Review of the Public Health Education and Research Program: Report to the Commonwealth Department of Health and Aged Care*, Commonwealth Department of Health and Aged Care, Canberra.

Pan American Health Organization 2000, *The 126th Session of the Executive Committee: Resolution CE126.R18*, 26–30 June, Pan American Health Organization, Washington, DC.

Roper, W., Baker, E.L., Dyal, W. & Nicola, R. 1992, 'Strengthening the Public Health System', *Public Health Reports*, vol. 107, no. 6, pp. 609–15.

Rychetnik, L. & Frommer, M. 2000, *A Proposed Schema for Evaluating Evidence on Public Health Interventions*, National Public Health Partnership, Melbourne.

Turnock, B. 1997, *Public Health: What It Is and How It Works*, Aspen Publishers, Maryland.

Voelker, R. 1997, 'IHI Views Collaboration versus Competition in Quality', *Journal of the American Medical Association*, vol. 278, no. 19, p. 1560.

6

Strategic Alliances in Public Health

Rae Walker, Heather Gardner, and Yvonne Robinson

Within any industry there are complex networks of informal linkages between individuals and organisations. In the health sector, informal linkages are important to and promoted by public health and community health organisations, medical colleges, health service managers, and allied health professional associations, among others. Health care providers establish referral patterns that are based on reputation and often on long-established patterns of interaction. Access to resources is facilitated by informal networks, which provide information and offer influence. Peers, who are often members of research networks, review health research grants. However, the capacity to transform informal linkages into strategic alliances is variable and influenced by the policy environment in which the organisations operate and the structural arrangements impacting on organisations (Lutz 1997). The changing policy environment in Australia (Yeatman 1990) has transformed the context in which strategic alliances develop and operate.

The policy environment of the 1990s reflects major influences from business (Osborne & Gaebler 1992) and from economics, especially in regard to the emphasis on funding mechanisms as instruments of control and markets as mechanisms of coordination (Powell 1990). Williamson (1975) views the relationships surrounding transactions between organisations as governed either by hierarchies using bureaucratic rules and procedures or by markets using contractual devices. Other organisational forms are considered to be a hybrid of markets and hierarchies.

The hierarchy–market dichotomy is perhaps unhelpful because it does not reflect the real world, as large organisations are changing. By opening up their boundaries and building relationships with other organisations

(Powell 1990; Osborn & Hagedorn 1997), organisations gain allies who provide better access to information and innovation, allow them to have stronger relationships with the people using their products and services, are better able to focus those products and services on market demand, and ultimately to gain market advantages. Partnership arrangements between organisations led to a different organisational form with its own dynamics, opportunities, and limitations. Alter and Hage (1993) argue that the interorganisational network is a new type of institution that will ultimately replace markets and hierarchies as forms of coordination and control. They argue that the network form is fundamentally different from anything that went before it and that its application in the private and public sectors challenges accepted beliefs that these sectors are fundamentally different.

The literature on partnerships in business and on theories of interorganisational network formation has provided new concepts by which to understand more about strategic alliances and linkages between health service organisations in market and policy contexts:

> it is these cooperative behaviours—the growing number of partnerships, alliances, joint ventures, consortia, obligational and systemic networks—that represent a stunning evolutionary change in institutional forms of governance (Alter & Hage 1993, p. 12).

What are strategic alliances?

The term 'strategic alliance' is used in different ways. Gulati (1995, p. 619) defines an interfirm strategic alliance as a 'voluntary arrangement involving durable exchange, sharing or codevelopment of new products and technologies'. The elements of voluntariness and durability in the relationship contained in this definition are useful for considering health sector interorganisational relationships. The criterion of codevelopment of new products and technologies is also helpful if it is understood to include service provision, the core business of health organisations, within products and technologies. Definitions of technology in health can easily accommodate health professionals and their practice; the current emphasis on outputs and outcomes and on services—such as community care—as products makes Gulati's definition even more pertinent. The definition would also accommodate joint research or teaching ventures between industries in the public and private sectors.

A strategic alliance can be 'any form of cooperative relationship between two or more firms, the purpose of which is to develop, design, manufacture, market or distribute products or services' (Barney & Hesterly

1996, p. 138). This definition emphasises cooperation for specific purposes and an explicit form of governance. The primary purpose of strategic alliances is the enhancement and utilisation of an organisation's productive resources (Lazonick 1991). The form of agreement that exists between the partners (Barney & Hesterly 1996) can also differentiate strategic alliances.

The trend to cooperation

During the 1960s and 1970s, businesses responded to 'inefficiencies in external markets' by internalising additional elements of production within a firm (Buttery & Buttery 1994). This strategy is described as vertical and horizontal integration. 'Where market imperfections exist, firms may take the opportunity to develop their own internal transfer mechanisms rather than deal in inefficient external markets' (Buttery & Buttery 1994, p. 16). The trend towards integration by internalisation occurred in an environment of fierce competition for market domination. The casualties of this strategy included many firms, product quality, and customer service. Further, the global markets and technologies of production were changing, with far-reaching implications for the organisation of economic activity. From the 1970s onwards the argument that the casualties of competition for market domination weakened Western economies in the global market became fashionable. The 1980s was a period of intense interest in cooperative ways of organising production. A key shift occurred when management learnt to differentiate between core activities (which should be retained within a firm) and noncore activities (which could be delegated to other firms) (Buttery & Buttery 1994). Delegation required working cooperatively with other firms, their partners in production, to achieve quality and service.

During the 1980s, Britain led a trend to introduce market principles into the redesign of integrated systems of health services that were financed and provided by government (Light 1997); from the late 1980s, Australia increasingly followed suit (Considine 1992; Gardner 1995; Owens 1995; Lin and Duckett 1997). There are positive and negative policy lessons to be learnt from market reform of the National Health Service (NHS), many of which are relevant to the Australian system:

> What the British are realising is that most of the benefits come from purchasing and most of the costs come from competitive contracting. If, then, purchases are made jointly via what might be called 'managed cooperation', information can be shared rather than hidden, thereby engendering and rewarding trust and promoting collaboration in meeting the health needs of communities. The British are now moving towards purchaser–provider partnerships (Light 1997, p. 303).

As early as 1993, the NHS Executive announced that partnerships and long-term agreements between agencies were the new order of the day. By 1996, competition was to be replaced with a preference for collaboration (Light 1997). In the White Paper, *The New NHS*, it is asserted that 'the internal market will be replaced by a system we have called "integrated care", based on partnership and driven by performance' (NHS Executive 1997, p. 1). There will be a 'new statutory duty of partnership placed on local NHS bodies to work together for the common good' (NHS Executive 1997, p. 26). Partnership, in this context, includes establishing joint planning structures for health and social care provision, multidisciplinary primary care groups for the provision of community care, and health action zones within which organisations will work cooperatively to implement a locally determined strategy for improving the health of local people. This is premised on staff in the NHS and other organisations developing a greater capacity to work in teams within their own organisations and across organisational boundaries.

Strategic alliances

The National Public Health Partnership (NPHP) and the North East Health Promotion Centre (NEHPC) are used in case studies 1 and 2 (see boxes 6.1 and 6.1 respectively) as examples of strategic alliances—one national, one state—to illustrate key principles relevant to the development of strategic alliances in the health sector in Australia.

Box 6.1
Case study 1—The National Public Health Partnership

The National Public Health Partnership (NPHP) had its genesis in discussions between the chief health officers of the departments of health in the Australian states and territories and with the Commonwealth about ways of approaching long-term, systemwide reform in public health. It was based on the concept of collaboration to develop a greater degree of coordination and clarification of roles and responsibilities. At the time of the NPHP development, the public health system was seen to be suffering from a number of fundamental weaknesses. These included the following:
- Most public health services were funded and delivered through vertical programs under which the Commonwealth provided

resources and the states and territories provided services. Vertical programs were thought to create barriers between the jurisdictions and problems for service delivery. In contrast, the most effective programs were those that had overcome these arrangements and developed in cooperative ways.

- Many public health issues transcended jurisdictional boundaries, so effective responses needed to be collaborative and complementary to have most effect.
- Some areas of public health were developing in ways that could create duplication and systemic inefficiencies because roles and responsibilities of the jurisdictions were not clear.
- There was an increasing need to link public health knowledge and skills into other health system developments, but the mechanisms were not readily apparent (NPHP 1998).

The NPHP was taken under the umbrella of the Australian Health Ministers Council and the NPHP Group (the governing committee) became a subcommittee of the Australian Health Ministers Advisory Committee in 1996. Effectively, the NPHP was linked into existing arrangements to facilitate political cooperation between governments. The NPHP Group is constituted by the chief health officer, or director of public health, from each state and territory and from the Commonwealth; representatives from the National Health and Medical Research Council; and the Australian Institute of Health and Welfare. This group acts as the prime coordinating structure for the partnership. The roles and responsibilities of the participating members of the NPHP and the operational arrangements and processes are outlined in a Memorandum of Understanding. The major work activities are structured through a rolling three-year work program in which priorities, working and monitoring arrangements are outlined.

NPHP is an intergovernmental coordinating arrangement. It is well placed to coordinate the major business of government between the states and territories, and between the states and territories and the Commonwealth. Public health services are provided within the states and territories by organisations including local councils, nongovernment organisations, general practitioners, community-based health services, and universities, among others. The means that these link other organisations into a coordinated effort with government are less clear.

Box 6.2
Case study 2—The North East Health Promotion Centre

The North East Health Promotion Centre (NEHPC) was an innovative network form of organisation embedded in the Victorian health promotion infrastructure. In contrast to the National Public Health Partnership (NPHP), the centre was a locally developed initiative. It grew out of existing alliances around coordination of health service delivery between community health centres, the acute care sector, general practice, local government, and a university with an interest in strengthening links between academics and practitioners. After several months of negotiation, discussion, and a situational analysis by the participating agencies, NEHPC commenced operating in May 1997.

The participating agencies comprised four municipalities (Banyule, Darebin, Nillumbik, and Whittlesea), four community health centres (Banyule, Darebin, Eltham, and Plenty Valley), two Divisions of General Practice (Northern and North East Valley), a hospital (the Austin and Repatriation Medical Centre), a health care network (North West Health), and a university (La Trobe University). The centre's catchment area was defined geographically by the boundaries of the four municipalities.

The local concerns that contributed to the creation of NEHPC were similar to those leading, at a national level, to the formation of the NPHP. There was, for example, a perceived need for greater clarity in the roles and responsibilities for health promotion between sectors. While health promotion has always been seen as part of the core business of community health centres, in Victoria an increasingly significant public health role has been played by local government through Municipal Public Health Plans. Commonwealth government grants for health promotion to Divisions of General Practice brought new players onto the scene. A health promotion role for hospitals has also emerged following the World Health Organization's (WHO's) 1995 Budapest Declaration.

The increasing diversity in the health promotion workforce raised concern about duplication of effort and resources. Health promotion activity commands only a small proportion of overall expenditure on health. The system can ill afford wastage of resources through duplication. Improved planning was seen as one way of ensuring the most efficient use of resources. Although there are national and statewide frameworks and strategic documents to direct health promotion effort, there has until recently been relatively little investment in health promotion planning capacity at the regional or subregional level in Victoria. NEHPC was created, in part, to address this issue.

From its early days, the NEHPC worked in an environment of increasing turbulence. In December 1998, 18 months after the centre began operating, the Victorian government announced its intention to create a more integrated primary health and community support system. In April 2000, a document issued by the Department of Human Services announced the new system structure based on primary care partnerships. In effect, the reform process created new linking structures and the integrating functions NEHPC had been set up to provide. In December 2000, it was decided to close the centre.

NEHPC was evaluated twice and the findings of the participating agencies' collaborative experience widely disseminated. The evaluations clearly showed that the centre had successfully developed a more integrated approach to health promotion and that the linkages were carrying over into the primary care partnerships.

When NEHPC was originally created by its participating agencies its aims were to
- provide a strategic planning framework for health promotion in the catchment area
- ensure coordinated and complementary health promotion activities between the participating agencies that met identified needs in the local population
- initiate innovative, high-quality health promotion activities among the participating agencies
- provide consultancy and support to the participating agencies on the development and evaluation of best-practice health promotion
- promote effective health promotion through teaching and research
- provide seed funding to carry out and evaluate health promotion programs
- develop a database to support the sharing of skills and resources across participating agencies.

Governance and accountability for NEHPC were provided through a steering committee, on which all participating agencies had representation, and an executive subcommittee, which included a representative from each sector (local government, community health, Divisions of General Practice, the acute care sector, and the university). Commitment to the centre was underpinned by a formal agreement with each participating agency.

The committee structure provided a mechanism for coordinated planning and activity for health promotion at the level of management. The centre also set up other networking structures to support improved collaborative activity between those working in health promotion in the participating agencies. These included working groups for three priority health promotion projects and for health promotion coordinators.

The centre provided a structure through which a diverse range of agencies—each of which has some role in health promotion—came to know and understand each other's contribution. It also helped to develop a shared understanding of health promotion, which is widely acknowledged to be a complex and contested concept. The centre then moved on to the challenge of creating a more systemic approach to coordinated planning and activity among the participating agencies. Agreement was reached to use the local government Municipal Public Health Plans as the appropriate planning machinery within which to set health promotion planning; processes have been set in place to achieve this. It is interesting to note the centre's pioneer role in building on Municipal Public Health Plans for local planning coordination. The primary care system reforms have adopted a similar approach. A network structure such as that of the NEHPC was challenging conceptually and practically. It was in some respects a virtual centre, which differs from a strategic business unit within an alliance. On the one hand, its two core staff provided a network coordinating function for its agencies rather than a direct health promotion service-delivery role. On the other hand, centre staff played a key role in initiating and framing discussion and managing externally funded projects. The centre was thus an active player in the network. Issues of leadership and of balancing what is gained and lost through partnerships were two of a number of dilemmas facing network participants in the new learning environment.

Although different in many respects, NPHP and NEHPC illustrate some key issues in the development and operation of strategic alliances.

The development of strategic alliances

Triggers for alliance formation

There are internal and external triggers that encourage businesses to form alliances (Buttery & Buttery 1994). The triggers for alliance formation internal to an organisation include

- production efficiencies
- market advantage
- access to knowledge, skills, and research capacity
- a reduction in competition.

External triggers include

- environmental pressures
- changes in government funding and market policy
- risk sharing
- creating opportunities in depressed areas
- gaining flexibility
- strengthening capacity.

Of the reasons given for the formation of NPHP, some are similar to the reasons for the formation of strategic alliances in business. There was clearly a sense that the capacities of the jurisdictions could be better used and that there were examples of this happening where cooperative arrangements had been established. Pressure to link public health knowledge and skills to other parts of the health system to support innovation was also perceived; however, the aspiration to prevent duplication developing between jurisdictions is not a usual reason for coordination between firms in a competitive environment. It appears that the jurisdictions, although formally independent of each other, have intersecting interests that create a shared purpose in regard to some public health matters. By means of NPHP, these shared interests can be acted upon in ways that create openings in organisational boundaries through which linkages between organisations can be formed. That NPHP emerged out of discussions between the chief health officers in the jurisdictions about common issues supports this view. Recognition that public health across Australia represents a problem domain (Gray 1989), within which the efforts of a number of key stakeholders are necessary for effective solutions to be found, is a sophisticated perception of the issues which might be found in the business or government sectors.

In terms of internal triggers for the formation of alliances, several are pertinent to NEHPC, although not all are stated explicitly in documentation relating to the centre's inception and purpose. For example, new money provided by the Commonwealth through the Divisions of General Practice to the system for health promotion initiatives meant that there was potential access, particularly for community health centres, to financial resources that would enable them to develop new joint health promotion services.

For some time both Commonwealth and state governments have used funding mechanisms to promote the development of partnerships in public health. Health promotion funding has been used in this way. NEHPC's participating agencies, through the relationships established in the centre, gained an enhanced capacity to respond rapidly to funding opportunities demanding partnerships between applicants. This provided the centre's agencies with a competitive advantage over other groups of organisations competing for the same tenders.

NEHPC could also be seen to be a consequence of a decision of some of its participating agencies to reduce the threat of competition. Vertical integration of community health services into hospital network structures was occurring in parts of Victoria at the time of the centre's inception. By setting up a partnership, North East Health Care Network (NEHCN) and community health centres created an alternative form of linkage. In Buttery and Buttery's (1994) terms, they were drawing boundaries around alliances rather than organisations, thus reducing competition.

External pressures have also been apparent in quality improvement initiatives in health promotion practice. A criticism frequently levelled at health promotion is that it is inadequately evaluated. Partnership with a university offered other participating agencies in NEHPC access to evaluation expertise as well as to possibilities of joint research ventures with a focus on practitioner relevance. In Victoria, the Department of Human Services has played an active role in producing documents for service providers about best practice in health promotion (for example, Deakin University 1996). These publications emphasise the need for a coordinated range of health promotion strategies covering all action areas of the *Ottawa Charter for Health Promotion* (World Health Organization 1986). A number of audits have noted a concentration of health promotion effort on individual and small group activities (for example, Lewis & Walker 1997). A similar finding emerged from an audit of the current health promotion work undertaken by the centre's participating agencies. Clearly, there is a need for service providers to develop more sophisticated health promotion programs that incorporate a greater diversity of strategies. No single organisation has the skills, resources, or mandate to deliver consistently programs with multiple strategies. Strategic alliances offer an obvious solution to the problem of developing and resourcing more complex programs.

Highly significant triggers for creating the NEHPC were concern about duplication and the need for coordinated planning. These issues have been raised as problems in a number of recent reports on health promotion and the broader infrastructure for health care and illness prevention in Australia. For example, the National Health and Medical Research Council (NHMRC) paper *Promoting the Health of Australians* (1996) noted that the 'Australian health promotion effort is poorly coordinated, fragmented and subject to inefficiencies due to duplication of effort' (1996, p. 12).

The issue of duplication can perhaps be seen as part of a larger problem that Gray (1989) describes as 'overlapping discretion'. All the NEHPC's participating agencies had an acknowledged—although not necessarily clearly specified—role in providing health promotion services. Gray argues that this type of situation results in interdependence between organisations and, where no single agency has the resources or mandate to dominate, creates conditions that call for collaborative solutions. The case for collaboration is even stronger where the problem or issue is ill defined and characterised by technical complexity and scientific uncertainty. This is certainly the case with health promotion, a multifaceted, underresearched, and contested concept. In these circumstances, collaboration can be understood as an attempt to create a 'negotiated order' in interorganisational relationships. Order is 'shaped through the self-conscious interactions of participants' (Gray 1989, p. 228). Viewed from this perspective, the NEHPC can be seen as a structure for enabling and brokering such interaction and negotiation. Similarly, the NPHP provides a structure through which governments can negotiate order, thereby reflecting principles described by policy network theorists such as Klijn (1997; see also Considine 1994; Colebatch 1998).

Processes of alliance formation

Not all alliances produce the benefits anticipated by the partners (Limerick & Cunnington 1993; Simonin 1997). An exploration of success and failure of strategic alliances requires an examination of issues in alliance formation, interdependence, and organisational learning and alliance management.

Gulati (1995) explores how social relationships influence the development of strategic alliances. He argues that organisations enter repeatedly into relationships with others whom they know and have worked with previously. Pre-existing ties that provide knowledge of capacities, and develop trust, increase the likelihood of the participants developing alliances when the opportunity arises. The issue of prior relationships arose at key stages in the development of the NPHP. The idea for a national public health partnership emerged from discussions between chief health officers who met regularly and had been doing so over many years, frequently, but not always, through NHMRC structures. Pre-existing relationships were important at a number of key points in the development of the NPHP.

Similarly, it is probable that the preexisting relationships in the sub-region contributed to the successful joint project that became the NEHPC. The agencies already had experience of collaborative activity and alliance building. For example, the community health centres in the subregion had formed an alliance and were also members of the North East Primary Health Care Forum. In 1996, the year in which the idea for the centre took shape and gained commitment, the former East Preston and Northcote Community Health Centre (now Darebin Community Health), with support from Darebin City Council, undertook a project to identify the major health needs in the municipality. They also jointly developed a three-year health promotion plan.

However, there is a limit on the number of alliances organisations will form with each other as potential benefits from additional cooperation appear to diminish and the issue of overdependence arises (Gulati 1995). In both the NPHP and the NEHPC, cooperation did not extend to all areas of activity. Although cooperation had been established in regard to certain activities, tensions remained in regard to others.

Strong relationships with particular organisations increase the likelihood of alliances forming with other organisations one step removed from the partners, between organisations that have access to information about the partners' track records or reputations:

> the social network of indirect ties is an effective referral mechanism for bringing firms together and that dense co-location in an alliance network enhances mutual confidence as firms become aware of the possible negative reputational conse-quences of their own and others' opportunistic behaviour (Gulati 1995, p. 644)

The network of organisations with which the NEHPC worked expanded substantially as externally funded projects were established. Through such projects, schools and community organisations entered the centre's network and, by association, those of the partners constituting the centre.

Key strategies adopted within the NEHPC were consistent with Klijn's (1996) description of an interactive management perspective. For example, in terms of 'managing aims and participating in the right games', the centre worked with its participating agencies to develop a shared understanding of health promotion and a joint vision for collaborative action based on WHO's Ottawa Charter. This process helped to clarify roles based on the differing skills, resources, and mandates of the network members. It also enabled identification of focused opportunities for synergy in health pro-motion where participating agencies can achieve better results together than alone.

Klijn also refers to the need to 'structure interactions' and 'activate par-ticipants'. The centre worked at developing a range of linkages between its participating agencies and actively involving individuals in centre initiatives. The steering committee and its executive subcommittee constituted formal channels for decision making and planning among agency managers. Working groups and short-term task groups provided opportunities for workers in the participating agencies to become involved in specific joint activities and to develop networks based on face-to-face interaction.

Interdependence

When organisations know each other's capacities they might recognise a degree of interdependence as complementarity of resources, or the capacity to achieve together what cannot be achieved alone (Kanter 1994). Organisations that recognise interdependence are more likely to seek each other out as alliance partners (Gulati 1995). Interdependence was recognised and offered as a reason for the establishment of the NPHP initiative.

Recognition of interdependence is not always a consequence of collaborative activity. In a study of general practitioner (GP) collaborative relationships, it became apparent that interdependence was often not recognised, irrespective of the qualities of the partners and their relationships (Walker et al. 1997). Realistically, potential interdependence alone is insufficient to support the development of strategic alliances.

Trust

Trust is considered a critical factor in interorganisational arrangements. In one view trust is predicated on confidence in predictability of expectations in a relationship and in the other is based on confidence in another's goodwill (Ring & van de Ven 1994). It reduces the 'perceived probability of loss' in an economic arrangement (Nooteboom et al. 1997, p. 329). However, trust alone is insufficient to control these relationships and perceived risk is further reduced by forms of governance that limit opportunism. Despite its fragility (Ring 1997), such trust can provide a basis for stability in interorganisational relationships that might simplify formal governance.

The second type emphasises resilience, 'faith in the moral integrity or goodwill of others on whom economic actors depend for the realisation of collective and individual goals as they deal with future, unpredictable issues' (Ring 1997, p. 122). It survives the occasional challenge, replaces some formal mechanisms of control with social norms and sanctions, and is the kind of trust that underscores stable, long-term relationships. Both kinds of trust may be present in a strategic alliance. As relationships develop, and the expectations of the actors are met, the more likely it is that fragile trust will evolve into resilient trust. What Alter and Hage (1993, p. 17) call a new 'culture of cooperation' has developed, which is an explanation for why more people are engaging in the apparently 'risky behavior of participating in a joint venture, strategic alliance, or production network'.

The issue of trust is particularly important—and difficult—in the inter-governmental alliance represented by the NPHP. In Australia, intergovernmental relations are typified by distrust and manifest disparities of interests. Through the NPHP a degree of trust is achievable, although it is most likely to be closer to the fragile form than the resilient. Even on the basis of fragile trust, members of health departments can make substantial progress on matters of shared concern, for example, to create consistency in public health legislation between jurisdictions.

Learning and adaptation

Simonin (1997) argues that strategic alliances only sometimes realise their potential benefits. Experience of undertaking alliances is, alone, insufficient to ensure that organisations make the best use of their opportunities. They must learn how to make them work and deliver the potential benefits. Organisations 'lacking proper know-how may multiply collaborative experience and rush into arrangements that are ill-conceived, poorly managed and, therefore, prone to early termination' (Simonin 1997, p. 1153).

When strategic alliances work effectively the participating organisations also change (Kanter 1989). Changes are found in the organisational power structure, which becomes a structure that supports the work of the alliance. The roles of staff are changed to support alliance goals and activities; changes also occur in the job skills of key staff, making them better able to 'juggle constituencies rather than control subordinates' (Kanter 1989, p. 152). Organisations that are good at working collaboratively contain people with the knowledge and skills to design and manage collaborations, to identify and resolve problems that emerge, to position their organisation strategically, and to conclude collaborations when it becomes appropriate.

In the NPHP the most senior public health officer in each jurisdiction sits on the NPHP Group, the senior operational committee. There is a relatively high degree of support for the NPHP at senior levels. In some jurisdictions structures have been established to shadow important aspects of the NPHP work—for example, the coordination of major public health strategies—but it is not yet clear how far the NPHP has penetrated the constituent jurisdictions.

Spreading learning from the collaborative activities within the NEHPC across its thirteen organisations, some of which are large, complex bureaucracies, was difficult. Communication existed at different levels across the organisations through committee structures (typically involving managers) and working groups (involving practitioners). Communication across these levels in organisations varied. In smaller organisations, team structures allowed those involved in centre activities to report back, consult, and make linkages with the ongoing work of the agency. In larger structures, such as local government, more extensive networks of individuals were created so that the work of the centre became the business of at least one person in a variety of team or divisional structures; however, the evaluation of the centre's first year of operation showed that knowledge and understanding of the activities coordinated through the centre varied greatly. Not surprisingly, this was coloured by the level and type of involvement. Those involved in more than one linking structure (committee, working group, advisory group, planning group) were those most likely to be aware of the range and extent of the centre's activity.

Strategic alliances in policy networks

Recently, there has been growing interest in ways that policy can be viewed in networked structures. Policy network members share a material interest that encourages regular contact, and participate also in a shared knowledge base that defines the broader policy community. In other words, a policy network is a subset of the policy community where the values (ideology, worldview, epistemology) are shared, but the policy network is a more continuously active group of people with shared interests (Howlett & Ramesh 1995).

When policy systems are viewed as networks, three main features can be identified (Klijn 1996). First, the form of interdependence itself is changed by the actors' interactions. Second, the policy network has many actors in a complex process of interaction. No single actor controls it and there is no single goal that can be used to evaluate success, as actors have diverse goals and interests. Third, the interdependencies and interactions form patterns of relations between actors that have a lasting character and are sustained by a set of consensual rules that emerge over time.

Issues in network management

O'Toole (1997, p. 116) is concerned with the problem of innovation, 'converting good ideas into steady, reliable streams of public action', and sees success as being particularly difficult to achieve when implementation develops 'in and through networks of interdependent actors'. Two key issues are uncertainty (including lack of trust) and lack of institutionalised rules for acting in the developmental stages of the network. Skilled management of the network processes can overcome both difficulties. Network management is different from management in and of separate organisations, as management of separate organisations suggests that management is a top down activity involving strategic planning, structuring and designing the organization (organizing), and getting the job done (leading). It is based on a view of policy and organization processes as orderly phased processes involving the formulation of problems, generating of alternatives, making decisions, and evaluating outcomes. In this classical perspective on management, the central questions of management—where to go and how to get there—are solved by hierarchical control and planning (Klijn 1996, p. 105).

In a network, where no single actor has the power to achieve a desired outcome alone, a different, more interactive perspective on management is appropriate so that

management stresses the unpredictability of (policy) processes. Managing aims and participating in the right games; making interorganizational arrangements to structure interactions, and activating participants for new games. In the network perspective on management, more attention is paid to the interaction process between actors and the ways these processes can be stimulated, sustained and changed when necessary (Klijn 1996, p. 105).

Key strategies adopted within the NEHPC were consistent with Klijn's description of an interactive management perspective. For example, in terms of 'managing aims and participating in the right games', the centre worked with its participating agencies to develop a shared understanding of health promotion and a joint vision for collaborative action based on the WHO's Ottawa Charter. This process helped to clarify roles based on the differing skills, resources, and mandates of the network members. It also enabled identification of focused opportunities for synergy in health promotion where participating agencies could achieve better results together than alone.

Klijn also refers to the need to 'structure interactions' and 'activate participants'. The NEHPC worked at developing a range of linkages between its participating agencies and actively involving individuals in centre initiatives. The steering committee and its executive subcommittee constituted formal channels for decision making and planning among agency managers. Working groups and short-term task groups provided opportunities for workers in the participating agencies to become involved in specific joint activities and to develop networks based on face-to-face interaction.

Of the cases used here to illustrate aspects of strategic alliances, the NPHP is the one most clearly trying to create coordinated action in a policy network so that issues in policy network management are of particular relevance to the NPHP. The NPHP has a membership consisting of state, territory, and Commonwealth public health divisions. All potential member organisations have signed the Memorandum of Understanding and all participate in the committees and working parties that have been established to further the work of the NPHP; however, members do not necessarily contribute equally. From time to time, two of the larger states and the Commonwealth have been very active, and at least one of the smaller states has reflected on the issues a small resource base raises for them. The organisational membership and committee structures have been stable and able to resist environmental stresses. In some cases, environmental turbulence has slowed progress on particular areas of the work plan, but other areas have been relatively unaffected. The role of policy subsystems, where knowledge is required on the feasibility of various options to address issue areas, is very different from agenda setting, in which a less detailed knowledge allows for involvement from a much broader membership.

The key actors in the NPHP are all senior members of government health departments. Parallel to the interactive processes of network management exist a set of committees, subcommittees and working parties that have an hierarchical relationship to each other. The apparent coexistence of two very different approaches to management locates the secretariat in a paradox. On the one hand it must facilitate horizontal linkages to further joint action, but on the other it must operate in a largely hierarchical set of relationships.

Conclusion

It remains to be seen whether, consistent with these two examples—one federal, the other state—a new climate of cooperation has been developing in the Australian health sector that will result in the formation of strategic alliances. It would appear that a common contributing factor in their formation—the possibility of accessing revenue from additional sources, which are multiple rather than single, and horizontal as well as vertical—will act as an incentive in many health areas at federal, state and territory, and local levels. Should governments wish to make this happen in the perpetual search for coordination, coherence, and control in the pursuit of outcomes, they will need to 'get the incentives right' (Owens 1995, p. 285). For the organisations themselves, in addition to the resource incentives, access to different skills and knowledge in pursuit of the achievement of objectives—such as the synergy in health promotion of the NEHPC—would appear to be as compelling; the one is a means to the other rather than an end in itself. For the NPHP the development of common policies should be enhanced from the interaction between many actors. Programs across jurisdictions would clearly strengthen Australia's capacity to address national public health issues.

Although the flexibility to move in and out of alliances is perceived to be positive it can, of course, have negative consequences for the alliance itself and for its individual members if it becomes too weak from uncertainty and instability. Commitment and trust could then be diminished. Their very reason for existence—that they are innovative, fluid, flexible, highly dynamic, provide new solutions, and promote new ideas—is in some ways the underlying reason that they are problematic. Alliances are threatened by the inequality of resources between the partners and their dependency on each other to achieve common goals. They are difficult to implement, difficult to manage, and difficult to maintain as lasting structures. To operate within policy networks and alliances, the participants must identify the key issues. What is it that they gain from this type of organisation? This would appear to be especially critical for those who are trying to manage the strategic alliance.

References

Alter, C. & Hage, J. 1993, *Organizations Working Together*, Sage, Newbury Park, California.

Barney, J. B. & Hesterly, W. 1996, 'Organisational Economics: Understanding the Relationship between Organizations and Economic Analysis', in S. R. Clegg, C. Handy, & W. R. Nord (eds), *Handbook of Organization Studies*, Sage, London.

Buttery, E. & Buttery, A. 1994, *Business Networks*, Longman, Melbourne.

Colebatch, H. 1998, *Policy*, Open University Press, Buckingham.

Considine, M. 1992, 'Policy: Managed or Expert?', in H. Gardner (ed.), *Health Policy: Development, Implementation and Evaluation in Australia*, Churchill Livingstone, Melbourne.

—— 1994, *Public Policy: A Critical Approach*, Macmillan Education, Melbourne.

Deakin University 1996, *Putting Best Practice into Practice*, Deakin University, Melbourne.

Gardner, H. (ed.), 1995, *The Politics of Health: The Australian Experience*, Churchill Livingstone, Melbourne.

Gray, B. 1989, *Collaborating: Finding Common Ground for Multiparty Problems*, Jossey Bass, San Francisco.

Gulati, R. 1995, 'Social Structure and Alliance Formation Patterns: A Longitudinal Analysis', *Administrative Science Quarterly*, vol. 40, pp. 619–52.

Howlett, M. P. & Ramesh, M. 1995, *Studying Public Policy: Policy Cycles and Policy Subsystems*, Oxford University Press, Toronto.

Kanter, R. M. 1989, *When Giants Learn to Dance*, Touchstone, New York.

—— 1994, 'Collaborative Advantage: The Art of Alliances', *Harvard Business Review*, July–August, pp. 96–108.

Klijn, E.-H. 1996, 'Analysing and Managing Policy Processes in Complex Networks: A Theoretical Examination of the Concept Policy Network and its Problems', *Administration and Society*, vol. 28, pp. 90–119.

—— 1997, 'Policy Networks: An Overview', in J. M. Kickert, E.-H. Klijn & J. F. M. Koppenjan (eds), *Managing Complex Networks: Strategies for the Public Sector*, Sage, London.

Lazonick, W. 1991, *Business Organization and the Myth of the Market Economy*, Cambridge University Press, Cambridge.

Lewis, B. & Walker, R. 1997, *Changing Central-local Relationships in Health Service Provision: Final Report*, Health Systems Research Reports no. 7, School of Public Health, La Trobe University, Melbourne.

Light, D. W. 1997, 'From Managed Competition to Managed Cooperation: Theory and Lessons from the British Experience', *Milbank Quarterly*, vol. 75, pp. 297–341.

Limerick, D. & Cunnington, B. 1993, *Managing the New Organisation: A Blueprint for Networks and Strategic Alliances*, Business and Professional Publishing, Sydney.

Lin, V. & Duckett, S. J. 1997, 'Structural Interests and Organisational Dimensions of Health System Reform', in H. Gardner (ed.), *Health Policy in Australia*, 1st edn, Oxford University Press, Melbourne.

Lutz, S. 1997, 'Learning Through Intermediaries: The Case of Inter-firm Research Collaborations', in M. Ebers (ed.), *The Formation of Inter-organizational Networks*, Oxford University Press, Oxford.

National Health and Medical Research Council 1996, *Promoting the Health of Australians*, AGPS, Canberra.

National Health Service Executive 1997, *The New NHS: Modern and Dependable*, National Health Service, London.

National Public Health Partnership 1998, *Background Paper*, National Public Health Partnership, Melbourne.

Nooteboom, B., Berger, H., & Noorderhaven, N. G. 1997, 'Effects of Trust and Governance on Relational Risk', *Academy of Management Journal*, vol. 40, pp. 308–38.

O'Toole, L. J. 1997, 'Implementing Public Innovations in Network Settings', *Administration and Society*, vol. 29, pp. 115–38.

Osborn, R. N. & Hagedorn, J. 1997, 'The institutionalization and evolutionary dynamics of interorganizational alliances and networks', *Academy of Management Journal*, vol. 40, pp. 261–78.

Osborne, D. & Gaebler, T. 1992, *Reinventing Government: How the Entrepreneurial Spirit is Transforming the Public Sector*, Addison Wesley, Reading.

Owens, H. 1995, 'Paying for Health Care Through Casemix', in H. Gardner (ed.), *The Politics of Health: The Australian Experience*, Churchill Livingstone, Melbourne.

Powell, W. W. 1990, 'Neither Market nor Hierarchy: Network Forms of Organization', *Research in Organizational Behaviour*, vol. 12, pp. 295–336.

Ring, P. S. 1997, 'Processes Facilitating Reliance on Trust in Inter-organizational Networks', in M. Ebers (ed.), *The Formation of Inter-organizational Networks*, Oxford University Press, Oxford.

—— & van de Ven, A. H. 1994, 'Developmental Processes of Cooperative Interorganizational Relationships', *Academy of Management Review*, vol. 19, pp. 90–118.

Simonin, B. L. 1997, 'The Importance of Collaborative Know-how: An Empirical Test of the Learning Organization', *Academy of Management Journal*, vol. 40, pp. 1150–74.

Smyth, J. D. 1997, 'Competition as a Means of Procuring Public Services: Lessons from the UK and the US Experience', *International Journal of Public Sector Management*, vol. 10, pp. 1–38.

Walker, R., Adam, J., & Lewis, B. 1997, *General Practice Projects: Collaborative Structures and Processes*, Health Systems Research Reports, no. 8, School of Public Health, La Trobe University, Melbourne.

Williamson, O. E. 1975, *Markets and Hierarchies: Analysis and Anti-trust Implications*, Free Press, New York.

World Health Organization 1986, *Ottawa Charter for Health Promotion*, WHO & Health and Welfare Canada, Ottawa.

Yeatman, A. 1990, *Bureaucrats, Technocrats, Femocrats: Essays on the Contemporary Australian State*, Allen & Unwin, Sydney.

7

Environmental Health Policy in a Time of Change

Valerie A. Brown AO, Rosemary Nicholson, and Peter Stephenson

Changing times

In Australia, as elsewhere, environmental health policy has only recently emerged from being in the policy background, where it had been subsumed under more general public health and environmental policies, into the policy foreground, where it is the primary vehicle for responding to the increasing environmental risks to health (Environmental Health Commission 1997; enHealth Council 2000). Global changes to the environmental systems of the planet and national increases in urban pollution and water and soil degradation require a strategic policy response. In 1999, the first National Environmental Health Strategy (NEHS) was formally accredited by federal, state, and territory governments, and acknowledged by a formal budget allocation, thus establishing a public policy direction for Environmental Health in Australia for the first time (enHealth Council 1999). This chapter explores the inauguration of environmental health policy in relation to its key stakeholders (the community, the professions, those in government, and those with the task of integrating environment and health) in the light of the new human–environment relationships of the twenty-first century. There are several significant elements of policy making, each with a different delivery point. It is important to recognise, too, that there is a difference between population-based environmental health policy—protecting the people from environmental risks—and practitioner-based Environmental Health policy, which governs practitioner education and training, and service delivery. Lower-case and upper-case initials are used to distinguish between these throughout this chapter.

The task of mitigating the effects of large-scale changes in human–planet relationships is not new to environmental health. Four successive major changes in human living conditions have been accompanied by matching sets of environmentally based risks to health. Table 7.1 lists the four 'natures' that have cumulatively shaped humans and the planet.

First came the long millennia of human evolution itself, with the creation of a human biology adapted to a particular combination of climate, air, and water. The move from hunter–gatherer lifestyles to small settlements meant further social adaptation to support growing populations under new physical conditions—perhaps the beginning of environmental health policy. In more recent times, the advent of large cities and the epidemics of infectious diseases saw urban planners, environmental engineers, and microbiologists brought into policy discussions to resolve each of these challenges to survival: having resolved the issues, humans are now faced with a fourth challenge—the impact of an expanding population on a finite planet. Recognition that policies supporting local solutions to global environmental change are now necessary is bringing into play a whole series of place-based policies ranging in scale from local through to state, national, and international.

Table 7.1 Cumulative health–environment relationships

Natures	*Years: before—present*	*Basis for environmental health*
First nature Evolution before humans	1 billion–2 million	*Human biology*: Physical conditions developed for human existence (air, water, soil, food supplies, biodiversity, climate)
Second nature Human evolution: Humans with tools	2 million–400	*Social adaptation* to different environmental conditions
Third nature Industrialisation: Humans with high technology	400–0 Phase 1 of Environmental Health	*Environmental adaptation* in response to different human needs
Fourth nature Globalisation: Humans with international connectedness	0–future Phase 2 of Environmental Health	*Human and environmental adaptation to changed environmental conditions*: Transition to sustainable development? Act locally, think globally

At the global level the current major policy initiatives are ecologically sustainable development from the environment side, and the World Health Organization (WHO) initiatives from the health side. At the local level, this requires the extension of traditional policies designed to ensure safe and adequate food production, control the risk of infectious disease, and police the control of industrial pollutants to include local actions with global effects.

The human-generated deterioration of global air, water, soil, and biodiversity that began in the nineteenth century continues, while population and human use of resources rise. *World Resources 2000*, issued jointly by the World Bank, United Nations Health and Environment agencies, and the World Resources Institute, confirms that the decrease in quality of each of these life-support systems is speeding up. A Cornell University study by Pimental and eight colleagues over five years estimates that 40 per cent of the world's disease burden is now environmentally based (Pimental, et al. 1998).

Environmental health policy is multidimensional

Environmental health policy, like all policy, is the socially negotiated response to the physical conditions and political agendas of the time. Environmental health enters fresh negotiations every time there is a change in the human–environment relationship, negotiations that have occurred regularly throughout human history. The nearest Australia has come to an environmental health policy is the National Environmental Health Strategy, in which environmental health is defined as 'those aspects of human health determined by physical, chemical, biological and social factors in the environment' (enHealth Council 1999, p. 3). The Strategy is defined as 'the combined efforts of a number of sectors throughout the community. No single organisation has the capacity to manage environmental health in isolation' (enHealth Council 1999, p. i).Environmental health policy is, hence, a multidimensional policy arena, overlapping public health, environment, urban development, agriculture, and law, to name but a few. It is more complex and harder to identify than the major policy areas with a definite government portfolio and responsible minister, lobby groups, and practitioners. While policy is often regarded as solely a government matter and only collect-on-shelf documents, in reality it goes far beyond that.

The range of Australian environmental health policies includes the following (cf. Brown et al. 2001).

- Broad field of activity (for example, environmental health fields may be sections of health policy, environmental policy, national food policy, industry policies).
- Statement of purpose or ideal goal (for example, Health for All by 2000, elimination of infectious diseases, a sustainable healthy future, clean and green industry, halting climate change).
- Generic planning principles and framework (for example, National Environmental Health Strategy—federal, Integrated Local Area Planning—all states, Air Quality Management Plans—New South Wales, Best Value Principles—Victoria, Cleaner Production—industry).

- Specific, issue-based strategies and sets of government decisions (for example, eliminating lead from petrol—federal, water quality objectives—New South Wales, Municipal Health Plans—Victoria, Health and Environment Plans—South Australia, lifecycle analysis of products)
- Programs of action (for example, Indigenous Environmental Health Forum, Community Environmental Health Action Plans, Landcare and Coastcare, health and environment monitoring, Healthy Cities, Local Agenda 21, Housing for Health in Indigenous Communities).
- Outputs that strengthen the policy process itself, such as allocating resources and drafting legislation that ensure strategies and programs are effective (for example, legislating the composition of petrol, funding the recommendations of the review of Environmental Health professional training, funding infrastructure programs for Indigenous communities).
- Outcomes—that is, policy directed towards making immediate, concrete advances towards an ideal goal (for example, rehabilitation of watercourses and water supplies, removal of pollutants from soils, basic infrastructure in Indigenous communities).

A distinctive element of environmental health in Australia is the need to address Indigenous Environmental Health, the greatest health risk in the Australian population (Australian Institute of Health and Welfare 1990–98). Indigenous environmental health involves all four different natures of the health–environment relationship at the same time. Aboriginal and Torres Strait Islander populations have at least 40 000 years of cultural adaptation to Australia's unique environmental conditions. After European settlement, the infectious diseases of the industrial era, now banished in almost all industrialised countries such as Australia, still give the Indigenous population the same health profile as if they were living in the Third World. More recently, the pressures of technological development have added industrial pollutants, dust from degraded ecosystems, and stress from separation from their cultural landscape, with which their identity is strongly linked (Read 2000).

The development of a national Environmental Health policy has accelerated recognition of the need for an Indigenous Environmental Health policy, particularly one that has significant Indigenous ownership. A first national consultation of stakeholders in Indigenous environmental health, held in Alice Springs in 1997, had the aim of developing an Indigenous response to the National Environmental Health Strategy (Indigenous Communities' Environmental Health Research and Development Program 1997). Four suggestions for such a strategy were

- to establish an Indigenous communities' environmental health strategy within the National Public Health Partnerships (NPHPs), based on extensive consultation with Indigenous communities

- to apply existing models of good practice in community environmental health in establishing locally appropriate benchmarks and monitoring systems
- to develop community-based environmental health strategies under the supervision of community leaders
- to set up a continuous education and career path from Environmental Health Worker to full professional Environmental Health Officer status.

The original workshop has now developed into an annual forum, in which the original four strands of an Indigenous environmental health policy have been further developed, and strategies proposed involving the full range of environmental health stakeholders (see National Environmental Health Forum 1999; enHealth Council 2000a). The enHealth Council and the Australian Institute of Environmental Health have ongoing working groups. Another contributor has been the Australian Army, whose presence and impact in developing environmental health infrastructure in Indigenous communities has been significant.

Environmental Health has many stakeholders

Contrary to the popular stereotype, policy is not created in a vacuum in an inner sanctum of government but is negotiated over time between the many interest groups that make up every community (Davis & Weller 1993). A policy community describes the full set of stakeholders as they debate the issues during the policy development process (Lindquist 1991). The policy community recently involved in developing sustainability goals in western Sydney included rural and urban and small and large communities; a range of age groups from children through to youths and older people; local, national, and international businesses and industries; local action groups on health and environment issues; Indigenous communities; professional services; education and research; government administrative departments and agencies; and elected representatives from the three spheres of government.

The interaction between so many expert sources and so many stakeholders is not going to be without conflicts of interest arising between the various sectors of the policy community. The wide range of potential stakeholders in a policy community, including the complex network of environmental health policy development, can be collected into four broad groups, each with their own legitimate goals, customary strategies, and avenues for action (figure 7.1).

The four sets of policy positions on environmental health are based on community members, professional practitioners and services, strategic planning groups, and on ideas and values, particularly those from people who are able to think in a holistic way. These are discussed below, each with appropriate examples from the field of environmental health.

Figure 7.1 Potential stakeholders in and sources for evidence in a policy community

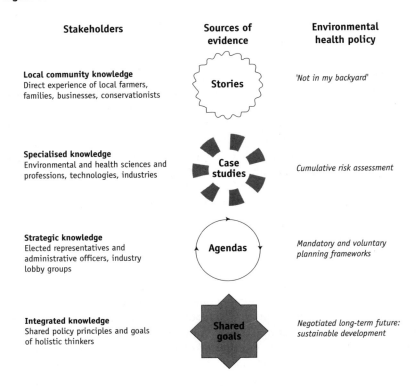

Stakeholders	Sources of evidence	Environmental health policy
Local community knowledge Direct experience of local farmers, families, businesses, conservationists	Stories	*'Not in my backyard'*
Specialised knowledge Environmental and health sciences and professions, technologies, industries	Case studies	*Cumulative risk assessment*
Strategic knowledge Elected representatives and administrative officers, industry lobby groups	Agendas	*Mandatory and voluntary planning frameworks*
Integrated knowledge Shared policy principles and goals of holistic thinkers	Shared goals	*Negotiated long-term future: sustainable development*

Community members

The community members are individuals and groups who are subject to the cumulative impact of local and global environmental pressures in their day-to-day activities and in their lived experience in a particular place. Their basis for policy development is largely local knowledge, driven by the so-called NIMBY 'not in my backyard' syndrome. Originally a term of contempt, it now helps us to recognise that global environmental risks can only be managed through the sum total of local solutions.

Example

Given the bioaccumulation of their toxins throughout natural systems, the reduction of risks from the pesticides known as persistent organic pollutants (POPs) can only be achieved if every nation and each locality ceases in their use. It is nearly four decades since the 1964 publication of Rachel Carson's book, *Silent Spring*, drew public attention to the effect of accumulation of twelve of the most dangerous organic pesticides in—among other places—eggshells and human breast milk. These pesticides have become known in the community as the 'dirty dozen'. Lobbying from local groups led first to local, then to state and national regulations controlling their use. Yet even now, their global elimination is the subject of contested international bargaining. A multilateral treaty remains to be negotiated (Brown 1999, 2000).

Professional practitioners and services

A highly detailed understanding of one dimension of environmental health is typically the case with most agencies, experts, and services that are involved in addressing environmental health issues. Each specialty has expert skills enabling it to calculate risks from its own information base and so contribute to its specialised policy area. The multidisciplinary solutions required to resolve environmental health issues require considerable negotiation and translation between these different specialisms.

Example

In the case of the public health risk arising from lead additives to petrol, the risk was not initially apparent from large-scale epidemiological studies, which originally reported no risk below 25 micrograms of lead per litre of blood. It took a combination of small-area studies, age-cohort studies, and educational tests to establish the deficit of 1 per cent in intelligence scores for each microgram of lead in the blood of 4-year-olds, a finding that resulted in national and international policy changes to eliminate lead from petrol (Greene et al. 1993).

Strategic planning groups

Political representatives and their local, state and territory, and national administrations have an important influence on policy and the planning strategies that might result. Planning frameworks in government and industry set short- and long-term goals and predetermine the types of strategies and programs to meet them. Planning frameworks might be mandatory, set in federal, state, or local legislation; or voluntary, as in municipal health and environment plans. They can be one-dimensional, as in Local Environment Plans in New South Wales, or integrated with social and economic dimensions, as in the Integrated Planning Act (Queensland). Although community priorities and specialist advice might inform each strategy, the final policy will also be required to satisfy political agendas.

Example

In the two examples outlined above, the moves to ban persistent organic pesticides and eliminate lead from petrol, it took more than thirty years before specialist evidence was accepted and policy developed. Community consciousness of the issues grew slowly over these years, with local services and authorities starting monitoring processes in order to protect their own populations. As local concerns became national concerns, pressures began mounting in other countries. Finally, the political agenda had to take notice of public pressures. Australia has by no means been in the vanguard of global environmental policy action. The USA lowered the permissible blood lead level from 25 micrograms per decilitre to 15, with a level of 10 in children, at least a decade before Australia dropped it to an average of 20 for adults and 15 for children. Australia joined with the USA to 'eliminate' pesticides from the environment after the event—that is, after they have become embedded in the soil—whereas the European Union proposed 'elimination' of their use before this could happen.

Holistic thinkers

Coordinators and change agents (such as Healthy Cities, Sustainable Communities, and Local Agenda 21) who are responsible for the increasing number of programs bringing together policy, strategy, and action, need a capacity for holistic thinking and skills in the integration of disparate interests. This policy group offers leadership and a focus on negotiating policy goals towards taking all the agendas, the evidence, and locally preferred sustainable futures into account. Developing shared goals and the agreed policy principles with mutual respect for all the contributors provides the integrative focus, rather than all players negotiating their separate piece of the action.

Example

Healthy Cities projects are based on the five principles of the so-called New Public Health (now more than a decade old), namely, integrated policy, supportive environments, strengthened communities, individual skills, and services reoriented from treatment after harm is done, to elimination of the source of harm. From their beginning in 1986, Healthy Cities projects have expanded to more than 5000 cities worldwide. In its 10-year anniversary redesign, the WHO project incorporated Local Agenda 21, the United Nations program for community-based environmental sustainability. For many human settlements—Vietnam, China, and the USA—Healthy Cities offers the best opportunity to address the complexity of environmental health issues as a whole and for the long term (Tsouros 1995).

Environmental health policy as a matter for negotiation

Establishing the ideal goals and agreeing on policy principles often takes years of negotiation within the relevant policy community; that is, between the groups in Australian society with an interest in the issue. No single group in the policy arena has sole rights to policy development. In some cases, the client community influences policy and industry against the wishes of government, as in the case of the labelling of genetically modified foods. In other cases, government maintains control of a policy position despite the strong lobbying of its constituency, as in the Australian government arguing against the elimination of the use of the dirty dozen POPs. Professional groups might compete with one another for policy seniority and the right to set standards.

Other players—such as the industry lobby groups, consumers, and related professions—might lock into opposing positions, as in the movement to remove lead from petrol, or they might form a partnership in spurring government to action, as did the beef cattle industry, consumers, and the chief government medical officer—in the Australian ban on European beef products in 2000. Or the policy change required may be more of a transformation than a rearrangement of existing systems, as in the principles and practice of sustainable development (table 7.2).

Table 7.2 Policy cycle framework for ecologically sustainable development and the new public health

A set of principles	
Ecologically sustainable development	New public health
• intergenerational equity	• intersectoral social justice policy
• conservation of biodiversity	• supportive environments
• intragenerational equity	• strengthened community
• dealing cautiously with risk*	• reorienting services to prevention*
• local/global accountability	• individual life skills
Source: ESD Executive Summary, 1992	Source: WHO, 1986

A set of strategies	
Local Agenda 21	**Healthy Cities**
Applying the precautionary principle*	Practising health promotion*
• reduce resource inequity, depletion, and degradation	
• eliminate health and environment risks from overconsumption	
• resolve issues of society and the human condition	
Source: Dovers, 1995	

A set of actions
Increased efficiency of resource use and decreased waste production by
• management practices that improve the resilience of social and natural resource systems*
• dealing cautiously with risk and irreversibility
• integration of social and environmental considerations into economic decision making
• community involvement in decisions.

* Principles linking health and environment around the policy cycle

Source: ESD Steering Committee, 1992

Each set of stakeholders addresses environmental health issues from a different perspective, based on different experiences and sources of evidence. Without respect for each other's interpretation of the issues there can be no negotiation, only a temporary truce. Without listening to and learning from the different experiences and evidence, the sets of stakeholders remain fragmented and so become part of the problem rather than part of the solution. Without a shared holistic vision of the future, the transition to long-term environmental health remains bogged down in the short-term needs of the present. Titmuss (1974, p. 12), the so-called father of social policy, defines an effective policy as 'principles directing actions towards a pre-determined goal', and suggests that policy development is always about change, since continuing along the same path does not require a policy directive.

Respecting the four sets of stakeholders and their construction of a sustainable human future is a necessary condition for a unified approach to successful policy development. Each has different but equally valid ways of constructing that knowledge. Community members share stories based on their own experience and personal observations. Scientists and professions collect their evidence from case studies or other structured sources of information. Political representatives and administrators work to a strategically determined agenda. A shared purpose provides the integrating, holistic overview, allowing everyone to move forward, an essential prerequisite for a multidimensional and crowded stakeholder field such as environmental health.

Environmental health policy as a decision making cycle

Since the environmental health practitioner is expected to bridge a number of elements, including government and community interests; policy, planning and action; the environment; and public health professions, and is subject to a stringent review of outcomes, the practitioner is involved at all stages of the change management cycle (see figure 7.2). In an environmental health principles–strategy–action–review cycle, the overarching goals and principles could be drawn from health policy, environment policy, or industry policy. The strategies can be developed by specialists from a wide variety of areas including microbiology, toxicology, urban design, environmental engineering, human physiology, and law. Many different members of the workforce, including health and community services, environmental management, local industries, and the resident community, might implement the programs in one locality.

Comparing the current position to the policy cycle in figure 7.2, there is still no Australian national environmental health policy as such, but a national strategy with guiding principles, from which policy principles have to be deduced. The NEHS Guiding Principles are based on

- protection of human health
- interrelationships between economics, health, environment
- sustainable development
- interrelationships between local and global organisations
- partnerships
- risk-based management
- evidence-based decisions
- efficiency
- equity.

Figure 7.2 Stages of the policy cycle

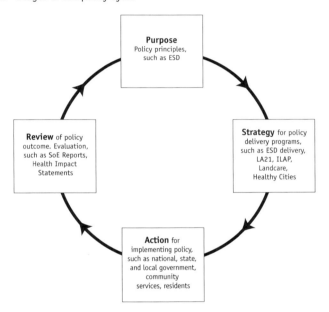

An Australian Charter for Environmental Health accompanies the guiding principles (enHealth Council 1999, pp. 6–7), which provides lists of the entitlements and responsibilities of three of the four stakeholder groups—communities, business and industry, and government—but somewhat surprisingly neither the expert advisers nor the integrative programs are specified. The NEHS is also strongly committed to action. The National enHealth Council, with membership from all four stakeholder groups, has produced a strong Implementation Plan (enHealth Council 2000b), and has a funding allocation in the federal Budget for the first time in history. The Implementation Plan falls under three main headings: environmental health justice, environmental health systems, and the human–environment interface.

In describing environmental health policy as multidimensional and multistakeholder, it becomes evident that the policy process will flounder without an integrative process linking stakeholders at each step of the policy cycle. Regardless of which stakeholder group initiates change in the policy process, it will need to include the full policy community; that is, accept contributions from all four groups represented in figure 7.1 and the full policy cycle in figure 7.2. The success of the policy process will depend on the cooperation of the communities in which the policy is implemented, the accuracy of the expert advice and support, the negotiating skills of governments, and the shared determination and focus at each of the stages of the policy principles–strategy–action–review cycle.

Environmental health policy changes over time

Dramatic changes in human–environment relationships over the past 200 years have generated major advances in health status and lifestyle for those in industrialised countries with high socioeconomic status, very little advantage for those with lower socioeconomic status or living in the developing nations, and major new waves of environmentally based risks to health (McMichael 1993).

Noteworthy is the magnitude of the changes and their cumulative effects. Table 7.3 outlines four eras of human health–environment relationships, with environmental health as an expert practice arising only in the last two eras. Looking now in more detail at the delivery of environmental health since its beginning in the nineteenth century, we can see that it falls into four phases: three in the industrial era and a fourth, still developing, in the era of globalisation (table 7.3).

The first major change in the human health–environment relationship of the scientific era, and so the first in which there were explicit environmental health considerations, came with the agricultural revolution. Marked increases in the quality and quantity of food production—due to the development of agricultural tools and more intensive agricultural practices—brought food security to some, but malnutrition and starvation to the many others who were dispossessed and displaced from their own land production. In phase 2 of environmental health practice, tool development escalated into the Industrial Revolution and inspired the mass movement of the increasing population into town centres, which were fast becoming the first major cities. Policy decisions lay in the hands of the civic authorities, which initiated urban renewal, sewerage, and hygiene practices on the advice of planners, engineers, and the first public health physicians. Public health and environmental health policies were synonymous, with the emergence of strategies restraining the freedom of some people—quarantine,

Table 7.3 Cumulative phases of environment and health relationships and environmental health policy

Era of industrialisation			
Phase	*Illness*	*Practical response*	*Policy response*
1 Agricultural revolution—population expansion			
1750–1870	Malnutrition	Intensive agriculture	Land enclosures
	Food safety	Supervised markets	Local autonomy
	Starvation	Poorhouses	Poor laws
2 Industrial revolution—Infectious disease epidemics			
1870–1930	Cholera	Sewerage	Urban infrastructure
	Diphtheria	Domestic hygiene	Public health
	Tuberculosis	Urban design	Urban development
3 Economic development—Environmental degradation			
1930–70	Polluted air, water	Standards, inspection	Public health
	Lung cancer	Industry controls, taxes	Occupational health
	Cumulative impacts	Environmental monitoring	Environment and health protection
Era of globalisation			
4 Sustainable development—global environmental stress			
1970–present	Melanoma (from ozone hole)	Eliminate fluorocarbons Reduce CO_2 emissions, increase renewable energy	Halifax convention Kyoto protocols
	Disease spread (from climate change)	Sustainable environmental	ESD&EH strategies
	Allergies, toxicity	management	

Adapted from V. A. Brown, J. Ritchie, & A. Rotem, 1992

condemned housing, resumption of land for sewerage, and controls on contamination of water sources and waterways—in order to safeguard the health of the greater community (see table 7.3).

By the beginning of the twentieth century, after the major epidemics of infectious diseases had been controlled in the developed countries through hygiene and public infrastructure, the third phase of environmental health policy emerged with the growing need to control the by-products and wastes of economic and industrial development (Brown et al. 1992). Environmental health became a subset of a wider public health agenda now giving a higher priority to lifestyle risks. Maintenance and inspection of the regulations introduced in phase 2 became the major professional strategies of environmental health practitioners in phase 3.

As the pressures of industrialisation continued, environmental health practice faced another significant change. Added to its existing responsibilities was the responsibility for protecting natural systems for now and for the future, for the local population, and for the greater regional, national and global communities. Environmental health has always been concerned with community protection from a long-term and local perspective, but now a locality cannot be protected in isolation. The long shadows of the major cities and the rapid interregional transport of goods and services mean that collaborative regional, national, and ultimately global action is required.

Redesigning the built environment and maintaining hygiene, key aspects of the second phase of environmental health policy, are both still requisites for responding to current global environmental pressures. One example is the design of energy-efficient buildings to reduce the carbon dioxide emissions that contribute to climate change (Southern Sydney Regional Organisation of Councils 1993). Reorganising vector (disease-carrier) controls as climate change allows them to spread into new areas is another (Ewan et al. 1991). In addition, the social change programs developed to change health behaviour in the second phase of public health are equally necessary to change environmentally damaging behaviour (Brundtland 1987).

Globally, international conventions have failed to arrest the escalating rates of environmental degradation. The global temperature is still rising, the ozone hole is widening, and soil salinity and shortages of water are the results of irrigation; soil salinity, contamination and the depletion of forests are all increasing. Food production per head is falling, species are disappearing. All these events are occurring at the same time as the population is rising (although the rate of population increase is slowing). Fossil fuel use is increasing, although the proportion of renewable energy used is rising. On a local scale, environmental health practitioners join with a wide range of other professionals in facing the local adverse effects of global deterioration (Brown 2001). A set of principles for sustainable development for the twenty-first century was developed at the United Nations Conference on Environment and Development (UNCED) in 1992 (UNCED 1992). Titled Agenda 21, a version was developed for delivery at the local level, and called Local Agenda 21. With the move towards implementation of the sustainable development principles, a new relationship has emerged between the environment and health, and formed a firm basis for policy development, strategic planning, and program delivery in environmental health practice.

Environmental health policy: finding the answers

The goal of environmental health policy in the era of globalisation (the fourth era of human–environment relationships) is to reduce social risks to environmental sustainability and environmental risks to social sustainability. Policy development would be on both a local scale and a global scale (as in the elimination of POPs, discussed previously). In the Australian context, this suite of activities would require marked changes in the problematic partnership between public health and environmental management, as highlighted in Brown et al. (2001). An influential paper relating to this nexus from an international perspective is 'Global Environmental Integrity: The Cornerstone of Public Health' (Soskolne & Bertollini 1998).

Environmental health is but one segment of a rapidly changing world, a world that is changing physically as well as socially. The changes are occurring on a long lead-time, so that it will be decades before we reverse them, even if we give their reversal the highest priority right now. Environmental health is not the only profession required to respond to these changes: they are equally significant for engineers, planners, health service providers, and educators. The changes that are required are so significant that we cannot deal with them using a step-by-step approach, changing things little by little.

What is required is a transformation of the policy development roles that the professions, governments, and communities have traditionally played, each servicing their own jurisdiction (Brown 1997). The new and broader role of environmental health policy and practice cannot be effective if it is locked into a fixed policy community and separate policy cycle for each issue. For policy to be implemented, when it might fall outside traditional boundaries of environmental health action, requires new and different strategies from those of the past.

On the one hand, the inclusion of sustainable development policy in environmental health policy might well seem radical to environmental health practitioners who might still be working in the second and third phases (described in table 7.3). On the other hand, the traditional regulatory and risk-reduction emphasis that grew out of the first three phases has been categorised by global agencies such as the United Nations Commission for Sustainable Development and the more active networks of Local Agenda 21 (International Council for Local Environmental Initiatives 1999) as unduly conservative in meeting twenty-first century issues. An integrative approach to environmental health issues and environmental health practice is one of the most important contributions environmental health policy can make.

The most hopeful avenue for lasting change—one that brings Australian health and environment policies together and offers the chance of a productive synergy between stakeholders—is a partnership between the precautionary principle (dealing conservatively with risk) and health promotion (acting before the risk appears). In table 7.2 the parallels between Local Agenda 21 and Healthy Cities provide examples that incorporate the full policy cycle in figure 7.2. Unless this wheel turns full circle, policy changes will remain simply volumes on a shelf.

Environmental health policy and practice of today combines precautionary and innovative strategies, links global and local scales, includes both the biophysical and the social, and draws together community, experts, and government. This is a complex agenda, but no more complex than the task that faced environmental health at the time of the creation of the first major industrial cities.

References

Australian Institute of Health and Welfare 1988 (*see also* 1990, 1992, 1994, 1996, 1998), *Australia's Health: The First Biennial Report of the Australian Institute of Health*, AIHW, Canberra.

Brown, L. 1999, 2000, *World Environment Report*, Worldwatch Institute, Washington DC.

Brown, V. A. (ed.) 1997, *Managing for Local Sustainability: Policy, Problem-Solving, Practice and Place*, National Office of Local Government, Canberra.

—— 1999, 'Top Down, Group Up or Inside Out? Community Practice and the Precautionary Principle', in R. Harding & E. Fisher (eds), *Perspectives on the Precautionary Principle*, Part VI, The Federation Press, Sydney.

—— et al. 2001, *Grassroots and Common Ground: Guidelines for Community Environmental Health*, RIMC Occasional Paper no. 2, University of Western Sydney, Sydney.

——, Ritchie, J., & Rotem, A. 1992, 'Health Promotion and Environmental Management: The Partnership for the Future', *International Journal of Health Promotion*, vol. 7, no. 3, pp. 219–30.

—— 2001, 'Planners and the Planet: Reshaping the People/Planet Relationships: Do Planners Have a Role?', *Australian Planner*, vol. 38, no. 2, July.

Brundtland, G. 1987, *Our Common Future, Report of the World Commission on Environment and Development*, Oxford University Press, Melbourne.

Davis, G. & Weller, P. 1993, *Strategic Management in the Public Sector*, Centre for Australian Public Sector Management, Griffith University, Brisbane.

Dovers, S. 1995, 'A Framework for Scaling and Framing Policy Problems in Sustainability', *Ecological Economics*, vol. 12, p. 93.

Ecologically Sustainable Development Working Groups 1992, *Final Report: Executive Summaries*, AGPS, Canberra.

enHealth Council 1999, *The National Environmental Health Strategy*, Commonwealth Department of Health and Aged Care, Canberra.

—— 2000a, *Indigenous Environmental Health*, report of the second national workshop, Commonwealth Department of Health and Aged Care, Canberra.

—— 2000b, *The National Environmental Health Strategy Implementation Plan*, Commonwealth Department of Health and Aged Care, Canberra.

Environmental Health Commission 1997, *Agendas for Change*, Chartered Institute of Environmental Health, London.

ESD Steering Committee 1992, *National Ecologically Sustainable Development Strategy*, Department of Environment, Sport and Territories, Canberra.

Ewan, C. et al. 1991, *Health Implications of Long Term Climate Change*, AGPS, Canberra.

Greene, D., Berry, M., & Garrard, J. 1993, *Reducing Lead Exposure in Australia: Risk Assessment and Analysis of Economic, Social and Environmental Impacts*, National Health and Medical Research Council, Canberra.

Indigenous Communities' Environmental Health Research and Development Program 1997, *Issues of Environmental Health in Indigenous Communities, Contribution to the Draft National Environmental Health Strategy, Report of a Workshop, Alice Springs*, 18 September, University of Western Sydney, Sydney.

International Council for Local Environmental Initiatives 1999, *Initiatives*, no. 22, 18 July.

Linquist, E. 1991, *Public Managers and Policy Communities: Learning to Meet New Challenges*, Canadian Centre for Management Development, University of Toronto, Toronto.

McMichael, A. 1993, *Planetary Overload: Global Environmental Change and the Health of the Human Species*, Cambridge University Press, Cambridge.

National Environmental Health Forum 1999, 'Indigenous Environmental Health', *Report on the First National Workshop*, National Environmental Health Forum Monographs, Adelaide.

Pimental, D. et al. 1998, 'Ecology of Increasing Disease: Population Growth and Environmental Degradation', *Bioscience*, vol. 45, pp. 815–26.

Read, P. 2000, *Belonging: Australians, Place and Aboriginal Ownership*, Cambridge University Press, Cambridge.

Soskolne, C. & Bertollini, R. 1998, *Global Ecological Integrity and 'Sustainable Development': Cornerstones of Public Health*, based on an International Workshop, WHO European Centre for Environment and Health, Rome Division, Rome, 3–4 December.

Southern Sydney Regional Organisation of Councils 1993, *Waste Management Movement Across Southern Sydney*, report.

Titmuss, R. M. 1974, *Social Policy: An Introduction*, George Allen & Unwin, London.

Tsouros, A. D. (ed.) 1995, 'The World Health Organization Healthy Cities Project: State of the Art and Future Plans', *Health Promotion International*, vol. 10, no. 2, pp. 133–41.

United Nations Conference on Environment and Development 1992, *Agenda 21: A Blueprint for Survival into the 21st Century*, United Nations Environment Program, Rio de Janeiro.

World Health Organization 1986, *Ottawa Charter for Health Promotion*, World Health Organization, European Office, Copenhagen.

World Resources Institute et al. 1996, *World Resources 2000*, Oxford University Press, New York.

PART 2

CASE STUDIES OF THE HEALTH POLICY PROCESS

8

Interest Groups and the Market Model

Eileen Willis

The chapter examines some of the social and political forces that shape health care policy in Australia. It is proposed that four groups influence health care policy: citizens, health professionals, the state (politicians and bureaucrats), and the private for-profit sector. Health policy in Australia is driven by the state, but the other three groups give shape to who and what is funded and how funding is organised. The conflict and contestation over the direction of health policy and funding in the last decade is reducible to tensions between those approaches that support the welfare state and those that support the market. Since power is unequally distributed between the four groups the outcome of this contest cannot always be predicted, although an underlying argument of this chapter is that currently the market tends to be in the ascendancy. In order to illustrate the argument, three case studies are provided to outline the power of the four groups to shape policy towards either the welfare model or the market model.

An analysis of the processes used by the four groups to influence policy requires an exploration of social movements and interest groups as agents of policy change. The desire of the state to maintain the welfare model is aptly illustrated through the first case study (box 8.1), the 1989 Factor 'f' Program, which was introduced by the federal Labor government to ensure that multinational pharmaceutical companies invested in Australia. The ability of health professionals to shape public health policy depends on their relative power within the system. Medicine is the ideal case study for illustrating the way in which a dominant interest group can capitalise on state-based reforms. The National General Practice Strategy and the National Rural Health Strategy in the second case study (box 8.2) illustrate the way in which medicine has effectively bargained with the government to maximise its own interests. However, the cost of this struggle to individual general practitioners (GPs) is evident in recent developments in the corporatisation of general practice. Women's health policy, the third case study (box 8.3), provides the opportunity to explore how policy can be influenced by a social movement, but then recaptured by a medical interest group.

Other chapters in this book have used Alford's structural model as a framework for understanding the interplay between various interest groups (see Creelman for a detailed outline of Alford's approach). Alford's model presents health care as a field on which the game is played out between a range of interest groups. It is recognised that the field is not level and that the rules shift and change for the various players: the state, the professions, consumers, and the private for-profit sector. One way to understand the game is to make a distinction between who the players and winners are, and who owns the stadium.

In the case studies discussed below there are winners and losers in the game, but a more important issue is who owns the stadium and who decides what game is being played. Is the game about the health of citizens (one group of players) or the health of the market (the other group of players)? These questions are important for understanding the shape of health care policy and the impact of shifts in ideology and practice. Opening up the welfare state to market forces can then make it difficult to control.

The health care policy context: the welfare state

Policy making for effective health care in any nation does not occur in a vacuum. Political parties are influenced by ideology, which in turn influences what is considered good policy and how it ought to be implemented. A number of chapters in this book have commented on the welfare state: Grbich, for example, notes that Medicare is an important part of the welfare state. Behind this universal and free health insurance scheme is the belief that all citizens have the right to health care regardless of their economic circumstances. Not only is health care a basic human right, but it also functions in strengthening citizenship and a robust economy, as do other welfare provisions such as pensions, rebates, and subsidies. Behind the ideology of the welfare state is the recognition that many citizens either cannot work or do not earn enough to provide adequately for themselves and their families, so that this need must be met by the state through a redistribution of taxes. The principle is essentially one of reducing class differences through redistribution.

Economic rationalism and health care policy

Economic rationalism is often presented as an alternative to the welfare state. Currently, both the Liberal–National Coalition government and the Labor opposition appear to favour economic rationalism—neoliberalism—with variations in how it is operationalised (Gardner 1997). Economic rationalism is an attempt to incorporate the principles of the market into the public sector. These principles include competition, privatisation, strategic policy making, incentives, program budgeting, and an orientation towards the product (Gardner 1997, p. 3). Two points can be made here. First, economic rationalism by definition puts economic considerations above welfare considerations. This is the very meaning of the term—the primary rationale is economic. However, while critics invariably accuse economic rationalism of being simply a cost-cutting exercise, it is also (as Gardner notes) about effectiveness, achieving objectives, best practice, standards, codes of conduct, and benchmarking (Gardner 1997, p. 3). Such processes are not of themselves antithetical to the welfare state. The process of privatisation and internal competition leads to a situation where governments might maintain a broad overview of welfare services but retreat from taking responsibility for the day-to-day welfare of citizens by leaving it to a third party or outsourcing. This does not mean that the government necessarily abandons welfare, which leads to the second point. Economic rationalism is sometimes confused with deregulation and lack of government control. In the area of social welfare, deregulation is not about lack of government control. It is, rather, about the government stepping back from the day-to-day provision of services, but bringing tighter control to how the funds are spent, what is funded, or what can or cannot be negotiated (Pixley 1999). This is not a reduction in power, but a redefinition of power, often with the two seemingly opposing goals of increasing efficiency and providing more resources or a better service to citizens.

At first sight this approach seems reasonable. However, critics argue that the state has moved from the role of arbitrator between civil society and the enhancement of democracy, to siding with the market. This is a harsh assessment given that the state has always had to interact with the market in the provision of health care. A further consideration is to ask whether it is possible for the state to open up health care to further market penetration, yet still maintain control.

The situation is further complicated by professional interest groups. Their agendas might not fit neatly with either economic rationalism or welfare ideology, but are, rather, linked to the status and independence of their members. These organisations desire independence from both the state and the market, so arguments that there has been a shift to the market state need to clarify whether this shift is merely a matter of degree or a radical change in the way health care in Australia is organised.

The role of interest groups and social movements in health policy

According to Doyle and Kellow (1995), interest groups can be divided into those that meet either the public or private interests of members. Interest groups include citizen groups such as the Consumers' Health Forum, professional associations such as the Australian Medical Association (AMA), unions such as the Australian Nursing Federation (ANF), or more broadly based lobbies such as the AIDS Council. Interest groups also include large multinational corporations or loose federations of business interests such as the Business Council of Australia, the Chambers of Commerce and Industry, or the Private Hospitals Association. In some cases interest groups receive direct funding from the government to further their agendas. The Divisions of General Practice and the National Rural Health Alliance are two such groups that have received significant funding over the last few years, while the Australian Community Health Association is an example of an interest group defunded in 1996. It does not have to be pointed out to the astute reader that this shift in funding to professional and consumer groups says something about the ability of government to control or influence the political process and, more importantly, about the power of funding to control such interest groups.

Public interest groups such as the loose coalition for the preservation of Medicare or the Conservation Association can become so powerful that they take on the characteristics of social movements or mass organisations that are able to influence the political process by the sheer weight of their numbers (Waters & Crook 1993, p. 212). However, the broadbased membership of public interest groups and social movements limits their bargaining power. People join such groups as part of active citizenship. Their commitment to these social movements—for example, to the environment, deinstitutionalisation, or disability rights—is usually additional to their need to work in paid employment, so meetings and political action must be done outside work time through the process of protests and lobbying. In some cases particular organisations represent the interests of these movements and might be able to bargain successfully with government; but their hold over members is tenuous, although their power to create a public mood or influence voting patterns might significantly influence policy makers.

Private interest groups

Private interest groups have more specific interests and are often professional associations. They might charge membership fees and seek compulsory membership for registration or unionisation. Private interest groups further the private interests of their members, might be exclusive, and are invariably highly organised and governed by bureaucratic laws and procedures. Examples of this sort of interest group are the Royal Australian College of Nursing and the AMA. Besides representing the professional and moral interests of their members, these organisations, federations, or unions might act as pressure groups, lobbying policy makers and politicians (Doyle & Kellow 1995). In fact, a number of interest groups employ professional lobbyists in Canberra to perform this role.

Private interest groups are usually formed to respond to a wide range of member interests: so, for example, the AMA could not be reduced to being merely a political lobby group, as it is also a professional association for doctors, a forum for continuing education and research, a clearing house for the production of professional journals, and a venue for member networking. Neither the AMA nor the Health Information Association of Australia (HIAA) are political parties. Their interests are distinct, although at times they might form close alliances with political parties, as do the various unions in Australia. Further, some professional elites within these interest groups might formally join political parties or seek election based on their high profile in the group. An example of this would be Brendan Nelson, who resigned from the presidency of the AMA to take up a federal seat with the Liberal Party. Similarly, members of the trade union movement might move on to safe Labor seats. Despite this, the focus of the professional associations and consumer and employer groups is on serving their members, not gaining a seat in government. Indeed, their members might differ in their party allegiances, although as Doyle and Kellow (1995) note there is a tendency for professional and employer groups to share the same class and voting patterns. If it suits their interests these organisations might work closely with the government of the day, while at other times they might be critical of government policy and attempt to influence it to change (Doyle & Kellow 1995).

The importance of these private interest groups cannot be overstated. They act as both conservative self-serving lobby groups and as forces for reform. As associations that are already well organised, they are able to respond immediately to the changes in government policy that invariably occur between elections. However, not all interest groups are consulted by the government in power. Those that are consulted are those with the most bargaining power. The relative power of some interest groups over others gives the lie to claims that Australia is a pluralist society. Power is not equally available to all interest groups, including within the profession of medicine, where power is unevenly divided and a number of political positions prevail.

General practitioners (GPs) are represented by a number of associations that act as quasi-professional and union bodies. These include the Royal Australian College of General Practitioners (RACGP), the Doctors' Reform Society, the AMA, the Australian Association of Academic General Practitioners, the General Practice Society of Australia, the National Association of General Practitioners of Australia, and the Rural Doctors Association of Australia. All these professional associations represent specific ideological positions on the role of medicine in Australia or a particular area of general practice. However, when politicians come to consult with the medical profession on broadbased issues, it is more likely to be with the AMA or the RACGP than with the other associations. While this is presumably a matter of efficiency, it is also reflective of the power of the AMA and the relative lack of power of other medical profession organisations. Under federal president Kerryn Phelps, the AMA had a difficult relationship with Michael Wooldridge, the Coalition Minister for Health. The relationship between the AMA and the minister might be eased with the appointment of Dr Kay Patterson as Coalition Minister for Health. Patterson's consensus style will mean that public differences are unlikely to arise, but negotiations will still be focused on health outcomes.

The leaders of these organisations are able to rally members to action or to be publicly critical of government, independent of whether members vote Liberal, Labor, or Democrat. This is possible because of shared professional and financial interests or the moral authority of their cause. Groups organised around protecting the private interests of members are usually highly organised and have access to resources through membership fees, or the high status and powerful networks of their members (Doyle & Kellow 1995, p. 119). Where they offer a key public service they are in a position to enter into bargaining with governments and political parties in order to safeguard the interests of their members. In many instances governments will not act without consulting these professional groups or organisations, whether it be directly or informally.

Wilson (1973, p. 282) defines bargaining as a process 'by which two or more parties seek to attain incompatible ends through the exchange of compensations'. A central argument of this chapter is that the process of bargaining results in an exchange of costs and benefits and in turn this alters or modifies health care policy in the interests of those at the bargaining table. The consequence is that policy change may appear to be incremental rather than radical or unpredictable. Private interest groups have expertise that the government must take into account for political reasons. They are able to make informed critical comment on government policy, which can be used by opposition parties to discredit the government. For this reason governments make a point of negotiating, consulting, and bargaining with powerful interest groups such as the AMA, or business interest groups such as the Australian Pharmaceutical Manufacturing Association. The first case study (see box 8.1) explores the difficulties experienced by the state in maintaining the welfare state against global, multinational, interests.

> *Box 8.1*
> *Case study 1—Business interest groups and the welfare state*
>
> *The pharmaceutical industry and the triumph of the market*
> Interaction between governments of the day and business interest groups is not necessarily a balanced affair. Many interest groups that represent large corporations and multinationals are in a position to hold the government to ransom, or at least to place the government in a position where it will act contrary to its own policies. An intriguing example of this is the Factor 'f' Program instituted by the Department of Labour and Industry in 1987 under the then Labor Minister, John Button (Lofgren 1997). A key element of the welfare state in Australian health care policy is the Pharmaceutical Benefit Scheme (PBS), established in the early 1950s to provide either free or subsidised prescription drugs to all Australians. Australian-based and multinational pharmaceutical companies operating in Australia must submit their products to the Pharmaceutical Benefits Advisory Committee (PBAC) for accreditation and listing on the PBS. Acting on advice from the PBAC, the government negotiates a price thereby to a large extent determining the profits to be made by the drug companies. The PBAC represents various professional interest groups made up of doctors, pharmacists, and academics from the AMA, the Doctors' Reform Society, and the Pharmacy Guild (Doctors' Reform Society 1999). Drug companies, through the Australian Pharmaceutical Manufactures Association (APMA), have argued that this arrangement unduly suppresses profits and is unfair given the high cost of research and development needed to bring new drugs onto the market. In 2001, the PBAC was restructured and a former executive member of the pharmaceutical industry association was included. In the late 1980s, the Labor government sought to stimulate the pharmaceutical industry in

Australia through a series of industry incentives known as the Pharmaceutical Industry Development Program (PIDP) and the Factor 'f' Program. The 'f' is merely the sixth factor impeding the maintenance of cost-effective prescription drugs in Australia and refers to the fact that the government does not allow drug companies to set their own price for drugs listed on the PBS schedule. This was seen by multinational companies to be a disincentive to investing in research and development in Australia, but is really a clear example of government regulation in the interest of citizen welfare. Lofgren (1997) estimated that between 1987 and 1999 over $1 billion dollars was awarded to a small number of multinational and local drug companies, such as Glaxo and Merck, Sharp and Dohme, Bristol-Myer, Squibb, the (by then) privatised Commonwealth Serum Laboratory, Faulding, Sigma, and SmithKline Beecham. (Since then, with the amalgamation of some of these companies, the number has become even smaller.) However, to be eligible for funding, the companies had to agree to increase their research and development activities in Australia. While the program aimed to compensate the companies for lower profits, its primary aim was to stimulate the industry in Australia. A robust industry was seen as conducive to the government's aim of maintaining a welfare-state approach to pharmaceuticals. As Lofgren (1997, p. 76) notes, 'The declared rationale was that low prices should not be an impediment to the development of an Australian-based, internationally competitive industry.' The success of the program remains contradictory. On the one hand, increased research and development did result in estimates suggesting that over $4338 million of value-added activity took place between 1989 and 1999, including the creation of 470 jobs and the retention of a further 390 jobs until 1990 (Lofgren 1997). Further, the number of multinational companies investing in Australia increased, as did the vertical integration between Australian and American or European companies, universities, and research institutes. However, by 1995 it became evident that more companies met the requirements for funding than there were available funds. This led to a shift in the allocation arrangements and to a number of companies missing out on expected subsidies. Unfortunately, by this time, companies had come to expect the financial allocation and to base their research and development output on the subsidy. This led in some instances to companies breaking agreements with universities for research and development projects and to the Australian Pharmaceutical Manufactures Association and pharmaceutical companies arguing that the program was a poor substitute for failure to pay a fair price for drugs. More important, these companies were now integral to the industry—part of a web of research and development activities—and the government was in no position to ignore them.

As Lofgren (1997, p. 67) argues, 'State interventionist industry policy does not necessarily imply measures which have the effect of preserving or extending the influence of state agencies vis-a-vis business. The bargaining process can in effect weaken the position of government to regulate the sector.' It illustrates also that policies directed at strategic bargaining are difficult to sustain. Factor 'f' did encourage multinational companies to come onshore and to invest in Australia, but once the program rules changed, companies were in a position to threaten to move offshore, to reduce or stop all research and development, or to change direction. For example, in an interview in *Business News*, Sigma's chief executive said it will diversify into wholesale and retail and away from research and development, which are seen to be high risk areas (de Cercq 1999). He blamed a fall in profits over the 1998–99 year on the PBS subsidy. More recently, drug giant Pfizer, makers of Viagra, took the PBAC to court over failure to be listed, while Orphan, makers of Naltrexone, threatened High Court action. The government agreed to list Naltrexone before the case went to court, illustrating the power of this business interest group to influence government decisions (Doctors' Reform Society 1999). Responses from the Minister for Health, Michael Wooldridge, to reform the PBS process had also been slow up to this point, but then suddenly accelerated. Multinationals are organised to maximise profits and they are used to governments offering them sweeteners to stay onshore. Factor 'f' remains in its new guise as the Pharmaceutical Industry Investment Program. Between 1999 and 2000, approximately $300 million was allocated to compensate pharmaceutical companies for low returns, and funding continues to those companies that engage in value-added activity or research and development.

In the 2000 Budget, consumers became subject to stricter controls on who would receive benefits, and a number of hay fever-related drugs were removed from the schedule, not because this is a rare condition, but because thousands of people suffer from hay fever in Australia. The rationale for the removal of these high-usage drugs is that they are for chronic, not acute, conditions; that is, the conditions they treat are not life threatening.

■

Balancing the demands of powerful multinationals against the desire to maintain the welfare state is a difficult task for any government working to a budget. In this case, it is difficult to argue that various interest groups, such as consumer groups and business groups, have equal opportunity to lobby the state. Clearly, power is not evenly divided between the consumer, the state, and business interests. In this case, the market has defeated the state and the consumer will pay. The price of drugs will remain low, but the number staying on the schedule will alter.

Box 8.2
Case study 2—Professional interest groups and
government fiddle while the welfare state burns

The General Practice Strategy as the catalyst for corporatisation
We turn now to explore the interactions of one professional interest group (general practitioners) and the state. The General Practice and Rural Health Strategies represent a fascinating case study in the complexity of market, professional, welfare, and state interest interactions in health care in Australia. In the 1970s the Whitlam Labor government attempted to reform primary health care services through the establishment of a network of community health centres where general practitioners (GPs) would be employed as salaried medical officers. The decade between Whitlam and Hawke—when Australia was governed by the Liberal–National Coalition led by Malcolm Fraser—saw the gradual erosion of funding to these centres, partly as a result of Coalition policy in response to the recession, but also as a result of the resistance of doctors to what they saw as socialist medicine. In many states community health centres were prevented from offering medical services because of resistance from the Australian Medical Association (AMA). Community health centres could not become one-stop shops for preventative and acute services (Swerissen & Duckett 1997). Also, during the Liberal–National Coalition period of federal government from December 1975 to 1983, the universal health insurance program was gradually dismantled. With the reintroduction of Medibank as Medicare under the Hawke Labor government, health care once again became part of welfare provision. Yet as cobeneficiaries with their patients of the public health insurance scheme, GPs remained private providers, operating largely within a culture of small business rather than in that of public service. Their payment was still based on piece work—that is, on numbers of

patients seen. As a consequence, the number of doctors in rural areas began to dwindle given that their incomes were dependent on fee for service or, in effect, population density. The second attempt by the state to reform primary health care services was instigated in the 1990s under the General Practice Reform Strategy and the Rural Health Strategy (see the chapter by O'Connor and Peterson for a more detailed discussion and analysis of the GP Strategy). Both the federal Labor Party and the Liberal–National Coalition government's agenda have been to attempt to improve access, quality, and efficiency for consumers; in effect, to extend the welfare state. A major strategy had been to link increases in funding to the reform programs, rather than increasing the Medicare rebate, which is now around 50 per cent less than fees received by medical specialists and which has only recently been indexed. In 1994, the (Labor) government announced that health insurance rebates for GPs would only be 50 per cent of the Consumer Price Index. The balance of the funds would be allocated to the GP Strategy. In effect, GPs could only gain extra funding by meeting the federal Labor government's reform agenda. In 1996 the (Liberal–National) government reduced the number of allocated Medicare provider numbers in an attempt to control the oversupply and maldistribution of doctors between urban, rural, and remote areas and as a cost containment measure. A further area of reform has been the ongoing Coordinated Care Trials. While the trials are not directly part of the GP Strategy, they are an example of the government's endeavour to seek efficiencies along with improved services and, if successful, will effectively make a number of GPs budget holders for designated populations. The AMA and RACGP have resisted budget holding.

Some authors have argued that these forces have resulted in the restratification of medicine (for example, White 2000). It is certainly true that some of the medical specialisations resisted GP accreditation and the differences in remuneration point to a stratified medical profession with GPs at the bottom. It is possible, however, to argue that organised medicine, through the AMA and RACGP, seized the initiative in the reform process and used it to advantage by ensuring GP dominance within the multidisciplinary team. Some of the directions of the reform process illustrate this. The Commonwealth publication *General Practice in Australia* acknowledges that GPs are the cornerstone of preventative health care in Australia (Department of Health and Aged Care 2000a, p. xxix). This is a major coup for medicine, which, at the ideological level, confirms the doctor's role as the head of any multidisciplinary team and of primary health care services and initiatives, hence justifying for the doctors their major share of funding.

In August 2000, the Rural Doctors Association of Australia wrote to the Rural Health Alliance, a government-funded interest group representing the interests of a number of health professionals and consumer groups, criticising it for not publicly supporting the increased role for medicine (Department of Health and Aged Care 2000c; Rural Doctors Association of Australia web page, 2000). The key to understanding this conflict is through examining the Alliance's attempts to broaden funding under the Rural Health Strategy beyond funding for medicine. The Alliance and the various allied professional groups have used a primary health care argument, only to have the government publicly announce that general practice is the key player in primary health care. The increased role is not simply at the level of ideology or rhetoric. One of the five funded programs of the GP Strategy is that of the Divisions of General Practice. Unlike the community health program, which sought consumer control, the Divisions are controlled by GPs themselves and have become the conduit for channelling much government funding, including funding the Divisions themselves (Department of Health and Family Services 1996; Swerissen & Duckett 1997, p. 18). This was an initiative of the AMA and the RACGP, and one that the government did not want to fund. It was organised medicine's solution to government attempts to get GPs to collaborate and coordinate their care with other health service providers in their area. Other initiatives for general practice include financial support for the amalgamation of solo practices, Medicare provider numbers for shared care, the demonstration projects in virtual amalgamation, and the establishment of a GP vocationally trained register. These initiatives have been funded by federal government and are examples where—once again—the reform process is paid for by the state. This time it is not for a multinational, but for quasi-small businesses. Similar successes are evident for rural health. Government funding for the 2000–04 Regional Health Strategy, aptly titled *More Doctors, Better Services*, is around $562 million (Department of Health and Aged Care 2000b). Of this, the majority goes to general practice through a range of initiatives. These include

• grants to university departments of medicine to establish rural health units

- increases in places for medical students, including the establishment of a new medical school, despite there being an oversupply of doctors
- scholarship programs for undergraduate medical students, with offers of reduction in the Higher Education Contribution Scheme to those doctors who work in rural areas
- bonded scholarships of $20,000
- funding for specialist medical support for GP services
- increases in the number of places in vocational training programs, in effect extending provider numbers
- financial grants for relocation and equipment (Department of Health and Aged Care 2000b).

Financial and educational support for allied health and nursing services is considerably lower, despite the fact that these health professionals outnumber doctors, and nurses have taken a leading role in rural and remote health care. With the exception of the Rural Pharmacy Allowance, the focus is on providing funding for the employment of allied health professionals, but not on giving these professionals additional incentives beyond their salary. This is despite the recognition that one of the impediments to maintaining GPs in rural areas is the lack of health infrastructure in rural and remote areas. Despite these gains it should not be presumed that medical groups are united in how best to maximise the interests of GPs. The AMA represents the interests of a broad range of doctors, while the RACGP represents more directly those of GPs. Conflict between the two groups has surfaced from time to time, reflecting a problem faced by many professional associations that enjoy close relations with the government but that must also serve the interests of members. In 1992, following the release of *The Future of General Practice: A Strategy for the Nineties and Beyond*, senior GPs in the AMA were dissatisfied with the Association's acceptance of GP accreditation, and broke away to form the Australian Association of General Practitioners (AAGP). In 1994, tensions between the AMA and RACGP heightened when the Labor government attempted to establish the Better Practice program as the method of accreditation. These tensions were further fuelled by other medical interest groups, such as the Rural Doctors Association of Australia, which formed as a result of dissatisfaction with the RACGP and the AAGP, of which the latter wished to be consulted directly by government on the reform strategy. The establishment of the GP Forum to bring these groups together highlights the fact that any GP can now belong to up to six-teen groups, each with a different agenda. It also highlights the fact that the government has had to respond to these divisions by funding successive committees established to coordinate the various groups (Department of Health and Aged Care 2000a; Rural Doctors Asso-ciation 2000; Rural Health Alliance 2000). It might be presumed that such divisions weaken the position of GPs in relation to the state; however, GPs continue to take the major share of the National Rural Health Strategy funding and the GP Strategy continues to take up government expenditure and has done so for the past decade. The 1996–97 federal Budget for the General Practice Strategy was $223.45 million. Funding continues to be a major issue, with the Relative Value Study (RVS) the latest issue under debate (PriceWa-terhouseCoopers 1999). GPs threatened to campaign on the RVS in the 2001 federal election. It could be argued that the very debate within general practice has been a strategy to stall government reform, enable general practice to shape the reform, and increasingly to shift the focus from quality primary care to funding. Consulting with the medical lobby is a costly but necessary process, with out-comes as unpredictable as recent events indicate. The struggle between general practice and the state over the GP Strategy has been about remuneration and practice reform. GPs have interpreted the struggle as one where they are sandwiched between hostile and arro-gant specialists above, demanding consumers below, and a govern-ment that wants reform without a concomitant increase in funding (Marjoribanks et al. 2000). This feeling is widespread, despite the fact that the mean billing for a full-time doctor for the period 1998–99 was approximately $189,332 per annum (Australian Med-ical Association 2000, p. 43).

◼

One response to this sense of being under siege has been a rapid accel-eration in the corporatisation of general practice since mid 1999 (Australian Medical Association 2000). A number of publicly listed companies, includ-ing Revesco, Foundation Healthcare, Sonic Health Care, and Health Care of Australia, as well as Macquarie and United Health Care (which is owned by entrepreneurial doctors), have purchased general practices. Under these arrangements the GP may remain with the practice, but now as an employee with a guaranteed salary and without the worry of small business overheads and the need to maintain an office and accounts. The AMA has expressed concern at the aggressiveness of some acquisitions, payments well above market value for goodwill, the vertical integration of these companies with radiology and pathology services, and the control over the doctor's work that these corporations can now command. As the AMA (2000, p. 5) paper says, 'If corporations control referrals from a substantial segment of the GP market they could well eventually control the cash flow through to radiologists, physicians, surgeons and private hospitals paving the way for USA style managed care.' Meeting the interests of consumers is now pitted against meeting the needs of shareholders (Australian Medical Association 2000). How GP interest groups and the state respond to these accelerating moves will significantly impact on all aspects of health care in Australia in the next decade.

Box 8.3
Case study 3—From social movement to interest group

The rationalisation of women's health policy
According to Waters and Crook (1993), social movements are characteristically a product of disenchantment with the rational and bureaucratic form of government, which is seen to represent the narrow interests of class groups. Social movements represent the interests of minority groups whose concerns are not simply based on class, but might involve equal rights for women (who are an exception, being a majority group) or Indigenous people, protection of the environment, disarmament, or antinuclear issues. Social movements might exercise power at the ballot box by shaping the way large numbers of voters act. Conversely, they might influence the policies taken up by particular political parties. However, while political parties might have sympathies with social movements and support policies in order to win elections, their interests do not always overlap. In the health arena there have been social movements concerned with women's health, public health and primary health care, pro-life and pro-choice, disability rights, and deinstitutionalisation for people with mental illness. Each of these social movements has impacted on health care policy by bringing particular ideologies to policy development. Social movements, such as the women's movement or the disability rights movement, serve very public interests. Doyal and Kellow (1995) refer to social movements as public interest groups, suggesting that their political clout is at the level of protest or ability to gain media attention and to pressure policy makers, but is limited at the level of specific day-to-day policy

---

formation. This is because they are broadbased networks and coalitions, often insistent on democratic forms of governance, so that it is difficult for political parties to identify the leaders. In many instances, key interest groups might move into the breach, serving as consulting groups to government on policy. The Women's Electoral Lobby (WEL) is an example of this, as is the Consumers' Health Forum. However, the ability of these organisations to represent the wishes of all women or consumers is tenuous. It becomes easier for governments and bureaucrats to talk directly with key professionals representing private interest groups, which might or might not share the same values as the social movement. Their own professional interest groups might have an agenda to maximise professional interests. Given this, it is often impossible to identify leaders of social movements who will be able to speak in the interest of citizens.

Women's health policy: from social movement to a 'body bits' approach

In Australia in the late 1970s and early 1980s, feminist activists, including feminist nurses and doctors, were successful in focusing attention on the uniqueness of women's health experiences. The primary focus of the women's health movement was on legitimating women's own experience of their bodies, their health and illness experience, and their encounters with predominantly male health practitioners. The critique was that the medical profession concentrated on women's reproductive conditions, treating their body parts isolated from women's social or emotional experience. This was despite the fact that it was known that women in their capacity as mothers and carers interact more with the health care system than men (Horsley et al. 1999). Doctors were predominantly male and worked in a system where there was little encouragement for consultations that focused on the social issues confronting many working class, Indigenous, and migrant women. Women felt their genuine complaints, such as those about domestic violence, were trivialised; or their biologically natural conditions, such as menopause, were medicalised. As Willis (1999, p. 51) argues, 'for feminist theorists, health status is inextricably linked with society, culture and the socioeconomic structures within which women live their lives'.

As a social movement the women's health movement was sufficiently powerful over the 15-year period from 1975 to 1990 for the

1983–96 federal Labor government to sponsor a nationwide consultation of women prior to the establishment of the National Women's Health Policy (Department of Health 1988). Liz Newbry headed the consultation, and more than a million women across all states and territories were invited to comment on the proposed draft and final document. The consultation brought together women from a wide range of organisations across a range of political persuasions. The National Women's Health Policy committed itself to a social view of health where the participation of women was a key factor within a health promotion framework. In effect, it aligned itself with the primary health care movement, which was also at its height during these years. Key elements of the women's health movement included a commitment to reducing sexism and sex-role stereotyping in the delivery of health care, and a focus on primary health care. Areas identified included 'reproductive health and sexuality, occupational health and safety, the health of ageing women, the health needs of carers, violence against women and the women's emotional and mental health needs, and the health effects of sex-role stereotyping' (Horsley et al. 1999, p. 217). A diversity of approaches was instigated. These included continued funding for stand-alone women's health centres as well as attempts to reform mainstream services through education and policies of positive discrimination at all levels of the health care system. One approach to reforming mainstream services was through encouraging more women into medicine and ensuring that schools of medicine developed strategies for achieving gender balance in student intakes. By the early 1990s some of the more radical approaches were under attack. Horsly et al. (1999) identify the Proudfoot case and the shift in funding encapsulated in the 1993–98 Medicare Agreement as contributing factors. Dr Alan Proudfoot challenged the legality of stand-alone women's health centres before the Human Rights and Equal Opportunity Commission, arguing that they were a form of discrimination against men, who could not access these centres. Although the commission found in favour of women-only health centres, the case symbolised a shift in the fortunes of the social movement, away from one of radical social change to a more conservative position for women in society in general and for women's health in particular. The 1993–98 Medicare Agreement, consistent with economic rationalism, moved to outcome-based funding and a population approach. This inevitably led to the funding of programs that could demonstrate outcomes in terms of numbers of admissions, discharges, or clients consulted, and away from those programs that focused on community participation and development or that had more nebulous outcomes to do with social and emotional wellbeing (Horsly et al. 1999). The shift in direction, along with a more conservative approach to women's issues and the concurrent rationalising of health funding in Victoria and South Australia, has led to various forms of structural incorporation of women's health centres into mainstream services (see chapters 1 and 2 for analyses of federal and state funding tensions). Although women's health centres remain and carry out a number of programs within a primary health care focus, their funding has been significantly reduced and their political impact within the overall system has diminished. At the same time, specific-purpose programs are more generously funded; as is general practice, where most practices now employ female GPs. The inclusion of female GPs does not of itself mean that mainstream services have been radically reformed. Although many female GPs are sensitive to women's health issues, they are themselves victims of male professional dominance (Pringle 1998). Further, female GPs are also members of medical interest groups and work within this framework. At the policy level the focus is now on body bits rather than social and emotional wellbeing (Horsley et al. 1999, p. 22; Willis 1999). A pertinent example of the focus on body bits rather than on empowerment and participation is the Breastscreen Program implemented in 1991. Karen Willis (1999) has argued that this program was seen as politically safe. It focused on a known gendered cancer, targeting a deserving group—rural women—at a time when the controversial HIV/AIDS was on the policy agenda and funding to women's health centres was being reduced or realigned. A focus on mammography screening of rural women, while necessary, shifted women's health into a conservative arena, away from more radical feminist issues such as sexuality, lesbian health, and domestic violence. Willis points out that the real health gains of mammography are debatable, but this is not conveyed to women. For example, detection rates are about 1 in 400 screens, yet women are encouraged to have regular checks as a matter of responsible and rational behaviour. In a policy climate in which outcomes are the focus, the number of women who present for mammograms or the percentage identified with cancer are seen as more important than informed decision making or public debate about the real or perceived benefits of this service. Current targets seek a 70 per cent participation rate (Breastscreen South Australia 1999). In her study, Willis found that much of the material presented to women that was part of the

> process of informed consent was misleading. A key aim of the National Women's Health Policy was informed consent. Willis (1999, p. 57) found that the 'language of the recruitment for a population-based program is very different to that of a women's health service adhering to the principles of the National Women's Health Strategy'. For Willis (1999) and Horsley et al. (1999) Women's Health policy has been recaptured by the acute services and the medical lobby—by private interest groups. This has occurred as a result of a shift away from social models of health and a robust welfare state to an outcome-based, population-focused, and a market-driven health care system.
>
> ■

It could well be asked where are the feminist activists of 15 years ago or the social movement that gave energy to women's health? Have they been captured by evidence-based medicine and economic rationalism? Social movements have difficulty airing their views where the prevailing rationale is economic, particularly so in cases like Breastscreen where it is difficult to challenge the efficacy of the program.

Conclusion

A key aspect of the arguments offered here is that the power of some interest groups has increased while the influence of others has waned as the ideological differences in policy between the two major parties has blurred and coalesced around the increased shift to a market state (Hancock 1999; Pixley 1999; Smyth & Cass 1999). In the case of the Factor 'f' Program, maintained under the newly created Pharmaceutical Incentive Program, the power of large multinationals to circumvent government attempts to maintain the welfare state are evident. Factors such as the ruling of the courts, manipulation of the media, share prices, and the impact of the global economy on the way in which the government negotiates with these companies are reasons for this move to more conservative policies. It is shifting ground, where the government's own policy has enabled pharmaceutical companies to strengthen their bargaining position rather than curtailing or regulating it.

In the case of professional interest groups, sometimes created or sustained through government funding, it is clear that policy is a matter of negotiation, but the outcomes cannot be predicted. What is achieved is what survives and emerges from the bargaining processes. In the case of the GP Strategy and the National Rural Strategy, the reform appeared at first sight to have enhanced the welfare state, yet we might well ask whether funding one professional group, as is the case for the Rural Strategy, or enhancing a professional group over a social movement, as is the case in the GP Strategy, is necessarily the best policy. However, given that the government had to negotiate with medicine, this might well have been the most pragmatic outcome.

What was not predicted was that the market was able to capitalise on GP disenchantment, offering them financial remuneration without the responsibilities of small business. The logic of capitalism has prevailed: successful small businesses have given way to amalgamation and corporatisation. It is no longer a matter of the state tempering further demands on GPs for fear of further corporatisation: the process has begun and will accelerate. Major efforts are now required by the state and the profession to stem the tide; however, this will depend on whether the state sees corporatisation to be in its interests or not. The AMA (2000) suggests that the government is currently playing a wait-and-see game, subscribing to the view that large corporations offer better economies of scale than can small business. As is pointed out in the case studies of the pharmaceutical industry and general practice, multinational and large corporation interest groups are operating with little resistance from the state.

The case study of the women's health movement raises the question to what extent do governments respond to the public mood by providing programs that will maximise their votes but not necessarily maximise democracy? It is also a case study of the rise and fall of a social movement. One of the processes of charismatic social movements is that they eventually become routinised and formally organised. Formal organisation includes special interest groups for women within professional associations, as well as moves by governments to bring the organisation under mainstream bureaucratic control. Feminist health professionals also belong to interest groups. Interests can be caught between the goals of the social movement and those of the professional association.

In the opening paragraphs of this chapter, Alford's structural model was mentioned, as was the fact that health care policy was influenced by the interests of professional groups such as medicine, the state, consumers, and the private for-profit sector—that is, the market. At first, it might be assumed that all four groups are playing the same game. The outcomes are merely a matter of which team is the strongest and has access to knowledge and resources. However, if there is a shift to a market model, where the market is now characterised by large corporations and multinationals rather than small business and professional interest groups, then the rules of the game have shifted, raising the question—of who owns the stadium and which game should we be watching—the one on the field or the one in the corporate box? For countries such as Australia, where the government is still determined to maintain a welfare state, the answer is not clear. As two of the case studies illustrate, even if the state still owns the stadium, it is clear that having invited the market into the game, a takeover could be imminent.

References

Australian Medical Association 2000, *General Practice Corporatisation*, AMA Scoping Paper, <http://www.domino.ama.com.au/Dir/103/Gebe5c4e76bc4a2569970016 fae3?Open>, 20 December.

Baker, P. 2000, 'Evaluation of the General Practice Amalgamations Incentives Program and the Demonstration Projects in Virtual Amalgamation: Request for Tender', *Weekend Australian*, 7 October, p. 47.

Bloom, A. (ed.) 2000, *Health Reform in Australia and New Zealand*, Oxford University Press, Melbourne.

Bollan, M. 1996, 'Recent Changes in Australian General Practice', *Medical Journal of Australia*, vol. 164, pp. 212; online version available at <http:www.mja.com.au/>, 6 October 2000.

Breastscreen South Australia 1999, *Breastscreen at 10 Years*, Breastscreen South Australia, Adelaide.

Commonwealth Department of Community Services 1988, *National Policy on Women's Health: A Discussion Paper*, AGPS, Canberra.

Commonwealth Department of Health and Aged Care 2000a, *General Practice in Australia 2000*, AGPS, Canberra.

—— 2000b, *More Doctors, Better Services, Regional Health Strategy*, AGPS, Canberra.

—— 2000c, *Regional Health Strategy, Budget 2000–2001*, Media Release <http://www.health.gov.au/budget2000/ruralmediaaindex.htm>.

Commonwealth Department of Health and Family Services 1996, *General Practice in Australia 1996*, AGPS, Canberra.

De Cercq, K. 1999, 'Strategy: For Ailing Profits, Sigma Prescribes a Spending Cure', *Business News*, vol. 21, p. 46; online version available at <wysiwyg://52// www.brw.com.au/stories/19991126/4284.htm>.

Doctors' Reform Society 1999, *Bitter Pill*, <http://www.drs.org.au/wwwboard/ messages/595.htm>.

Doyle, T. & Kellow, A. 1995, *Environmental Politics and Policy Making in Australia*, Macmillan Education, Melbourne.

Duckett, S. 1997, 'Doctors and Healthcare Reform', *Medical Journal of Australia*, vol. 167, pp. 184–5; online version available at <http:www.mja.com.au/>, 6 October 2000.

Gardner, H. (ed.) 1997, *Health Policy in Australia*, Oxford University Press, Melbourne.

General Practice Branch 1999, *Synopsis of the Reports of the General Practice Reviews*, Commonwealth of Australia, Canberra; online version available at <http://www.health.au/hsdd/gp/finlrprt.htm>.

Hancock, L. (ed.) 1999, *Health Policy in the Market State*, Allen & Unwin, Sydney.

Horsley, P., Tremellen, S., & Hancock, L. 1999, 'Women's Health in a Changing State', in L. Hancock (ed.), *Health Policy in the Market State*, Allen & Unwin, Sydney.

Leeder, S. 1999, *Healthy Medicine: Challenges Facing Australia's Health Services*, Allen & Unwin, Sydney.

Lofgren, H. 1997, 'Industry Policy to Set the Market Free: Drug Pricing and the Factor 'f' Program', *Labour and Industry*, vol. 8, no. 2, pp. 67–84.

Marjoribanks, T., Lewis, J., & Pirotta, M. 2000, 'General Practitioners' Experiences: Theorising Changes in Professions', in *Sociological Sites/Sights: Multiple Locations, Multiple Knowledges, Multiple Visions*, Papers from the Sociological Conference, Flinders University, Adelaide, 6–8 December.

National Rural Health Alliance 2000, *National Rural Health Alliance*, <http://www/ruralhealth>, 10 October 2000.

Pixley, J. 1999, 'Social Movements, Democracy and Conflicts over Institutional Reform', in P. Smyth & B. Cass (eds), *Contesting the Australian Way: States, Markets and Civil Society*, Cambridge University Press, Cambridge.

PriceWaterhouseCoopers 1999, *A Resource-based Model of Private Medical Practice in Australia: The Practice Cost Study, Preliminary Findings*, Medicare Schedule Review Board, vol. 1, Royal College of General Practitioners; online version available at <http://www.racgp.org.au>, 10 October 2000.

Pringle, R. 1998, *Sex and Medicine: Gender, Power and Authority in the Medical Profession*, Cambridge University Press, Cambridge.

Royal Australian College of General Practitioners 1999, *Medical Leaders Agree to GP Cooperation*, <http://www.racgp.org.au/news/media/cooperation>, 10 October 2000.

Rural Doctors Association of Australia 2000, <http://www/rdaa.com.au/gpcentre.html>, 13 October 2000.

Smyth, P. & Cass, B. (eds) 1999, *Contesting the Australian Way: States, Markets and Civil Society*, Cambridge University Press, Cambridge.

Swerissen, H. & Duckett, S. 1997, 'Health Policy and Financing', in H. Gardner (ed.), *Health Policy in Australia*, Oxford University Press, Melbourne.

Waters, M. & Crook, R. 1993, *Sociology One*, 3rd edn, Longman Cheshire, Melbourne.

White, K. 2000, 'The State, the Market, and General Practice: The Australian Case', *International Journal of Health Services*, vol. 30, no. 2, pp. 285–308.

Willis, K. 1999, 'Compromise, Country Women and Cancer: Women's Health Policy in Australia', *Annual Review of Health Social Sciences*, vol. 9, pp. 51–61.

Wilson, J. 1973, *Political Organisations*, Basic Books, New York.

9

Workplace Reform in the Public Health Care Sector

Pauline Stanton

The public health care sector is a major area of public expenditure, and governments throughout the world have introduced cost saving policies into their health care budgets due to concerns about rising costs. There are various explanations for increasing costs, but most include ageing populations, increased use of advanced technologies, and consumer and supplier induced demand (Twaddle 1996). In Australia, as in many other developed countries, the health care workforce represents the largest single component of costs in the health sector (Australian Institute of Health and Welfare 1998a). As labour costs are such an important component of total costs, policies that include cost containment strategies targeting the workforce are increasingly attractive for governments (Thornley 1998).

At the same time, the health care sector has been subject to continuing innovation and change. Over the past few years there have been major advances in and increased use of medical diagnostic and treatment technology and services. New systems and processes, including new information systems, have similarly seen rapid development. In Australia, there has been growth in the numbers of specialist medical practitioners and nursing specialists, and an increased emphasis on community care (Australian Institute of Health and Welfare 1998b). These changes require new ways of working and different forms of skill development. Coping with the increased pace of change requires more flexible work practices, in terms of both service delivery and employment relations.

Workplace reform is a significant policy concern at state, territory, and Commonwealth levels, not only in the health sector but also in other sectors. Industrial reform through the decentralisation of industrial relations has been a major feature of successive Australian governments throughout the 1980s and 1990s (Wooden 2000). However, in the health care sector, there are a number of barriers to change, some of which are beyond the scope of the industrial arena; there has been no comprehensive approach to workplace reform in the health sector in Australia.

This chapter focuses on the strategies employed by the Victorian Liberal government under Premier Kennett from 1992 to 1999 in the context of federalism, including the decentralisation of industrial relations through the introduction of enterprise bargaining. Reforms to the health sector during this period also included financial restraint, new systems of funding, privatisation, and outsourcing. The chapter utilises data from a study into employment relationships in public hospitals in Victoria.

The Kennett government's strategies had a number of objectives, one of which was productivity improvement, but it focused mainly on cost control and represented a cost reduction approach to the management of the workforce. Such cost reduction strategies can lead to work intensification, increased job insecurity, poorer conditions of employment, and labour shortages. They can undermine trust and commitment. Also, they tend to focus attention on the hotel and support services, which are often the easiest sectors in which to achieve savings, but do little to engage clinicians to make more extensive workplace reform in terms of clinical practice.

It is time for a more inclusive and comprehensive approach to workplace reform in the public health care sector. Such an approach is essential for achieving more efficient and effective work practices and for creating a capacity for continuing change in health care structures and processes, as technological change accelerates.

Improving productivity in the public health sector

The Australian public health sector is an industry in which responsibility for industrial relations has traditionally been located well away from the workplace through a reliance on centralised processes of conciliation and arbitration. This has meant a greater emphasis on centralised award provisions than in other industries and, apart from senior management, less flexibility at the local level over remuneration and nonwage forms of compensation (Braithwaite 1997). As health sector resources became tighter in the 1990s there was greater pressure for workplace reform. Health service managers were forced to become more strategic and less operational in their practice as the industry was faced with major change due to pressures of increasing demand for services at a time of shrinking resources. Braithwaite (1997, p. 133) concluded that the industry's centralised and rigid industrial structures made such changes difficult and argued that 'the health sector's relatively inflexible and award bound working conditions and compensation structures need alteration'.

Changing these structures in the health sector is not simple. The health sector is one of the most highly unionised industrial sectors. Australian Bureau of Statistics (ABS) figures from 1999 show trade union density in the health and community services sector was 30.7 per cent compared to 25.7 per cent for all industries (ABS 1999). In some hospitals, union membership among nurses is estimated to be 60 per cent (Stanton 2001c). The Australian Nursing Federation (ANF) is increasing its membership at a time of union membership decline in most other sectors (Stanton 2001c). Also, nurses provide an essential service to the community (Fox 1998).

Labour inflexibilities are not just industrially based. The health care sector is a highly educated, highly professionalised sector with a number of different professions and paraprofessions, each with its own particular history and features (Gardner & McCoppin 1995). Features of professionalism include long training, specialised knowledge, independence, clinical autonomy, and a certain amount of mobility (Gunderson 1982). The control and restriction of entry to professions is managed by the professionals themselves, often supported by government regulation. Professional groups, in particular doctors, use claims based on clinical autonomy to defend practices that might be necessary but that can also be used to protect their own self-interest. The stronger professions have managed to translate such practices into regulations concerning service delivery. The health sector has been described as having 'a very tribal craft-oriented professional structure' that undermines change and can lead to conflict between professional allegiances and organisational allegiances (Stanton 2000, p. 9). The power of the health professions and trade unions is often cited as a barrier to change in the health industry (Harrison & Pollitt 1994; Alexander 2000).

A human resources director of a large hospital network in Victoria argued that similar practices and rigidities in many other industries have been overcome (Stanton 2000, p. 8) and that 'People have recognised the stupidity and futility of those [rigid frameworks] and how damaging it is to the relationships of people who have to work together and have found better ways of doing things'. He believed that the health sector is so rulebound and institutionalised that 'You end up with situations, quite literally, where groups of employees ... work out a better way of doing things and have to hide it from both the unions and the Department of Human Services, and other structures in case someone finds out and stops them'.

The method by which public health services are funded also impacts on employment relationships and can promote or hinder organisational change. Gunderson (1982) argues that, historically, increases in health-sector labour costs were passed directly on to third parties, either governments or insurers. In a system where funding has no direct relation to results, the pressure on health care managers to contain costs is not so great and therefore managers might be less motivated to improve the efficiency of labour utilisation.

Finally, the general governance and funding approach in the health sector has traditionally supported a view that employees in the industry are not responsible for how they spend money (Stanton 2000). In other words, clinicians are responsible for patient care; where the money comes from is someone else's problem. This is an important point, as, similarly, Braithwaite (1997) found an industry with an unclear locus of workplace managerial control. Although within the workplace the financial, business, and strategic performance rests with management, patient care processes rest with health professionals and in particular with doctors, who largely control the production process in health organisations. Compared to their counterparts in manufacturing, health care managers have relatively little control over the production process.

Workplace reform and the Kennett government

Australian governments have been increasingly influenced by neoliberal approaches to policy making in the public sector. This includes a commitment to the use of market forces in the allocation of resources, utilisation of corporate sector management models, and a decreasing role for government in service delivery, with a consequent cutback in government spending (Gardner 1995). Underlying these approaches is a search for improved efficiency and effectiveness. This is in part fuelled by fears of rising costs in the public sector and a set of beliefs that traditionally organised public services do not manage costs, improve quality, or meet appropriate standards of service. Neoliberals argue that public services are captured and dominated by powerful interests, such as trade unions, professional associations, and special interest groups (Dawson & Dargie 1999).

Neoliberal policies had a particularly strong impact in Victoria. The Kennett government accelerated change with policies that included a commitment to small government through outsourcing and privatisation, the introduction of private sector managerial practices through the development of performance reviews, audits, contractual relationships, and a 'steering not rowing' approach to service delivery (Osborne & Gaebler 1992, p. 30; Alford & O'Neil 1994). Barraclough and Smith (1994) have pointed out significant continuities between the neoliberal policies of the Kennett administration and the policies of the previous state Labor government.

Industrial reform

The Kennett government was committed to controlling industrial reform and the power of trade unions. Teicher and Gramberg (1999) argue that the aim of the Kennett government was to create a malleable and compliant workforce for reasons that were not just ideological but also economic. These reasons included the perceived need to cut expenditure, reduce debt servicing, and to increase the competitiveness of the state's economy.

The Victorian government's industrial legislation, the *Employee Relations Act 1992* (Vic.), came into effect in March 1993. This Act was introduced along with the *Annual Leave Payments (Public Sector) Act 1992* (Vic.), which abolished the annual leave loading, the *Public Sector (Union Fees) Act 1992* (Vic.), which stopped the practice of deducting union fees from pay, and the *Public Sector Management Act 1992* (Vic.) (Teicher & Gramberg 1999). The Employee Relations Act abolished the Victorian Industrial Relations Commission and existing state awards and introduced individual and collective agreements with basic minimum conditions (Creighton & Stewart 2000). The Public Sector Management Act mainly affected public servants directly employed by the state, rather than hospital staff. It was a step towards modelling the public service on the private sector managerial approach (O'Neil 1999) and sent a managerialist message to the rest of the public sector.

In December 1992, the federal Labor government introduced amendments to federal legislation to allow the transfer of state employees who had no recourse to compulsory conciliation and arbitration to the federal arena (Creighton & Stewart 2000). These amendments began to be acted upon almost immediately by all branches of the Health Services Union of Australia, but the Australian Nursing Federation was pursuing its own federal award, which it had been given leave to do by the Australian Industrial Relations Commission (AIRC) in June 1992. The ANF had been seeking a federal award for Victorian nurses since 1983 (ANF 1992).

Through the courts, the Kennett government fought hard to prevent the transfer of Victorian awards to the federal jurisdiction. In February 1994, after a series of challenges, a full bench of the AIRC ruled in favour of the nurses (Gardner 1994). However, the Victorian government continued to attempt to reverse the decisions of the Commission in making interim awards covering other state employees. Finally, in *re Australian Education Union and others: ex parte the State of Victoria and another* in 1995, the High Court ruled that the AIRC could make an award binding the states and their agencies in relation to minimum wages and working conditions. It did, however, preclude the Commission from making an award binding the states in relation to qualifications and eligibility for employment, at least on the ground of redundancy (CLR 1994–95).

Although the Victorian unions were successful in transferring their awards to the federal jurisdiction, they did not escape enterprise bargaining. In the federal arena the Labor government was committed to managed decentralism, which meant a move from centralised conciliation and arbitration to a greater role for collective bargaining at the enterprise level (Dabscheck 1995). In 1993, the Australian Hospital Association (AHA) debated whether enterprise bargaining was suited to the special conditions in the health sector. Some argued that the emphasis on productivity achievements in the enterprise bargaining process was not possible in the health care sector because of the difficulties of measuring output.

Laurie Brereton, then federal Minister for Industrial Relations, expressed another concern, arguing that collective bargaining in the health sector was less appropriate than in other areas. 'An unfettered right to strike and immunity in the bargaining stream can never be the sole preserve of those in essential services like health. Bargaining can therefore never be their provider' (AHA 1993, p. 11). The Australian Council of Trade Unions, which supported enterprise bargaining (AHA 1993), took a different approach, arguing that the health sector could not be out of step with the rest of industry and that solutions could be found to manage the enterprise bargaining process in that sector.

Managers at the forum described the complexities of managing staff in the health sector. They saw the need for further workplace change and were willing to examine enterprise bargaining as a vehicle of change; however, they stressed that there are other tools of change open to managers. They reported that workplace change and reform was already happening in the health sector with or without bargaining (AHA 1993). In fact, as Fox (1998) has argued, there has always been an element of bargaining in the health care sector, but this was largely in tandem with conciliation and arbitration.

Since 1993, there has been in Australia an increasing emphasis on enterprise bargaining. In Victoria from 1993 onwards, there was a dramatic increase in the number of enterprise agreements registered in the public health and community services sector in Victoria (Stanton 2001b). However, despite a policy commitment by the state government to enterprise bargaining and an increase in the numbers of such agreements, in practice the impact has been limited. There is evidence that industrial relations in the Victorian public health sector, even under the Kennett administration, were ultimately centrally determined even though bargaining has mainly replaced conciliation and arbitration (Stanton 2001b). Reasons given for this include

- the role of government as funder of the sector and therefore as the effective employer
- the strength of the health professions
- the political nature of the sector.

Employers in the Victorian hospital sector have argued that industrial action is so sensitive in the health sector that the minister for health has to become involved very quickly in any industrial dispute. One director of human resources (HR) argued that: 'The political nature of industrial relations in the health area meant that it was difficult for the Minister to remain as detached from things as the Minister would have liked.' Another HR director who had also worked in the manufacturing area thought the health sector had a 'lower breaking point' than other industries (Stanton 2001b, p. 318).

Health policy-driven workplace change

O'Brien argues (1997) that public sector industrial relations is as much a political process as it is an industrial process, as governments are fiscal guardians and policy generators as well as service providers and employers. Governments certainly have a number of tools available to them, not just industrial reform, and the Kennett government introduced a range of policies into the health sector including stringent Budget cuts, casemix funding, outsourcing, and privatisation, as well as an emphasis on arm's length government.

In the early years of the Kennett government there were substantial Budget cuts—11.9 per cent over two years and no adjustments for increased hospital costs. Managers had discretion about where to cut, but cuts still had to be made; often, the easiest way to reduce costs was to reduce the numbers of staff. The state Department of Health and Community Services made voluntary departure packages (VDPs) available to public sector health staff. Estimates vary, but John Paterson, the then Secretary of the Department of Health and Community Services, estimated at the time that 8000 jobs could be lost in the sector (Minogue 1993). Harkness (1999) suggests that 10 per cent of state hospital employees lost their jobs, and one union official estimated job losses of 10 000 across the sector (Stanton 2001b). The easiest areas to cut back in staff or to outsource were initially in the nonclinical areas such as the hotel services, cleaning, and catering, but these services were not the only areas to feel the impact of Budget cuts. The management and administrative sections of hospitals were also decimated as organisational restructuring forced by financial restraint led to flatter management structures as layers of management and administrative staff were made redundant.

The Victorian Hospitals' Association (VHA) saw some benefits in the cuts but worried about how far they would go, arguing that

> The availability of voluntary departure packages has enabled hospitals more recently to make massive reductions in staff numbers to deal with the work practice issues, which were 'untouchable' in years gone by. To date these staff reductions have

concentrated on the nonclinical staff. While efficiencies have improved, the strain reveals itself, for example, in less than adequate levels of cleanliness in hospitals. If this strain is to be extended to the clinical staff, then the impact on the quality and quantity of care is likely to be marked (Hughes 1993, p. 1).

The impact was already affecting laboratory work. This applied particularly to pathology and other medical science areas covered by the Medical Scientists' Association of Victoria (MSAV). This was an area ripe for reduction because of the developments in new technology in medical science. Restructuring had been taking place in the area since 1991 (Kearney & Whitfield 1991), however, the pace picked up with the availability of VDPs. The MSAV argued that sizeable numbers of medical scientists accepted VDPs and, because of the fact that VDPs were structured to be most attractive to those on higher salaries, the public health sector lost many of its most skilled and experienced scientists at this time (Bremner & Kelly 2000).

It is difficult to understand the full impact of the 1993 Budget cuts without also examining casemix funding. Duckett (1995) argues that although the government came into power with a commitment to cut government spending, it was soon understood that in the health portfolio the size of the proposed reduction meant that a simple flat rate cut across the board would be unachievable in efficient hospitals and generous to inefficient ones. Another approach was necessary. The introduction of casemix funding in July 1993, focusing as it did on funding outputs, gave the potential for hospital performance in key areas to be measured and compared. Not everyone saw the benefits, as the ANF argued: 'The inherent danger of the simultaneous introduction of casemix and the execution of Budget cuts will mean that casemix will be the mechanism by which vulnerable areas are identified and cuts are made' (Minogue 1993, p. 26).

Lin and Duckett (1997) argue that casemix funding was an equitable way to achieve savings, with the most efficient hospitals benefiting at the expense of the more inefficient ones. The Victorian Hospitals' Association (VHA) also supported the introduction of casemix funding, although it had reservations about the speed with which it was introduced and the severity of the Budget cuts (VHA 1992).

From the government's perspective, casemix funding had a number of benefits: for the first time outputs that were to be funded could be identified, defined, and measured, thus giving the government a useful monitoring and arm's length management tool for measuring productivity. Also, core acute health business had to be identified. Noncore business included such items as the provision of staff cafeterias and pathology services to private patients. These services were transformed into business units, which could be run on business lines with hospitals accountable for their financial performance (Duckett 1995). They also became discrete services that had the potential to be outsourced, leaving someone else to manage those services, perhaps in a way more subject to market discipline.

At the time, casemix funding was severely criticised for its potential to shift costs to the community through early discharge, and reduce quality of care due to an emphasis on throughput and discharging people 'quicker and sicker' (Draper 1992). However, casemix funding was a major tool in arm's length management. It gave the government the added bonus of having a much better awareness of exactly what it was buying from the hospitals and it provided clearer benchmarks against which hospitals could be judged.

Outsourcing and privatisation were two other policy developments that had a major impact on employment relations. Unlike local government, health organisations were not forced to outsource their operations in the early years of the Kennett government. However, the impact of Budget cuts and the identification of noncore business meant that a number of hospitals found it in their interests to outsource areas such as hotel functions and some support services. This was one area over which management had total discretion.

A number of organisations put services up for tender, many of which were won by inhouse bidders. The introduction of contestability in 1995 took outsourcing one step further, forcing those who had not yet taken part to consider it and test their services against others (Phillips Fox and Casemix Consulting 1999). This again had a particular impact on the Health Services Union of Australia and the MSAV.

The tendering process had in itself led to new work practices and technical efficiencies, regardless of whether the service was eventually contracted out through the requirements of lower cost structures and improved systems of responsibility (Phillip Fox and Casemix Consulting 1999; Stanton 2001b). Some employers saw the process more strategically. As one HR director argued,

> In our organisation we quite consciously did not pursue competitive tendering as simply a cost reduction exercise. We pursued competitive tendering or contestability as a mechanism to achieve structural reform. We weren't actually interested, necessarily, at an ideological level, in giving our hotel services over to a private company. What we were interested in doing was working with the staff and unions to actually get improvements in the quality of service that was delivered from these. The net result was that at the end of the contestability process we haven't outsourced anything to an external proprietor (Stanton 2001b).

Another advantage of the outsourcing process was that hospitals could keep any savings made and steer them elsewhere, usually to direct patient care (Stanton 2001b).

The unions had a different view of outsourcing, seeing it as a threat to their members' employment conditions (Stanton 2001b). Young (2001) reports that in the public health sector most unions had made agreements with employers so that outsourced workers would take their existing terms and conditions with them. Even so, union officials argued that, although they managed overall to negotiate a transfer of terms and conditions of employment to new businesses, jobs were lost in this process; often, continuity of service provisions and superannuation entitlements were lost too. In other words, the tendering process had led to greater job insecurity (Stanton 2001b).

The impact of policy change

The Australian Institute of Health and Welfare (AIHW) argues that the health workforce is now more efficient and productive than ever. In 1996, fewer hospital staff treated significantly more patients at a much higher rate of patient turnover and declining average length of stay (Australian Institute of Health and Welfare 1998b). Measured productivity in the Victorian health sector increased rapidly in the Kennett years, presumably in part due to the policies outlined previously (Australian Institute of Health and Welfare 1998b; Phillips Fox and Casemix Consulting 1999).

There is also increasing evidence that competitive policies have had a detrimental effect on the workforce. Allan et al. (1999) argue that the patterns of labour utilisation in Australia have changed in three major ways over the past twenty years. These are

* job broadening or multiskilling
* an increase in employment insecurity
* work intensification.

The effects on staff of increases in productivity and efficiency in the health sector have not been measured, although there is some evidence of an increasing intensification of work. For example, Allan's (1998) study into a Queensland public hospital found increased work intensification as the state government sought to contain health care expenditure through Budget cuts and the setting of activity targets leading to a decline in staff motivation and morale. A study into medical scientists in Victoria found increasing work intensification in the industry leading to workers complaining of greater stress levels and ill health (Weekes et al. 2001). A report commissioned by the ANF into nursing labour shortages in 1999 found increases in nursing workloads as a result of staffing shortages, and argued that nurses had left the industry because they were no longer willing to put up with worsening working conditions (Considine & Buchanan 1999).

There is evidence from other countries that have followed similar policy directions. In New Zealand, the nurses' union argued that while productivity increased rapidly, the impact on working conditions for employees was dramatic (Blake 1997). Penalty rates were replaced by a 10 per cent increase in the base rate, the hours of work changed, annual leave was cut back, sick leave was reduced, and meal allowances were taken away. At the same time there was a deliberate increase in the use of casual staff at the expense of permanent staff.

Thornley (1998), in the UK, was interested in the impact of the decentralisation of pay determination on the processes of bargaining. She found that there were very low pay increases, and that management often argued an inability to increase pay due to financial constraints, and sometimes tried to impose settlements on staff. She found that significant amounts of staff and management time were absorbed in negotiations over fairly small amounts of money. This had an impact on morale, leading to increased potential for conflict, and undermining staff motivation and trust in management. This last point demonstrates that competitive policies often have a less obvious impact on the workforce. One of the poorly researched sites of structural change in the health sector is the impact on professionalism, trust, and commitment of staff.

One of the fundamental features of professionalism in the health sector—particularly for medical professionals—is that of clinical autonomy and clinical judgment. Health professionals are trained to exercise independent judgment in an uncertain and complex environment. Southon and Braithwaite (1998) argue that the recent health reforms take a simplistic view of such realities of health service delivery, leading to fundamental problems for health professionals. 'The implicit rejection of the centrality of professionalism will provide stress for committed professionals, irrespective of the level of remuneration provided to them' (p. 27).

Braithwaite (1998) argues that policies such as casemix funding reflect a simplistic view of the hospital as a factory and can alter the way relationships are structured from one of collegiality to one of contract. There is a danger that, as hospitals get paid only for what they do, they will neglect the intangible or invisible aspects of service delivery. Duckett states that 'there are many aspects of health care which should be valued but can't be priced' (Duckett 1995, p. 132).

A study into the introduction of policies such as competitive tendering into community health centres found an increase in a culture of secrecy and mistrust. Staff were becoming more and more excluded from decision making in case they shared information with colleagues in other agencies who were now their competitors (Stanton 2001a). Similarly, Peacock (1997) found that outsourcing in the National Health Service (NHS) in the UK had led to decreased trust between organisations, as each was competing against the other for funding. Other critics of market approaches and their impact on professionals would argue that 'notions of duty, rights, collegiality, service, obligation, care, compassion or even need ... are eliminated' (Davis 1995, p. 127).

A number of health service managers (Stanton 2000, p. 8) have argued that Kennett's cost reduction policies did force some useful changes on the industry:

> The fundamental change has been brought by simply unrelenting expenditure restraint on the industry and this health care group, which has forced management in to taking hard decisions about staffing profiles in the group, and as a consequence that has been the vehicle for change, and the change has largely been to attempt to downsize, to increase flexibility in our rostering and similar kinds of moves (HR Director).

There was also an awareness of the limitations of such policies. One human resources director (Stanton 2000, p. 6) commented:

> I think that the whole government's structure for health has been basically driven by accountants. It's basically around dollars and cents and that is not what is required to get reforms in the health sector. It's about partnerships, it's about relationships, it's about getting learning processes established in the workplace. It's about people; it's about more effective problem solving and it's about all of those things. When you get those things happening I think that the dollars and cents will look after themselves. So there's been a series of signals and a series ... of management parameters that take the system in a particular direction and it's not the direction that it needs to be going in.

There has been little done to address such issues in any comprehensive way at either the central or the local level. One point of view is that over the years the human resource function in the health sector had been significantly undervalued.

> There has not been a recognition that you have to make an investment in your workforce in order to reap the benefits that a workforce can bring. In the nature of such investments they tend to be medium to long term and the whole ethos, the whole cultural base of public hospitals is a nine month to twelve month financial horizon. It's not uncommon for hospitals not to know what their annual budget is until October and November; this creates a profound preoccupation with a focus on costs (employers' association interviewee, Stanton 2000, p. 6).

If hospitals are not diverted and distracted by industrial campaigns then there is, theoretically at least, an opportunity to give greater attention to organisational issues. However, under the Kennett government, health policy was focused on cost reduction; consequently, the human resource management practices in the sector also tended to focus on cost reduction. Although hospital managers might know they need to ask questions about their organisational health they are afraid of the answer because of the cost implications.

> There is a subconscious focus on cost, cost, cost, throughput, throughput, through-put. Without particular regard to the sustainability of their present staffing level or their present staffing mix or the correct skill mix. Is the skill mix optimal for the targets they have, or not? (employers' association interviewee, Stanton 2000, p. 6).

To carry out policies that focus on long-term strategic development requires not only a new way of thinking, but also time and ability to focus on the future rather than just reacting to the present. Policies that focus on cost control and competition by their very nature focus on the short term. What is missing in the public health sector services is a longer-term perspective.

Working with people to achieve workplace reform

As well as the criticisms of the short-term focus of competitive policies there is also the question of the appropriateness of using industrial mechanisms as a means of reform in the public health care sector. Encouraging decentralised wage bargaining in public health care contains a number of fundamental problems.

The first problem relates to the relationship between the legal employer and the effective employer. As Fox argues (1998), in the public health sector, although the legal employer may be a hospital, the effective employer is the funding body; that is, government. She argues that he who pays the piper calls the tune. Through her analysis of five major industrial disputes in the health sector and the complex relationships between the employers and employees involved in the disputes and the government, Fox concludes that 'Centralised bargaining is inevitable when significant financial costs are involved and funding is controlled from a central source, the effective employer, as distinct from the legal employer, (Fox 1996, p. 27).

The question is, how much real control does the legal (the local) employer have over employment relations? When significant new costs are likely, for example, due to a wage demand, there will be pressure to involve the effective employer, the central government. Here lies another problem for government. Universal access to publicly funded health care is highly valued by the general public; if a government keeps out of the bargaining process but still controls the purse strings, it runs the risk of being forced to accept ultimate responsibility as the public comes to believe that the government, through its intransigence, is undermining their access to health care.

Another problem is the transaction costs in localised bargaining. Decentralisation is time consuming, complex, and can be wasteful; a number of health care managers believed that, under the Kennett government, they made few if any productivity gains (Stanton 2001b).

A final concern about enterprise bargaining as the avenue for workplace reform is that productivity bargaining focuses on enterprise and not on system problems. Kyle argues that:

> There is no way devolved processes, even at state level, can wholly or effectively address broader issues such as nurse labour force planning, portability of entitlements, national competency standards or qualitative and quantitative patient/client focused industry benchmarks and practice standards (Kyle 1993, p. 3).

Australia was not the only country experimenting with the decentralisation of industrial relations in health in the 1990s. In the United Kingdom the Conservative government commenced the decentralisation of the National Health Service through the establishment of hospitals as trusts. A key aim of the 1990 NHS Act, which established the trusts, was the encouragement of local pay determination and the creation of health care attendants, a new grade of staff whose pay was determined outside existing national arrangements (Thornley 1998). The logic behind this was that by bypassing national negotiating machinery, hospitals could gain greater control of labour costs and labour utilisation at the local level, with or without unions. Local bargaining largely failed; in 1997, only 11 per cent of nurses were on local contracts (Whitehead 1997). The Blair government has since returned to a system of national pay determination matched with local flexibility over human resource issues (Department of Health and Social Service 1997).

However, there are some advantages to decentralisation and managers: union officials in the Victorian study identified benefits such as greater flexibility of the process and the encouragement of employers to take responsibility for the management of their staff. Union officials also saw enterprise bargaining as an organising and marketing tool that increased their dialogue with members and gave their members more ownership of a claim (Stanton 2001c).

The fundamental industrial relations question here is the balance between central and local decision making. In the Victorian study there was a constant tension—in relation to changes in work practices—about how much can be changed centrally and how much needs to be changed locally. There was much discussion on the reality that, although as funder government has a fundamental role in setting wage levels in the industry, there are many issues that need to be resolved at a local level.

The election of the Bracks Labor government in Victoria in 1999 saw a return to centralised industrial relations in the Victorian health care sector. Employers in the Victorian study became concerned about the danger of inflexibility in a centralised system. They feared that agreements between central agencies might not relate to individual and local issues and problems, that this one-size-fits-all approach could squeeze out a lot of local initiative and local ability to achieve change. From the employers' perspective an example of this was the decision by the AIRC in 2000 regarding the reintroduction of centrally determined nurse:patient ratios. This decision has had a direct effect on employers and the government.

First, the AIRC decision was made at a time of an acute nursing labour shortage, which left the government and employers having to embark on an extensive recruitment and retraining strategy to meet the requirements of the ratio. Nurses are desperately needed, so the Bracks Labor government's campaign targeted the estimated 14 000 registered nurses who had left the public health system over the years (Davies 2001).

Second, it can be argued that this is exactly the kind of centralised decision-making process that undermines flexible labour utilisation in the workplace and does nothing to engage management and staff within the workplace to achieve a staffing profile that enhances service delivery.

One solution to deal with the central–local balance is to completely decouple wage determination from the enterprise bargaining process through a pay review board model for the industry-based wages and conditions alongside local bargaining on work practices and other issues. The advantage of this approach is that an independent body can deal with the difficult question of wages. The problem with this approach is that once pay and conditions are removed from a bargaining process there is little else for management to bargain with. Another solution is that each year in the funding round there could be an agreed additional amount of funding provided for wages, or wage increases, and then individual employers could negotiate with employees to work out how that should be put into practice at the local level.

However, the real difficulty is that wages in the health industry are inextricably bound up with conditions of employment, career structures, and so on, and it is not so easy to pull them apart. Also, as stated above, many of the problems regarding inflexibility in the health sector are system problems to do with professional regulations that cannot be bargained away in an industrial framework. These regulations are also integrally tied up with service delivery issues, so it might be that the most fruitful avenue of achieving change in work practices is to focus at the level of service delivery.

There is some room for optimism for such a focus. In the Victorian study (Stanton 2000) there was recognition by everyone interviewed that it was time for a change and a different approach to workplace reform. In particular, one view was that a move away from an emphasis on competition back to a collaborative approach was needed in the public health field. It was also felt that people in the health industry can and do adapt to change, as one of the representatives from the Department of Human Services (DHS) in the Victorian study (Stanton 2000, p. 13) stated:

> Industrial relations is made far more complex than it really needs to be. At the end of the day, people want reasonable conditions of employment, they want certainty, they want more money, of course, more money but they will allow some changes if it's skilfully handled.

The union officials interviewed (Stanton 2000) also supported this point; although they wanted a return to a greater centralisation of wages and conditions they also believed there was some room for local agreement making. They had a number of issues on their wish lists for improvement—benefits that the unions believed improved staff commitment and motivation. These included educational and professional development, better career opportunities, and more job security. Some union officials also emphasised that their members were interested not only in themselves but also in developing new ways of delivering care to people, particularly in rural areas, and giving a good standard of service to the community.

One departmental officer argued that Australia needs to have a vision for health care; the effect of a change of government in Victoria in 1999 presented a chance to take stock and 'change the emphasis, back towards community of interest, back towards service planning and away from whatever it was we went through, in terms of highly aggressive, competitive entities, each one doing its own thing and often a large scale removed from any sense of community' (Stanton 2000, p. 9).

Management and organisational theorists argue that, in order for any change to be effective, people need to feel in control of the process and involved in its planning and implementation. Research on clinicians and health reform in New South Wales, the United Kingdom and New Zealand found increased enthusiasm for their work in hospital specialists who were involved in management decision-making processes, but decreased enthusiasm in hospital specialists who felt excluded from the process yet still had to work within restrictions on resources (Perkins et al. 1997).

One HR director in the Victorian study (Stanton 2000) described how attempts to bring in change often met with passive resistance from both management and staff, who felt that they had been through this before. People felt that change had been done to them, not with them. Alexander (2000, p. 173) argues that successful engagement of clinicians in health sector reform needs a change in culture in many institutions and that hospitals with a 'them and us' culture will not survive in a rapidly changing environment. An approach that focuses on involving people in different ways of doing things can be more effective than bargaining over incentives. For example, one HR director (Stanton 2000, p. 11) suggested that: 'If you can get people to actually decide to deal with each other as individuals who have a mutual interest in achieving something you might end up with a fundamental basic change in attitudes.' He believed that exploring continuums of care for people and focusing on patient outcomes as opposed to health industry inputs as the appropriate measures was a more appropriate strategy for reform. Practitioners then started to focus on the end result; that is, the outcome for the patient.

> Once they really start to look at that they really need to look at a whole spectrum of things from how they're treated in the community through to how they get treatment in a hospital or post-hospital and it doesn't, if you think beyond it, that depends not on nursing care or doctor care, it depends on how the patients get treated and perhaps we need to concentrate on that issue, rather than just my small professional sector of that (Stanton 2000, p. 11).

In 1993 Marilyn Beaumont, the ANF's federal secretary, argued that nursing was already looking at efficiency and effectiveness in service delivery. She pointed to the potential of a Keating Labor government initiative, the Best Practice in Health Program, which she believed encouraged people to work together. 'The Best Practice Program is about those in the workplace agreeing on what needs to change and all sharing the benefits arising from that change' (Beaumont 1993, p. 18).

Developments in best practice are good examples of engaging clinicians in focusing on improvements in patient care that can lead to work practice reform. Also, by focusing on outcomes for patients, professionals can be encouraged to work more collaboratively and overcome barriers at the local level in a manner that can never be achieved at a central level. However, to take such an approach needs time, resources, goodwill, and the removal of incentives that encourage perverse outcomes—all of which need commitment and support by both state and Commonwealth governments.

Conclusion

The public health sector workforce is such a large component of costs in the public health sector that any attempt at health sector reform will have a major impact on the workforce. Also, the changing nature of the health sector means that workplace reform is inevitable and necessary. Australian governments do not have a comprehensive approach to workplace reform in the sector. Instead, they have utilised industrial reform and competitive and cost-focused policies that do not take into account the special features of the sector and the people who work within it.

Such policies, while having some benefits in forcing change into the industry and improving measured productivity in the short term, lead in the long term to other problems, including work intensification, labour shortages, and the undermining of commitment and trust.

An approach that focuses on the best outcomes for patients is needed and the way to do this is to encourage staff to work together. Drawing on their knowledge and expertise can lead to collaborative change. While this approach can only be achieved at the local level, it has to be recognised and supported at the central level by governments that can provide the necessary resources and encourage organisations to take the time to develop this approach. Governments can also focus on the removal of perverse incentives within their policies and create an environment in which best practice is not only valued but also shared throughout the industry.

References

Alexander, J. 2000, 'The Changing Role of Clinicians: Their Role in Health Reform in Australia and New Zealand', in A. L. Bloom (ed.), *Health Reform in Australia and New Zealand*, Oxford University Press, Melbourne.

Alford, J. & O'Neil, D. (eds) 1994, *The Contract State: Public Management and the Kennett Government*, Deakin University, Centre for Applied Social Research, Melbourne.

Allan, C. 1998, 'The Elasticity of Endurance: Work Intensification and Workplace Flexibility in the Queensland Public Hospital System', *New Zealand Journal of Industrial Relations*, vol. 23, no. 3, pp. 131–51.

—— O'Donnell, M., & Peetz, D. 1999, 'More Tasks, Less Secure, Working Harder: Three Dimensions of Labour Utilisation', *Journal of Industrial Relations*, vol. 41, no. 4, December, pp. 519–35.

Australian Bureau of Statistics 1999, *Employee Earnings and Benefits and Trade*, ABS, Canberra.

—— 2000, *Union Membership*, ABS, Canberra.

Australian Hospital Association 1993, *Reform in the Health Workplace*, Proceedings from the AHA Industrial Relations Seminar, 23 September, Australian Hospital Association, Canberra.

Australian Institute of Health and Welfare 1998a, *Australian Hospital Statistics 1996–97*, AIHW, Canberra.

—— 1998b, *Australia's Health 1998: Sixth Biennial Health Report of the Australian Institute of Health and Welfare*, AIHW, Canberra.

Australian Nursing Federation 1992, 'Federal Award Decision for Victorian Nurses', *Australian Nursing Journal*, vol. 22, no. 3, September, pp. 6–7.

Barraclough, S. & Smith, J. 1994, 'Change of Government and Health Service Policy in Victoria 1992–3', *Australian Health Review*, vol. 17, no. 4, pp. 7–21.

Beaumont, M. 1993, 'Enterprise Bargaining and the Nursing Industry', *Australian Nursing Journal*, vol. 22, no. 11, June, pp. 17–18.

Blake, N. 1997, 'Awards on the Blink', *Australian Nursing Journal*, vol. 5, no. 3, September, pp. 19–22.

Braithwaite, J. 1997, *Workplace Industrial Relations in the Australian Hospital Sector*, Studies in Health Service Administration, No. 80, University of New South Wales, School of Health Services Management, Sydney.

—— & Hindle, D. 1998, 'Casemix Funding in Australia: Time for a Rethink', *Medical Journal of Australia*, vol. 168, pp. 558–60.

Bremner, J. & Kelly, R. 2000, 'The Medical Scientists' Association of Victoria: A Case Study of Professional Trade Unionism in the 1990s', in G. Griffin (ed.), *Trade Unions 2000: Retrospect and Prospect*, Monograph No. 14, National Key Centre in Industrial Relations, Monash University, Melbourne.

Considine, G. & Buchanan, J. 1999, *The Hidden Costs of Understaffing: An Analysis of Contemporary Nurses' Working Conditions in Victoria*, Australian Centre for Industrial Relations Research and Training, University of Sydney, Sydney.

Creighton, B. & Stewart, A. 2000, *Labour Law: An Introduction*, 3rd edn, Federation Press, Sydney.

Dabscheck, B. 1995, *The Struggle for Australian Industrial Relations*, Oxford University Press, Melbourne.

Davies, J. 2001, 'Numbers Up as Strategy Cuts in', *Age*, Melbourne, 7 April.

Davis, A. 1995, 'Managerialised Health Care', in S. Rees & G. Rodley (eds), *The Human Costs of Managerialism*, Pluto Press, Leichhardt, NSW.

Dawson, S. & Dargie, C. 1999, 'New Public Management: An Assessment and Evaluation with Special Reference to UK Health', *Public Management: An International Journal of Research and Theory*, vol. 1, no. 4, pp. 459–81.

Department of Health and Social Service 1997, *The New National Health Service*, Government Stationery Office, London.

Draper, M. 1992, *Casemix, Quality and Consumers*, Health Issues Centre, Melbourne.

Duckett, S. J. 1995, 'Hospital Payment Arrangements to Encourage Efficiency: The Case of Victoria, Australia', *Health Policy*, 34, pp. 113–34.

Fox, C. 1996, *Enterprise Bargaining and Health Services: A Special Case?*, National Key Centre in Industrial Relations, Melbourne.

—— 1998, 'Collective Bargaining and Essential Services: The Australian Case', *Journal of Industrial Relations*, vol. 40, no. 2, June, pp. 277–303.

Gardner, H. 1995, 'Interest Groups and the Political Process', in H. Gardner (ed.), *The Politics of Health*, 2nd edn, Churchill Livingstone, Melbourne.

—— & McCoppin, B. 1995, 'Struggle for Survival by Health Therapists, Nurses and Medical Scientists', in H. Gardner (ed.), *The Politics of Health*, 2nd edn, Churchill Livingstone, Melbourne.

Gardner, P. 1994, 'Full Bench Rejects Victorian Government Attempt to Cancel Nurses' Federal Award', *Australian Nursing Journal*, vol. 1, no. 7, February, p. 21.

Gunderson, M. 1982, 'Health Sector Labour Market: Canada, USA and UK', in A. S. Sethi & S. Dimmock (eds), *Industrial Relations and Health Services*, Croome Helm, London.

Harkness, A. 1999, 'Prognosis Negative: Health Care Economics and the Kennett Government', in B. Costar & N. Economou (eds), *The Kennett Revolution*, University of New South Wales Press, Sydney.

Harrison, S. & Pollitt, C. 1994, *Controlling Health Professionals*, Open University Press, Buckingham.

High Court of Victoria 1995, 'Re Australian Education Union and Others; Ex Parte the State of Victoria and Another, CLR 1994–1995', vol. 184–8, High Court of Victoria, Melbourne.

Hughes, A. 1993, 'Budget Strain: The Pressure Increases', *Report of the Victorian Hospitals' Association*, No. 40, April, Melbourne.

Kearney, B. & Whitfield, J. 1991, *Review of Pathology Services in Inner North and West Melbourne*, Health Department Victoria, Melbourne.

Kyle, F. 1993, 'Productivity Bargaining in the '90s: Seeing the Forest or the Trees?', *Australian Nursing Journal*, vol. 1, no. 3, September, p. 3.

Lin, V. & Duckett, S. 1997, 'Structural Interests and Organisational Dimensions of System Reform', in H. Gardner (ed.), *Health Policy in Australia*, Oxford University Press, Melbourne.

Minogue, K. 1993, 'Health Funding Changes Spell Disaster for Victoria', *Australian Nursing Journal*, vol. 1, no. 1, July, p. 12.

O'Brien, J. 1997, 'Occupational and Professional Identity as an Industrial Strategy in the New Zealand State Sector', *Journal of Industrial Relations*, vol. 39, no. 4, December, pp. 499–517.

O'Neil, D. 1999, ' "The Quiet Revolution": Public Service Reform in the Kennett Era', in B. Costar & N. Economou (eds), *The Kennett Revolution*, University of New South Wales Press, Sydney.

Osborne, D. & Gaebler, T. 1992, *Reinventing Government*, Addison Wesley, Massachusetts.

Peacock, S. 1997, 'The UK Experience of a Managed Competition Environment', *Healthcover*, vol. 7, no. 4, pp. 53–5.

Perkins, R., Petria, K., Alley, P., Barnes, P., Fisher, M. & Hatfield, P. 1997, 'Health Service Reform: The Perceptions of Medical Specialists in Australia (New South Wales), the United Kingdom and New Zealand', *Medical Journal of Australia*, vol. 167, pp. 201–4.

Phillips Fox & Casemix Consulting 1999, *Health Services Policy Review*, Victorian Department of Human Services, Melbourne.

Southon, G. & Braithwaite, J. 1998, 'The End of Professionalism', *Social Science and Medicine*, vol. 46, no. 1, pp. 23–8.

Stanton, P. 2000, 'Valuing the Intangible: Building Trust and Commitment in the Public Health Sector', Paper presented to *Trust in the Workplace: Beyond the Quick-fix*, University of Newcastle, Newcastle.

—— 2001a, 'Competitive Health Policies and Community Health', *Social Science and Medicine*, vol. 52, no. 5, pp. 671–9.

—— 2001b, 'Enterprise Bargaining in the Victorian Public Hospital System 1992–99', Crossing Borders, 15th AIRAANZ Conference, Association of Industrial Relations Academics of Australia and New Zealand, Wollongong.

—— 2001c, 'The Impact of Enterprise Bargaining on Trade Union Organisation and Membership in the Victorian Public Health Sector 1992–99', Ten Years of Enterprise Bargaining, 3 and 4 May, University of Newcastle, Newcastle.

Teicher, J. & Gramberg, B. V. 1999, ' "Economic freedom": Industrial Relations Policy under the Kennett Government', in B. Costar & N. Economou (eds), *The Kennett Revolution*, University of New South Wales Press, Sydney.

Thornley, C. 1998, 'Contesting Local Pay: The Decentralisation of Collective Bargaining in the NHS', *British Journal of Industrial Relations*, vol. 36, no. 3, pp. 413–34.

Twaddle, A. 1996, 'Health Systems Reforms: Toward a Framework for International Comparisons', *Social Science and Medicine*, vol. 43, no. 5, pp. 637–54.

Victorian Hospitals' Association 1992, *Report of the Victorian Hospitals' Association*, November/December, Victorian Hospitals' Association, No. 92.

Weekes, K., Peterson, C., & Stanton, P. 2001, 'Stress and the Workplace: The Medical Scientists' Experience', *Labour and Industry*, vol. 11, no. 3, April, pp. 95–120.

Whitehead, M. 1997, 'NHS Trusts "abandon" Local Pay Bargaining', *People Management*, vol. 3, no. 19, September, p. 25.

Wooden, M. 2000, *The Transformation of Australian Industrial Relations*, Federation Press, Sydney.

Young, S. 2001, 'Outsourcing in the Public Hospital Sector', in D. Kelly (ed.), *Crossing Borders: Employment, Work, Markets and Social Justice Across Time, Discipline and Place*, Proceedings of the 15th AIRAANZ Conference, Association of Industrial Relations Academics of Australia and New Zealand, Wollongong.

10

Globalisation, Complementary Medicine, and Australian Health Policy: The Role of Consumerism

Heather Eastwood

The road to regulatory reform in the area of complementary medicines started with consumer demand.

Senator Grant Tambling, 28 April 1999 (Tambling 1999e)

This chapter deals with consumerism and its influence on structural change in the Australian health system. It examines the ways in which Australian consumer demand for complementary medicine (CM) has influenced national health policy reform, service provision, tertiary education, research priorities, and industry. Exploring the phenomenon of consumerism within a globalised, market-based economic system, the chapter uses the burgeoning of CM in Australia as a case study to illustrate the power of consumerism to effect social change. Worldwide, CM is a multibillion dollar industry. Even in Australia, which constitutes only about 2 per cent of the world economy, CM accounts for some $2 billion annually (MacLennan 2000).

Consideration of consumerism involves the economic, cultural, and political implications of globalisation. The paradoxes inherent in globalisation and the changing nature of governmental policymaking under globalised market economies are problematic. On the one hand, consumerism is the driving force of globalised capitalism, producing a market that promotes commodification and consumption. As an ideology, consumerism is underpinned by consumer choice, rights, and empowerment, which some writers argue creates an allegiance to capitalism that increasingly displaces the notion of political citizenship (Yeatman 1998; Hancock 1999a). On the other hand, because consumerism is underpinned by the notion of individual rights, other writers regard consumerism as the basis of a social movement that encourages equality and social justice, which is quite contrary to capitalism (Niva 1992; Irving 1999). Accordingly, this chapter explores the concept of consumerism within the broader context of globalisation and the shift in late Western societies towards neoliberal government and New Right thinking which, *inter alia*, encourage market reforms in health care. It then examines the market-dominated health reform agenda of the current Australian Liberal–National Coalition government and uses CM as a case study to examine consumerism as the marketing of health.

The Australian government's rationale for health policy reforms in CM emphasises consumer choice and empowerment by promoting increased knowledge, product safety, and proven efficacy through government regulation of industry. These reforms assume the desirability of individuals taking greater responsibility for their own health. This chapter argues, however, that CM reforms are part of a broader economic rationalist agenda in health care to shift health care costs back to the consumer and thereby achieve economic efficiency in the health care system. CM as a case study shows how 'health reform is now one of the principal avenues redefining the boundaries between states, markets, and civil society' (Drache & Sullivan 1999, p. 5).

Consumer use of complementary medicine in Australia

Australian trends in CM are similar to those in other Western countries, such as the USA, the UK, and Canada. These trends include
- increased consumer demand for CM
- increasing provision of CM by orthodox medical practitioners
- increasing government regulation of CM and its practitioners
- increased tertiary education in CM
- moves towards a stronger scientific research base for CM.

As in other Western countries, the term CM covers both products and therapies. The products include vitamins, minerals, herbs based on naturally occurring substances, and therapies such as chiropractic, acupuncture, naturopathy, homoeopathy, and aromatherapy (Tambling 1999a).

Government estimates indicate that over 60 per cent of Australians use CM, that one in two Australians use at least one nonmedically prescribed CM, and that one in five Australians visit at least one CM practitioner a year (Wooldridge 1998). Currently, researchers estimate that Australians are spending $2 billion annually on CM, about two-thirds of that amount on complementary medicines and one-third on practitioners (MacLennan 2000).

The reasons for the exponential growth of CM in Australia and other Western countries are poorly understood. A review of studies on Australian use of CM (Eastwood & Correa 2000) found that people resort to CM for various reasons, including the failure of conventional biomedical treatment to alleviate symptoms or cure disease and an increasing attraction to holistic disease prevention, whereby health is viewed as entailing a continuum of mind, body, and spirit. Many consumers see prevention and self-help strategies as more compatible with the holistic health model that informs CM than with the biomedical model, which relies on disease management rather than prevention. Moreover, according to the Australian government, Australians are increasingly prepared to assume responsibility for their own health (Tambling 1999b). Demographically, the most prominent CM users in Australia are middle-class, educated women (MacLennan 2000).

Australian consumer interest in CM is often attributed to our ageing population and an increase in lifestyle and chronic diseases that seem unresponsive to biomedicine. With the advent of the Internet and the proliferation of consumer advocacy groups—for example, the Australian Complementary Health Association (ACHA)—the Australian public is confronted with a welter of health choices in which CM is prominent.

Reasons for CM use canvassed in the literature are associated with lifestyle factors, including a consumer attraction to holistic health practices. These practices emphasise natural medicines, self-responsibility for health, and a holistic view of the body (Eastwood & Correa 2000).

The increasing popularity of CM among Australians has also been associated with the effects of globalisation (Bensoussan 1999; Eastwood 2000a). In Western countries, the small-planet syndrome has enhanced ecological awareness as well as appreciation of nonWestern cultures, including their traditional, eco-friendly health practices, which eschew synthetic pharmaceuticals and invasive surgery. Moreover, through economic globalisation, the market is promoting and selling CM to Australian consumers (Eastwood & Correa 2000). Internationally, the market in complementary medical products is growing at a rate of more than 15 per cent each year. Surveys indicate that Australians spend more on complementary medicines than on pharmaceutical medications (MacLennan 1996).

Globalisation and definitions of consumerism

Globalisation processes

Globalisation is commonly defined as the shrinking-planet phenomenon, caused by advances in transportation and communications and by increasing ecological and economic interdependence, encouraging the perception that the world is but a single—albeit very large and complex—community (Eastwood 2000a). Waters (1994, pp. 230–1) identifies three dimensions of globalisation: economic, cultural, and political. Consumerism is a significant aspect of all three dimensions of globalisation. The following sections discuss the role of consumerism in each of these dimensions.

Economic globalisation and consumerism

Economic globalisation is associated with the ascendancy of deregulated markets in international trade and investment, and with the philosophy of neoliberalism that applauds the self-interest of market-based economies (McMichael & Beaglehole 2000). Janes (1999) attributes the influence of economic globalisation and neoliberal policy on health to an influential World Bank report, *Investing in Health* (World Bank 1993), which argued for a cost-efficacy approach to health services as commodities relegated to the market sector (Janes 1999, p. 1808). McMichael and Beaglehole (2000, p. 495) note the mixed impact of globalisation on public health. On the one hand, they note that economic globalisation has encouraged the growth and dissemination of technologies, which, they argue, has widely extended life expectancy. On the other hand, they note that aspects of globalisation are jeopardising health by eroding social and environmental conditions, widening the divide between rich and poor, and disseminating consumerism.

Within the context of economic globalisation, consumerism is widely regarded as the driving force of late capitalism. Sklair (1994, p. 95) argues that consumerism is the 'culture-ideology' of global capitalism whereby

> consumerism serves the interests of the global capitalist system, engaged in increasing the consumption of the products of capitalist enterprise through the profit maximising practices of each individual unit to the system as a whole, irrespective of the consequences upon the planet in which it is located.

Further to his argument, Sklair (1994, p. 96) points out that consumerism is based on induced wants; that is, 'the creation of an inducement of an almost limitless variety of wants, as opposed to needs', creating a culture of consumption in advanced Western societies (see also Featherstone 1991).

Commodification is a central characteristic of the culture of consumption and of global capitalism. Harvey (1998) describes commodification as the extension of capitalist rationality and profit motive into more areas of personal and social life and into more regions of the globe. In particular, globalisation theorists note the relationship between global capitalism, cultural change, and commodification. For example, Robertson (1992) argues that global cultural trends, such as the return to place, indigeneity, tradition, nature, and forms of the sacred, are commercialised and sold in the marketplace. Many of these cultural trends are a rejection of secular modernity that are, paradoxically, simply marketed by the global capitalist system, itself an outcome of modernity.

Cultural globalisation and consumerism

Closely linked to economic globalisation is cultural globalisation, a phenomenon that intertwines Western and nonWestern cultures and societies. Writers such as Waters (1996) characterise this phenomenon humorously as Americanisation, McDonaldisation or Coca-colonisation. Other writers (for example, Robertson 1992) note the reciprocal influence of non-Western cultures upon Western societies. These trends include

- a return to nature, particularly in response to the ecological crises
- a resurgence of the sacred, often involving New Age or Eastern religions
- a return to tradition and indigeneity, evidenced, for example, by the increasing use of traditional medicines.

Robertson (1992), Featherstone (1991), and others note that cultural trends are commodified in a consumer-driven global capitalism. For example, Crook, Pakulski, and Waters (1992) argue that these trends are being commodified in a postFordist capitalism that aggressively markets environmentally friendly goods, traditional health practices, and New Age products (see also Robertson 1992; Lash & Urry 1994). Consumer culture, according to Waters (1996), accompanies globalisation and exhibits a diversity of cultural forms, preferences, and experiences, as do, for example, the global commodification of tourism, exotic food, and multicultural entertainment. As a result, a welter of choices becomes available to consumers in Western cultures. An outcome of this is the expectation that the individual in consumer culture will exercise their choice by purchasing an ever-widening variety of products (Waters 1996).

Waters (1996, p. 15) notes that the globalisation of consumer culture has paradoxical effects, in that the commodification of culture is 'simultaneously homogenising and differentiating'. Thus, in Western societies, there is a proliferation of choices, but increasingly the same choices become available to everyone (assuming they have enough money). The result is a homogenisation of choice, creating the experience of conformity amid the appearance of diversity. Waters (1996, p. 13) sums up such homogenising trends with the phrase 'consumer global culture.' As noted above, these popular terms can obscure the fact that Eastern options are also becoming more widely available in the West. Increasingly, consumers in Tokyo, Delhi, Sydney, Beijing, and Chicago face the same array of options; increasingly, too, even as each place changes, every place starts to look and feel the same.

In response to the sameness created by global consumerism, consumerism itself by default becomes the primary medium through which people attempt to create individual and group identity (Miles 1996).

Consumerism as understood within the context of consumer culture is thus characterised by identity creation through the pursuit of lifestyle options. Cultural consumption and the cultivation of particular lifestyles go hand in hand (Featherstone 1991), even as real variation among lifestyles declines as a direct result of the commodification of culture. According to Robertson (1992), 'identity declarations' are inherent in the general process of globalisation, with globalising cultural trends resulting in identity crises and, in turn, identity reformation. Many theorists argue that this phenomenon results from the uncertainties inherent in the new global economy—for example, uncertainties arising from deregulation and the demise of welfare capitalism (Beck 1992; Turner 1995). Whatever its causes, there is widespread recognition of a pervasive cultural alienation that is simultaneously brought about by economic globalisation and combated through it by attempting to purchase identity.

In addition, cultural commodification and consumerism have spawned new perceptions of the relationship between the body and self (Featherstone 1991). In late modernity, advertising, health, and lifestyle literature emphasise body maintenance, holistic health, and the enhancement of the inner self through, for example, meditation and relaxation, and the use of holistic products such as herbs, vitamins, and mineral supplements. Featherstone (1991) claims that these types of activities are bringing about a change in the moral climate, so that individuals are assuming more active concern and responsibility for their health, happiness, and appearance.

These become moral issues when one accepts that one has only oneself to blame for inadequacies in any of these aspects of body and self. Once, this mindset was characterised as blaming the patient for their illness. Increasingly and subtly, the mindset is becoming one of blaming the consumer for their failure—or inability—to access the remedial options available in the marketplace.

Historically, consumerism as a lifestyle originated in the age of affluence that began in the USA with the end of the Second World War. At this time, retailing analyst Victor Lebow declared, 'Our enormously productive economy ... demands that we make consumption our way of life, that we convert the buying and use of goods into rituals, that we seek our spiritual satisfaction, our ego satisfaction, in consumption. We need things consumed, burnt up, worn out, and discarded at an ever increasing rate' (in Sklair 1995, p. 87).

The close relationship between market and culture supports Sklair's notion of consumerism as the culture ideology of capitalism. In late capitalism, consumerism both promotes and is conditioned by cultural homogeneity and cultural heterogeneity (Robertson 1992). The production and consolidation of difference and variety is an essential ingredient of contemporary capitalism, which itself becomes the connective tissue and final arbiter underlying cultural diversity across the globe. In the past, empires attempted to mediate and manage diversity through centralisation. Now, all roads lead to the bank, and the sun never sets on the global market. Transnational corporations, through globalisation processes, have begun to supersede nation states, rendering their boundaries less relevant. As a result, writers such as Yeatman (1998) and Hancock (1999a, b) argue that democracy and fundamental citizenship rights are under threat from global capitalism.

Political globalisation and consumerism

As the preceding discussion implies, consumerism can be viewed politically, either as a form of allegiance to capitalism or as informing consumer movements that challenge the inequalities inherent in capitalism. The discourse of consumerism imparts a political dimension to both capitalism and consumer movements that rely on an ideology espousing consumer choice and rights. Feldberg and Vipond (1999) and others (Yeatman 1998; Hancock 1999a) argue that consumer rights are overriding citizenship rights, whereby the market displaces the state. Feldberg and Vipond (1999, p. 48) further note that: 'Consumerism is a symptom of the crises of citizenship, with most political rhetoric addressing the electorate not as citizens but as consumers, as if the market were determining the very language of political community.'

Miller (1993) also highlights the potential for contradiction in the concept of 'capitalist democracy'. Capitalism encourages people to behave in ways that will maximise their individual wealth and consumption, while democracy urges people to give selflessly to their community, to participate for the public good. The two messages create tension in contemporary society, where, according to Miller (1993), the idea of citizen as activist, campaigner, or lobbyist has been replaced with the notion that the consumer discharges these traditional roles of citizenship. Therefore, consumerism as a behaviour that seeks maximum acquisition—the culture-ideology of capitalism—conflicts with consumerism as a political ideology that seeks to address and protect individual rights. The rhetoric of consumerism as a political ideology thereby goes against the fundamental characteristics of capitalism, manipulation of markets, and consequent inequality driven by the profit motive, and goes against those of consumerism as a culture-ideology espousing consumption, commodification, and acquisition of wealth and products.

Thus, consumerism can be viewed as a dissident political discourse that empowers consumer movements to challenge market power (Niva 1992).

Arguably, consumer movements can be viewed as new social movements in which consumers are mobilised through seeking consumer rights, satisfaction, and participation in decision and policy making. Through these movements, consumers become political as well as economic actors, thus shifting the focus from the economic attributes of consumerism to its social and political attributes (Irvine 1999). The new social movements provide a further political dimension to globalisation, with writers identifying the feminist, environmental, peace, human rights, and AIDS movements as globalising forces (Crook et al. 1992; Giddens 1991, 1994).

The addition of consumer movements to the ranks of the so-called new social movements serves to illustrate the paradoxes inherent in globalisation, which on the one hand encourages economic rationalism, but on the other hand creates sentiments that are value-based rather than market-based (Crook et al. 1992; Giddens 1991, 1994). Values of social justice, empowerment, and equity of access are espoused by consumer movements as consumer rights, but access to the global market entails access to goods of ideologically dubious origin, for example, exploited developing- world labour or ecologically damaging manufacturing (McKay 1995).

To summarise, the political dimension of consumerism, as analogous to citizenship, creates a tension with traditional notions of citizenship entailing rights and responsibilities in a state. Numerous sociological theories address this tension. Among these theories, however, the fundamental question remains: Does capitalism serve consumers or vice versa? In the present political climate of neoliberalism and globalisation, there is a tendency in late Western societies to avoid this question by adopting small government— government that is content to regulate without controlling the free rein of the market. Even education, the *sine qua non* of equal opportunity, is increasingly regarded as a commodity for sale in the global market. Health care, however, as the very bedrock of social justice, remains somewhat sacred; while not immune to the effects of economic globalisation, it provides a unique window upon the tensions and interactions among the economic, cultural, and political aspects of globalisation and consumerism.

According to Feldberg and Vipond (1999), the global restructuring of health care employs and invokes consumerism and consumerist models. Irving (1999, p. 90) astutely points out that the motive force behind market reforms in health is 'an intense focus not simply on "consumer interests" but on the management of health care costs and the related demand for greater economic efficiency within the health care sphere'.

Chernichovsky characterises consumer satisfaction and consumer choice as key features in an emerging paradigm for health system reform in industrialised countries where, despite the wide variety of health care systems in industrialized democracies, a universal paradigm for financing, organization, and macromanagement has been emerging through reforms of the past decade. The policies within this paradigm attempt to promote equity, social efficiency, and consumer satisfaction by combining the advantages of public finance principles—universal access and control of spending—with the advantages of competitive market principles—consumer satisfaction and internal efficiency. This paradigm is characterized by three systemic functions: (1) financing of care, based on public finance principles, not necessarily carried out by government; (2) organization and management of publicly funded care consumption by either competing nongovernmental entities or noncompeting public administrations; and (3) provision of care based on competitive market principles. The institutional arrangement of these functions lends itself to the creation of two internal markets for consumer choice and, of the three [systemic functions]; the second function is a key component of the emerging paradigm (Chernichovsky, 1995, p. 339).

Globalisation, consumerism, and health market reforms in Australia

Contemporary health care reforms in developed countries such as Australia are based on both a new managerialism, involving a shift towards entrepreneurial management and a push for contractualism and privatisation, and the marketisation of health, involving market principles aimed at ensuring efficient resource allocation and consumer choice (Hancock 1999b). These reforms are part of the market state and can be located within the ideological context of neoliberalism and economic rationalism. According to Hancock (1999b), the shift to entrepreneurial government and the market state draws on the dominant paradigm of economic rationalism and neoliberal forms of governance that illustrate Australia's interconnectedness to similar global shifts and reforms, particularly in New Zealand, Canada, the USA, and the UK.

An outcome of market reforms in health has been a shift in emphasis and power from provider to consumer. Consideration of consumer rights and consumer choice underlies current health policy, which is informed by the market model. According to information provided in the Commonwealth government publication *Reforming the Australian Health Care System: The Role of Government* (Department of Health and Aged Care 1999), consumer rights and consumer choice are the market forces that provide the impetus for a shift in focus from providers to consumers in the Australian health system.

According to this document, the shift in focus from providers to consumers entails the following points.

- The system is increasingly dedicated to patients rather than providers.
- A patient focus offers an opportunity to measure and monitor what the system provides for consumers in terms of quality of health care and outcomes.
- Empowering patients with information to inform choice will encourage rational decision making and partnership between doctor and patient.
- Consumer democracy in health care guarantees reforms in the system that will be soundly based.
- The shift from providers to consumers is potentially a better means to control costs, particularly through better management of chronic conditions (Department of Health and Aged Care 1999).

The market reforms in progress focus on increased competition and consumer choice as a means of promoting efficiency. In the past, the medical profession has determined the supply of health services. Now, consumerism, weighing in on the demand side of health service, is a market force that has increasing wherewithal to influence supply factors. As theorised previously, consumerism drives the logic of global capitalism, with the concomitant commodification of traditional health practices and medicines, and the sale of natural remedies and holistic health practices as part and parcel of lifestyle choices and identity formation. Like any other commodity, health becomes a service to be bought and sold, and is subject to market rules and discipline (Drache & Sullivan 1999). Also, consumers are theorised not only as economic and social actors, but also as political actors in a market state that is displacing citizenship rights with consumer rights. Nevertheless, writers such as Hancock (1999a) have argued that because health is recognised as a fundamental human right, health debates should be framed within the context of citizenship rights rather than of consumer rights. The former provides a more accountable framework within which to address issues of equality and social justice, while a global market that encourages consumers to exercise their rights by voting with their credit cards governs the latter.

The following sections examine the proliferation of CM in an Australian case study that illustrates the economic, cultural, and political power of consumerism—as the culture-ideology of capitalism—to bring about health policy reform and structural changes in service provision, education, research, and industry. As Hancock (1999a, p. 4) points out,

> Structural changes to the public sector, the blurring of public and private sectors and the dominance of the market transpose new issues onto ongoing ones of power and interests in relation to health policy, traditional relationships within hospitals and medical encounters, and in relation to access, equity, rights and citizenship.

Australian government responses and structural change

Complementary medicine consumerism

Australian government responses to the exponential increase in consumer use of CM include policy reforms and new legislation, with concomitant structural changes in education, service provision, industry, and research capacity. Analysis of policy responses from government support the contention that consumerism is the economic driver for CM health policy reforms in Australia. Clearly, the government rationale for these reforms is market based and aimed at placating both consumers and industry.

A review of Commonwealth government media releases and ministerial speeches reveals the prominence of the role of consumerism in the introduction of a raft of CM reforms in the Australian health care system. In 1996, recognition of the extent of consumer use of CM led the Australian government to hold the country's first National Alternative Medicines Summit in Canberra. The then Parliamentary Secretary for Health, Senator Bob Woods, noted that the government could no longer ignore the increased consumer demand for alternative medicine, now a billion–dollar industry in Australia alone (*Integrative Medicine Association Newsletter* 1996).

Responses to the growing popularity of CM have led the federal government to introduce policy initiatives, that it claims will provide consumers with safe health choices through regulation of the CM industry. Government speeches on CM reforms incorporate frequent reference to the ideal of choice in health care, as exemplified in the address of the then Minister for Health and Aged Care, Dr Michael Wooldridge, at the launch of the Southern Cross University Natural and Complementary Medicine Teaching Clinic. 'I have worked hard as Australia's Health Minister to support the right of Australians to freely choose natural therapies as a complement to conventional medicine and to ensure that the choice of health care remain as wide as possible while delivery remains as safe as possible ... I am working to make health a safer choice' (Wooldridge 1998).

References to consumer choice are prominent in the government's rationale for CM reforms, which, according to Senator Tambling, the Parliamentary Secretary to the Minister for Health (1999d), 'acknowledge the choice of a growing number of Australians to use complementary medicines in their health care and to ensure the continued safety of products'. It is inescapable that consumer choice is a dominant market force driving health reform in Western industrialised countries. It is equally obvious that consumerism is a major driver of global capitalism (Sklair 1994; Harvey 1998). As a consequence, the Australian government identifies consumer choice as a market mechanism impelling a shift of attention from providers to consumers in the Australian health system.

Health reforms in Australia claim to promote not only consumer choice but also insurance of safe choices. In the same speech as the one just quoted, the Minister for Health (Wooldridge 1998) emphasised consumer safety and product efficacy, proclaiming that,

> At the end of the day, finding safe and effective ways to treat sickness and pro-
> mote good health are all goals that every health practitioner is working towards
> … We have made a strong commitment to ensuring that any proposed remedy
> or drug is tested and shown on the basis of clinical evidence to work and be safe
> and have shown we are open to examining remedies that have traditionally
> fallen under the umbrella of natural therapies.

Government consideration of consumer choice—and directly consequent of the risks associated with CM—have led to regulatory reform, specifically through the creation of the Office for Complementary Medicine within the Therapeutic Goods Administration (TGA). Although complementary medi-cine is now a major part of the Australian health care industry, the government is demanding more evidence from CM suppliers regarding quality, safety, and efficacy (Therapeutic Goods Administration 1999).

In 1999, Senator Tambling claimed that

> while many countries around the world are struggling to balance the burdens of
> regulation and the obligation to safeguard consumer confidence in medicines,
> new Australian complementary medicines legislation strikes the right balance
> and will be a model for regulation of complementary medicines in other parts
> of the world.

He argued further that 'the new legislation shows that industry, consumers and the government can work together to enhance the health choices available to all Australians' (Tambling 1999c).

The Australian government's response to the CM industry has involved several policy reforms, notably including the establishment of an Office of Complementary Medicines within the TGA to regulate CM and to moni-tor its successes and adverse effects, and the establishment of a number of committees within the Office of Complementary Medicine—for example, the Complementary Healthcare Council of Australia and the Complemen-tary Healthcare Consultative Forum—to oversee regulation and reform.

The Commonwealth government's establishment of the Office of Complementary Medicines is a clear response to consumer demand. The government has undertaken that 'consumers will not be put at risk by com-plementary health products, will have access to information about these products, and will not be misled by promises made about the therapeutic benefits of these products' (Tambling 1999e). As Senator Tambling (1999e) noted in his opening speech for the launch of the Office of Complementary Medicines: 'Consumers demand of government a high degree of safety and confidence in the marketing approval process ... Consumers will not forgive a government that breaches its obligations to maintain optimal standards of public health and safety.' CM reforms include more accurate labelling to reflect increasing scientific evidence regarding CM, advertising restrictions on CM manufacturers, and requirements for reporting adverse effects of CM.

However, the government is also quick to recognise that complementary health care is a growth industry (Tambling 1999f), so has established committees such as the Complementary Medicines Evaluation Committee (CMEC) and the Complementary Healthcare Council of Australia (CHCA) to represent an important cross-section of industry, including manufacturers, suppliers, retailers, consultants, health care professionals, practitioner associations, and health patients and users. Government publications indicate that, through these types of reform measures, 'the Government wants to ensure that industry is not weighed down by unnecessary or lengthy approval processes, which might put Australia at a competitive disadvantage with the rest of the world' (Tambling 1999e).

Again resorting to consumerist ideology, the Commonwealth provides an additional rationale for reforms in the Australian health system by attempting to identify reasons for consumer use of CM. Significantly, the government has employed these reasons to support its current economic rationalist approach to health care, which, as argued above, involves a shift in policy emphasis from provider to consumer. According to Tambling (1999b), 'the focus of Commonwealth health programs and management has shifted towards the people they serve and the outcomes they are meant to achieve rather than the providers of services and their inputs'.

As a consequence of its commitment to ensure that a diverse range of complementary health care products is available to Australian consumers, the government claims that consumers are prepared to accept greater responsibility for their own health, estimating that consumers manage about 75 per cent of their own health problems without recourse to professional help. Part of the government strategy towards this so-called self-help involves approval of over-the-counter (OTC) medications that serve to reduce health costs to government by reducing doctor consultations and prescriptions (Tambling 1999b).

In addition, Tambling (1999g) notes that 'probably one of the most important factors in the growing demand for herbal medicines is the search by many consumers for products to enhance well-being'. Thus, CM is seen by government as preventative medicine and as providing promising treatments for chronic and lifestyle diseases. This, the government argues, has the potential to save lives and cut health care costs. As Wooldridge claimed in 1998,

> Chronic and lifestyle disease is costing the government a lot. There is enormous scope for natural and complementary therapists in areas of medicine such as controlling pain for those people with arthritis.

Moreover, he argues,

> The more we can ground natural and complementary medicine in science and find out through research and education what works and use that then the better off and healthier we will be. That's all the more important when you realise that one of the deficiencies of our health system is that it has become skewed towards treating illness after it occurs, rather than finding ways to prevent illness before it happens or promote good health generally.

Senator Tambling notes further that reforms acknowledge the role of the Internet in providing consumers with 'improved access to information on health care ... with thought given to ways of working together to help consumers be better-informed about health care ... particularly for consumers in remote areas' (Tambling 2000).

The reasons given by government for reforms in CM illustrate the shift in focus from provider to consumer, placing an emphasis on consumer choice, rights, self-responsibility, and empowerment through increased consumer access to CM, industry regulation, and reliable consumer information regarding use, effectiveness, and safety of CM.

The government's position reflects a consumerist ideology that supports capitalism through a political rhetoric of choice, rights, and empowerment. Its reforms are based on the culture-ideology of consumerism as a market mechanism that is fundamentally profit driven. It seeks to promote efficiency and cost saving in health—for example, through emphasis on self-responsibility for health, particularly self-medication and preventative medicine.

The government is also keenly aware that the use of OTC, including CM, medications benefits the pharmaceutical industry. Senator Tambling states that 'with exports and domestic sales of more than $1.6 billion per year and jobs for over 3000 Australians, the very important presence and role of the pharmaceutical sector is acknowledged by Government' (Tambling 1999b). There is, then, a real question regarding the relationship between the state, capitalism, and consumerism. As Hancock (1999a) points out, there are also questions regarding the relationship between health market reforms and issues of power relations, equity, and structural change. The following sections examine some of these issues in relation to structural changes in CM service provision, education, and research initiatives.

The role of CM practitioners in health policy reforms

The government's rationale for reforms in CM suggests that they are part of the Commonwealth's broader cost-cutting policy shift from acute to primary care, exemplified in primary health care initiatives such as the Enhanced Primary Care Packages and Coordinated Care Trials. CM is seen by the federal government as a significant part of the preventative medicine that has the potential to extend lives and cut costs in health care, and as providing promising treatments for chronic and lifestyle diseases. As the then Minister for Health claimed in 1998,

> These [CM] reforms in fact are a sign of change in health, in an area where change is fast happening. One of the greatest signs of this change is the ways new teams are forming in health that are fast leaving behind the traditional divides of conventional and complementary medicine, and forming instead teams comprising GPs, psychologists, physiotherapists and natural therapists (Wooldridge 1998).

While the reforms reflect the government's desire to save money and to protect consumers, they are also indicators of the power of consumerism to initiate broader structural change in the health care system.

Indications of consumer power to initiate structural change were evident at the Alternative Medicines Summit, organised by the Commonwealth Department of Health and Aged Care. Medical doctors as well as nonorthodox practitioners attended this summit, which was the first of its kind. The following quote, which comes from the Summit's representative for medical practitioners, illustrates its significance in the re-positioning of orthodox and alternative practitioners in the Australian health system. The doctor reported that

> I felt the tone of the day's proceedings was one of 'us versus them'. Inasmuch as 'natural and complementary practitioners' were seen as a distinct alternative to orthodox practitioners, particularly in cases of serious illnesses. Indeed, one speaker during the day indicated that as it was an Alternative Medicines Summit, orthodox doctors present should really be in only an observer capacity. In other words, there was no integration going on, rather the attitude was one of them seeking status as practitioners of the 'new medicine', and control of their therapies. This will of course bring forth the need for a 'Vocational Registration' for such 'approved practitioners', together with all control and the bureaucracy that that entails. I worry that this divisive stance, encouraged by the Government it seems, will further denigrate the position of 'orthodox' practitioners in the public's eyes, and leave real 'wholistic' doctors that the IMA [Integrative Medicine Association] represents, out in the cold, between these polarised camps.

In effect, the doctor concludes that alternative practitioners are attempting to establish themselves, with the aid of the Commonwealth, as the harbingers of a new medicine. Moreover, the same doctor recognised that government recognition of consumer demand for CM had broad implications for the health system and the health market by claiming that

> there is a paradigm shift occurring in health from within, that reflects a societal evolution, unstoppable by anyone. How to integrate all these practitioners, or even if it is desirable to, is a question that still perplexes me. There seems to be no one universal model, thus it becomes an exercise in lobbying for market share, and seeking for example, inclusion in Medicare.

For its part, the Commonwealth has implemented reforms in CM practice primarily through the Complementary Healthcare Consultative Forum, an initiative formed to discuss complementary health care research, regulation, and education as well as industry, consumer, and practitioner issues (Tambling 1999h). There has been considerable interest in practitioner accreditation and registration, particularly following the government announcement that suitably qualified complementary health care practitioner groups will be GST free for 3 years—provided they move towards regulation (Tambling 1999a). These types of initiatives give credence to the government's stance that 'alternative health practice has an integral role to play in providing a full range of health care options to Australia' (Wooldridge 1998).

In 1999, legislation in Victoria paved the way for registration of traditional Chinese medicine (TCM) practitioners, and the inclusion, alongside scientific evidence, of evidence based on tradition. As Dr Fiona Cummings (2000), Director of the Office of Complementary Medicines, explains:

> If you've got a herbal product that ... has been used for hundreds of years in a particular culture, one of the ways in which you can support your claim is with evidence of traditional use. So ... you could refer to the Chinese *Pharmacopoeia* or something along those lines ... you would also need to qualify that this is a traditional claim, rather than being based on scientific evidence.

These changes are significant. Until recently, orthodox medical practitioners have maintained hegemony by claiming a monopoly over a 'scientific' medicine. This is particularly true in Australia, which has a powerful physicians' lobby group, the Australian Medical Association (AMA). Nonetheless, one of the reactions by doctors to consumer demand for CM has been a dramatic increase in general practitioners' incorporation of CM, particularly TCM, into their service delivery. This too is an indication of the triumph of consumerist ideology.

Integration of CM into orthodox medical practice

Extrapolation from studies of general practitioner (GP) provision of CM indicate that approximately one in five Australian GPs provide some form of CM (Pirotta et al. 2000), one metropolitan study finding that 75 per cent of the GPs surveyed referred patients to CM practitioners (Hall & Giles-Corti 2000). The most common modalities used or recognised by GPs are acupuncture, manipulation, meditation, and nutritional and herbal medicine. An Australian study, which relied on 1996 Australian Health Insurance Commission data, shows that approximately one in seven GPs use acupuncture (Easthope 1998). Acupuncture is a peculiar case in Australia in that it is funded by our public Medicare system if administered by a licensed physician. This provides rebates to doctors and allows consumers greater access to acupuncture, but it is disadvantageous to traditional practitioners, who do not qualify for the Medicare rebate.

Exploratory research on reasons for Australian GPs' increasing provision of CM shows two major trends. The first is that GPs are responding to consumer demand for CM. GPs link this consumer demand to
- the clinical effectiveness of CM
- a better-educated public
- consumers' wariness of synthetic drugs associated with consumer beliefs that 'natural' medicines are safer
- consumer demand for greater choice and autonomy regarding health.

The second trend is that GPs themselves are increasingly critical of biomedicine, commonly noting the limitations of biomedical practice for treating many commonly presented ailments. GPs who provide CM are characteristically interested in a more holistic and preventative approach to medicine and thus are seeking new approaches to primary health care, including CM (Eastwood 2000a, b).

Orthodox ambivalence towards integration

Despite the fact that some GPs embrace CM, the orthodox medical profession as a whole is ambivalent towards integration of CM. On the one hand, doctors recognise the consumer demand for CM and acknowledge its clinical legitimacy—that is to say—it works, regardless of how or why. *AMAQ News*, a publication of the AMA, reports AMA policy on CM as recommending that 'we equip our current doctors and future GPs and specialists with working knowledge of the products and therapies' (McFie 2000, p. 15). On the other hand, the medical establishment recognises the potential of CM to undermine its hegemony over health provision. This same *AMAQ News* article goes on to note that 'their [general practitioner] patient numbers will be affected over time as the finite allocation of family health funds is being eaten up by paying for these supplements and unorthodox forms of medicine that have no proven effectiveness' (McFie 2000, p. 16). Accusing the government of accepting CM solely to attract votes, the article goes on to claim that 'it's up to the medical profession to undertake extensive research into the drugs and therapies and evaluate their usefulness' (McFie 2000, p. 16).

This kind of ambivalence has resulted in an evidence-based medicine movement (EBM) which, though expressed through the rhetoric of concern for consumers and the requirement that medicine is scientific, is arguably a defensive strategy deployed by orthodox medicine to maintain its hegemony over health care, and thus its market share. Ironically, EBM has turned out to be a double-edged sword, and it has been noted that 'there is simply no rigorous evidence for many of the daily clinical decisions in general practice', indicating that 'clinical legitimacy' is part of everyday practice, with or without the incorporation of CM (van der Weyden 2000, p. 534; see also Coleman 1994).

On top of this, the current Australian government, the Liberal–National Coalition, is critical of the medical establishment for restrictive practices that disadvantage health consumers. To the chagrin of much of the medical fraternity, the Australian Competition and Consumer Commission (ACCC), the government's consumer watchdog, has begun a searching and highly critical investigation of the medical profession's allegedly anti-competitive practices. According to Allan Fels, Chairman of the ACCC, the medical profession is artificially restricting entry into some specialisations and then acting as a monopoly by driving up prices for these specialised treatments (Fels 2000). In the midst of these controversies, the Commonwealth government is moving ahead with the institutionalisation of CM by encouraging more tertiary education in and research into CM.

Education and research initiatives

With regard to education, courses on CM are being incorporated into Australian tertiary institutions. Acupuncture, naturopathy, chiropractic, and TCM are taught at several universities in a number of states. The University of Queensland's Centre for the Evaluation of Complementary Health Practices is a new research centre that is incorporating teaching programs in complementary health practices to

- educate graduating health practitioners in the use of complementary practices

- improve understanding of the philosophy and practice of complementary health practices
- establish postgraduate teaching programs in CM.

Senator Tambling (1999a) has noted the need to develop strategies 'to stimulate research in the complementary health care fields', and has recognised the role research can play 'in promoting greater recognition and acceptance of complementary health care modalities in the array of health care choices to consumers'. With regard to research initiatives, close alliances between Australian industry and research institutions have been formed. For example, two corporations, Fauldings and Blackmores respectively, are sponsoring research centres at the University of Queensland and Southern Cross University (New South Wales). The University of Western Sydney has established a Traditional Chinese Medicine Unit, and there are CM research units at the University of Melbourne and Adelaide University. In addition, the Minister for Health and Aged Care has announced the establishment of a $2 million fund to be administered over three years to enable further research and development in CM (Tambling 2000).

It should be noted, however, that the majority of this CM research and education is funded by large corporations and institutions with a vested interest in outcomes, and carried out by members of the orthodox scientific and medical establishment with similar vested interests. Essentially, these vested interests result in what amounts to lobby groups, which may influence policy one-sidedly if not balanced by similar representation of consumer interests; hence the importance of CM consumer movements.

Complementary medicine consumer movements

CM consumer movements are active in Australia. The Australian Complementary Health Association (ACHA), headquartered in Victoria, is a typical example. Some of this organisation's stated goals are to create equity of access to complementary medicines and to empower consumers through informed decision making (see <http://home.vienet.net.au/~acha/welcome.htm>).

In line with the new social movements, the ACHA espouses values of social justice, empowerment, equity of access, and participation. The impact of these types of organisations, however, remains to be seen. As Irving (1999) points out, there are conflicting arguments over the level, type, and extent of evidence needed to evaluate the impact of consumer health movements on the Australian health system. For example, although the Consumers' Health Forum (CHF), established in 1987, was able to achieve representation on government committees, writers such as Willis (1988, cited in Irving) have argued that such representation amounted to little more than tokenism. In the intervening years since the publication of Willis's paper, however, things have changed. Now, government health policy explicitly endorses a shift in emphasis from provider to consumer and encourages consumer participation in the policy making process. No doubt much of this consumer participation will occur through organisations such as ACHA and CHF.

Conclusion

Already widespread in Australia, CM is steadily gaining acceptance by government, industry, education, the medical profession, and the consuming public. At present, however, the tax-funded Medicare system covers CM only when licensed, orthodox medical practitioners administer these therapies. While traditional practitioners of CM are increasingly subject to government regulation, so far their services are not rebatable under Medicare. No doubt, entirely traditional, stand-alone alternative medicine will survive in Australia, but the pervasive financial realities of the tax-funded Medicare system encourage the development of a hybrid form of practice emphasising the complementarity between Western and traditional medicines. Government policy initiatives and intensified research into CM are serving to hasten the integration of CM into Australian life and health by providing increasing evidence and assurance of CM's safety and efficacy.

The Australian government's involvement in CM is thus on the one hand serving to integrate CM into the mainstream health system through industry and practitioner regulation. On the other hand, however, government reforms in CM are part of broader market reforms in health that are aimed at treating chronic illness and promoting preventative medicine, part of which entails individuals accepting greater responsibility for their own health. While having obvious appeal for consumers, these types of reforms also enable governments to shift some of their health costs back onto the consuming public.

But there are limits on the ability of some segments of the population to pay out of pocket for CM, however desirable these services are to them. Recognising the demand for such treatments, private insurers already pay rebates for CM, even if administered by traditional practitioners outside the licensed medical establishment. Naturally enough, the expenses incurred are passed on to the consumer in the form of premiums paid. In light of the remaining inequality of access to CM, there are calls from policy makers and the public to consider inclusion of CM in the tax-funded Medicare system. This, of course, would greatly increase CM's financial attractiveness for patients and practitioners alike, and it might well increase the overall health of the populace, but it would probably also increase government health expenditure. This is the point at which consumerism, with its inherent ambiguities, takes centre stage. Will consumerism demand what is best for the consumer, what is best for the market, or what is best for society as a whole?

This chapter has explored the ambiguous role of consumerism in the development of Australian health policy regarding CM. On the one hand, it examined consumerism as an economic phenomenon, as the 'culture-ideology' of emergent global capitalism, the engine that drives the global market to commodify cultural change and to usurp the political boundaries of nations and states. The chapter also examined consumerism within the bounded nation state of Australia as a political mechanism, which, though supportive of capitalism, also encourages equitable health reforms. The rhetoric of consumer rights and choice is shared by all forms of consumerism, but the goals of the various forms of consumerism are divergent, if not contradictory. In the context of globalisation, the intersection of consumerism as an economic, cultural, and political phenomenon raises serious questions regarding the fundamental nature of democracy, the state, the market, and human rights. In all these areas, the ambivalent adoption of CM in Australia involves all of these intertwined issues, and might serve to illustrate the broader implications of globalisation.

References

Australian Complementary Health Association, <http://home.vienet.net.au/~acha/welcome.htm>.

Beck, U. 1992, *Risk Society*, Sage, London.

Bensoussan, A. 1999, 'Complementary Medicine: Where Lies Its Appeal?' *Medical Journal of Australia*, vol. 170, pp. 247–8.

Chernichovsky, D. 1995, 'Health System Reforms in Industrialized Democracies: An Emerging Paradigm', *Milbank Quarterly*, vol. 73, no. 3, pp. 339–72.

Coleman, V. 1994, 'Betrayal of Trust', *British Medical Journal*, vol. 42, pp. 96–102.

Complementary Health Council 2000, *Complementary Medicines Evaluation Committee's Guide to Levels of and Kinds of Evidence to Support Claims*, Commonwealth Department of Health and Aged Care, Canberra.

Crook, S., Pakulski, J., & Waters, M. 1992, *Postmodernisation: Changes in Advanced Society*, Sage, London.

Cumming, F. 2000, *Alternative Medicine, Part 3, Health Matters* <http://www.abc.net.au/rn/talks/.30/helthrpt/stories/s176462.htm>.

Department of Health and Aged Care 1999, *Reforming the Australian Health Care System: The Role of Government*, Occasional Papers, New Series no.1, Publications Production Unit, Canberra.

Drache, D. & Sullivan, T. 1999, 'Health Reform and Market Talk', in D. Drache & T. Sullivan (eds), *Market Limits in Health Reform*, Routledge, London.

Easthope, H. L. et al. 1998, 'Acupuncture in Australian General Practice: Practitioner Characteristics', *Medical Journal of Australia*, vol. 169, no. 4, pp. 197–200.

Eastwood, H. L. 2000a, 'Complementary Therapies: The Appeal to General Practitioners', *Medical Journal of Australia*, vol. 173, no. 17, pp. 95–8; online version available at <http://www.mja.com.au/public/issues>.

—— 2000b, 'Why are Australian General Practitioners Using Alternative Medicine? Postmodernisation, Consumerism, and the Shift towards Holistic Health', *Journal of Sociology*, vol. 36, no. 2, pp. 105–11.

—— & Correa, I. 2000, 'The Appeal of Complementary and Alternative Medicine to Australian Consumers: A Review of the Literature, *TASA Refereed Conference Proceedings*, Australian Sociological Association, Adelaide.

Featherstone, M. 1991, *Consumer Culture and Postmodernism*, Sage, London.

Feldberg, G. & Vipond, R. 1999, 'The Virus of Consumerism', Part I, in D. Drache & T. Sullivan (eds), *Market Limits in Health Reform*, Routledge, London.

Fels, A. 2000, 'Doctors Have No Cause for Complaint', *Australian*, 19 December 2000, p. 11.

Giddens, A. 1991, *Modernity and Self-Identity: Self and Society in the Late Modern Age*, Polity Press, Cambridge.

—— 1994, *Beyond Left and Right*, Polity Press, Cambridge.

Hall, K. & Giles-Corti, B. 2000, 'Complementary Therapies and the General Practitioner: A Survey of Perth GPs', *Australian Family Physician*, vol. 29, no. 6, pp. 602–5.

Hancock, L. 1999a, 'Rights and Markets: What Makes Sustainable Health Policy?', in L. Hancock (ed.), *Health Policy in the Market State*, Allen & Unwin, Sydney.

—— 1999b, 'Health: Public Sector Restructuring and the Market State', in L. Hancock (ed.), *Health Policy in the Market State*, Allen & Unwin, Sydney.

Harvey, D. 1998, *The Condition of Postmodernity: An Enquiry into the Origins of Cultural Change*, Blackwell, Oxford.

Integrative Medicine Association 1996, *IMA Newsletter*, Issue 6, December.

Irving, R. 1999, 'Losing Patients: Health Care Consumers, Power and Sociocultural Change', in C. Grbich (ed.), *Health in Australia: Sociological Concepts and Issues*, Longman, Sydney.

Janes, C. R. 1999, 'The Health Transition, Global Modernity and the Crisis of Traditional Medicine: The Tibetan Case', *Social Science and Medicine*, vol. 48, pp. 1803–20.

Lash, S. & Urry, J. 1994, *Economies of Signs and Space*, Sage, London.

MacLennan, A. H. 2000, *Alternative Medicine*, Part 1, Health Matters, <http://www.abc.net.au/rn/talks/.30/helthrpt/stories/s176462.htm>.

—— Wilson, D. H. & Taylor, A. W. 1996, 'Prevalence and Cost of Alternative Medicine in Australia', *Lancet*, vol. 347, pp. 569–73.

McFie, T. 2000, 'Complementary Medicine: The Future', *AMAQ News*, July, pp. 14–17.

McKay, J. 1995, 'Just Do It: Corporate Sports Slogans and the Political Economy of "Enlightened Racism" ', *Discourse: Studies in the Cultural Politics of Education*, vol. 16, no. 2, pp. 191–200.

McMichael, A. J. & Beaglehole, R. 2000, 'The Changing Global Context of Public Health', *Lancet*, vol. 356, pp. 495–9.

Miles, S. 1996, 'The Cultural Capital of Consumption: Understanding Postmodern Identities in a Cultural Context', *Culture and Psychology*, Sage, London.

Miller, T. 1993, *The Well-tempered Self: Citizenship, Culture and the Postmodern Subject*, Johns Hopkins University Press, Baltimore.

Niva, M. 1992, *Changing Cultures: Feminism, Youth, and Consumerism*, Sage, London.

Pirotti, M. V. et al. 2000, 'Complementary Therapies: Have They Become Accepted in General Practice?', *Medical Journal of Australia*, vol. 172, pp. 105–9.

Robertson, R. 1992, *Globalisation: Social Theory and Culture*, Sage, New York.

Sklair, L. 1994, 'The Culture-Ideology of Consumerism in Urban China: Findings from a Study in Shanghai', in R. Belk & C. Schultz (eds), *Consumption in Marketing Societies*, JAI Press, Connecticut.

—— 1995, *Sociology of the Global System*, 2nd edn, Johns Hopkins University Press, Baltimore.

Tambling, G. 1999a, *Better Understanding of Complementary Medicines*, Commonwealth Department of Health and Aged Care, Canberra; online version available at <http://www.health.gov.au:80/mediare1/yr1999/gt/gt99023.htm>, 1 July.

—— 1999b, *Health from the Shelf: The Consumer's Choice*, Commonwealth Department of Health and Aged Care, Canberra; online version available at <http://www.health.gov.au/archive/mediare1/yr1999/gt/gtsp990804.htm>, 4 August.

—— 1999c, *New Complementary Medicine Legislation Passed by Parliament*, Commonwealth Department of Health and Aged Care, Canberra; online version available at <http://www.health.gov.au/archive/mediare1/yr1999/gt/gtsp99007.htm>, 29 March.

—— 1999d, *New Partnership with Complementary Healthcare Industry*, Commonwealth Department of Health and Aged Care, Canberra; online version available at <http://www.health.gov.au:80/mediare1/yr1999/gt/gt99001.htm> 29 March.

—— 1999e, 'Launch of the Office of Complementary Medicines', Speech delivered to the Therapeutic Goods Administration, Parliament House, Canberra; online version available at <http://www.health.gov.au/mediarel/yr1999/gt/gtsp990428.htm> 28 April.

—— 1999f, 'Senator Tambling Strengthens Expert Committee on Complementary Medicines', Media release, Commonwealth Department of Health and Aged Care, Canberra; online version available at <http://www.health.gov.au:80/mediarel/yr1999/gt/gt99013.htm>, 30 April.

—— 1999g, 'Mediherb: Regulatory Reform for Herbal Medicines', Speech delivered at the Brisbane Conference Centre, Commonwealth Department of Health and Aged Care, Canberra; online version available at <http://www.health.gov.au:80/mediarel/yr11999/gt/gtsp990903.htm>.

—— 1999h, *Complementary Healthcare Consultative Forum Opening Address*, Commonwealth Department of Health and Aged Care, Canberra; online version available at <http://www.health.gov.au:80/mediarel/yr11999/gt/gtsp990701.htm>.

—— 2000, 'Complementary Healthcare Forum Examines Key Issues', Media release, Commonwealth Department of Health and Aged Care, Canberra; online version available at <http://www.health.gov.au/mediarel/yr12000/gt/gt20010.htm>, 14 April.

Therapeutic Goods Administration 1999, *Introducing Therapeutic Goods Administration*, <http://www.health.gov.au/tga/docs/html/intro.htm>.

Turner, B. S. 1995, *Orientalism, Postmodernism and Globalism*, Routledge, New York.

van der Weyden, M. 2000, 'General Practice Research and Communication', in *General Practice in Australia: 2000*, Commonwealth Department of Health and Aged Care, General Practice Branch, Health Services Division, Canberra.

Waters, M. 1994, 'Globalisation, Multiculturalism and Rethinking the Social', *Australian and New Zealand Journal of Sociology*, vol. 30, no. 3, pp. 229–4.

—— 1996, *Globalisation*, Routledge, New York.

Wooldridge, M. 1998, 'Launch of Southern Cross University Natural and Complementary Medicine Teaching Clinic', Commonwealth Department of Health and Aged Care, <http://www.health.gov.au/archive/mediarel/1998/mwsp980219.htm> 16 February.

Yeatman, A. 1998, *Activism and the Policy Process*, Allen & Unwin, Sydney.

11

General Practice in Australia: The Effects of Reforms and the Process of Privatisation

Debra O'Connor and Chris L. Peterson

According to the Department of Health and Aged Care (2000), there are 24 176 (nonspecialist) general practitioners (GPs), other medical practitioners, and medical specialists of whom 17 101 are vocationally registered GPs. The number of vocationally registered GPs has increased by 8 per cent since 1995–96. Since 1985, the number of nonspecialist medical practitioners billing Medicare has risen nearly 60 per cent. General practitioners are the primary point of contact for health care and are paid, in most cases, on a fee for service basis. A smaller number of GPs, some of whom work in community health centres, are paid a salary. GPs also operate as gatekeepers to the health system for a large proportion of the population; about 90 per cent of Australians see a GP at least once a year (Department of Health and Aged Care 2000).

General practice has undergone substantial changes since the beginning of the General Practice Strategy in 1989, through which the Commonwealth government introduced the possibility for GPs to become vocationally registered and encouraged them to take part in formal and ongoing education and training. However, since the late 1990s, with the increasing corporatisation of medicine, there have been structural changes to the face of the organisation and service delivery of medical practice, not unlike those that occurred over the last decade and a half in the USA. Corporatisation and other structural changes have affected the foundation on which many GPs have traditionally practised their profession.

This chapter reviews changes that have taken place since the development of the General Practice Strategy and provides an overview of the funding and operation of general practice in the community. Structural changes resulting from corporatisation and changes to the way that general practice is delivered are also identified. White's (2000) argument that general practitioners are moving from small business owners to employees of large corporations, thereby fundamentally changing their status, is considered. The implications for the future of general practice in Australia are then discussed.

General practice and its activities

Within Medicare, a general practitioner is defined as

> a recognised general practitioner (that is a vocationally registered practitioner [VRGP]; a Fellow of the Royal Australian College of General Practitioners, or equivalent; or a general practice registrar in a training placement) who had at least half of the schedule full value of his/her Medicare billing from nonreferred attendance items (Department of Health and Aged Care 2000, p. 42).

This definition focuses on the GP's qualifications and experience. By contrast, the Royal Australian College of General Practitioners' definition emphasises the daily role of a GP. A general practitioner 'is a doctor who provides primary, continuing, comprehensive whole-person care to individuals, families and the community' (Department of Health and Family Services 1996, p. xxvii).

In 1998–99 the federal government spent $2873 million for nonspecialist medical attendances. Additional costs arising from these consultations, including medications prescribed, were $4235 million. Costs have been increasing and, according to Britt et al. (2000), in the five years prior to 1998–99 primary nonspecialist services had risen by 9.3 per cent, while secondary costs had risen by some 40 per cent.

Rural GPs are generally trained to provide additional services in the following areas:
- anaesthetics
- triage
- obstetrics
- operations in relation to trauma and emergency medicine.

In many cases they will have completed subspecialty training in each of these areas. The areas for which GPs have traditionally had least time in Australia are psychological, psychosocial, and public health. In fact, GPs rate their competence in public health as being lower than in most other areas in the Royal Australian College of General Practitioners (RACGP) training program (Goldman et al. 2000).

The GP is generally regarded as a gatekeeper, as well as the coordinator and major provider of primary health care (Peterson 1996). The main reasons in Australia why people visit the GP are for respiratory and cardio-vascular diseases and musculoskeletal and skin diseases. For men, respiratory conditions are the main reason, followed by musculoskeletal and connective tissue conditions, then injuries. For women, respiratory conditions are the most common reason for a consultation, followed by tests, and reasons not associated with specific conditions. Seventy-five per cent of a GP's work time is spent in consultation; even those working in community health centres now focus mainly on consultations, the result of problems with financial remuneration for other than one-to-one services. The majority of GPs work in group practices; the number of GPs working on their own is decreasing. Only 1.2 per cent of urban GP time is spent in hospital work, compared with 3.1 per cent spent by GPs with rural posts (Department of Health and Family Services 1998).

In a recent survey of GPs, 60 per cent of practices had one or two GPs and 14 per cent had over six GPs. The number of solo practices is decreasing, with a concomitant 10 per cent increase in the number of practices of five or more practitioners since 1997–98 (Department of Health and Aged Care 2000, p. 56). Women GPs are more likely to work in a large practice. There is no discussion of this fact reported in the survey, but it could be assumed that, as women tend to prefer part-time work at certain times in their lives, larger practices can accommodate part-time work more easily. There is also an increasing number of part-time GPs.

In a survey of 1048 GPs in Australia by Britt et al. (2000), a series of data was gathered on the activities of GPs. On average, 147 problems were managed in each 100 encounters with patients; of these problems, 45.3 per cent were regarded as new problems for patients. On average, 110 medications were prescribed per 100 encounters. Clinical treatments such as psychotherapy, counselling, or advice were provided in 33.5 per cent of encounters, while physical therapies and excisions were provided for 6.9 per cent. For each of the encounters there were 11 per cent of referrals, 7.3 per cent of specialist referrals, 26.3 per cent of pathology test orders, and 7.5 per cent of imaging tests ordered.

The Australian Institute of Health and Welfare (AIHW) (1998) demonstrates that between 1994–95 and 1996–97 the volume of items per person increased by 1.5 per cent per year, and between 1986–87 and 1996–97 average consultation rates rose 2 per cent per year for males and 2.7 per cent per year for females. The AIHW maintains that this increase could partly be due to the 27 per cent increase in the number of practitioners during that period. Other factors include the increase in health promotion programs and increased awareness about chronic illnesses in the community.

The development of general practice

According to Bollen and Saltman (2000), the concept of general medical practitioners in Australia is as old as the first British settlement of 1788, and yet it is one of the most recently accepted disciplines in Australian medical practice. With the increasing development of medical specialisation since the Second World War, GPs were progressively excluded from hospital practice. Graduates were attracted to specialties and entered general practice—by default rather than design—as specialist courses became more difficult to enter.

Under Australia's federal system of government, health services were a state responsibility until 1946. After the Second World War the federal Labor government sought to establish a national health scheme similar to the National Health Service in the UK. This attempt was thwarted in 1946 by the Australian branches of the British Medical Association (BMA); these branches became the Australian Medical Association (AMA) in 1962. The BMA succeeded in ensuring that the Constitution ruled out the possibility of civil conscription for medical practitioners; that is, it ruled out a system of enforced salaries from the public purse. The RACGP was formed in 1969 to support GPs and to create recognition for the community and family basis of their work as well as to provide postgraduate education.

Initially, Australian medical schools were unwilling to recognise general practice as a specific discipline and refused to accept funding to establish departments of general practice in universities. Eventually, most schools were established with titles reflecting community medicine, although the focus was almost exclusively on general practice (Department of Health and Aged Care 2000).

The two-tiered universal health insurance rebate scheme introduced by the federal Labor government in 1972 ensured that GPs were fiscally differentiated from specialists. GP service rebates are based on time, whereas specialists' rebates are content based. The fee differential between GPs and specialists created antagonism between the two groups; GPs felt disadvantaged by their rate of pay for procedural work. Matters were partially resolved through the implementation of a registration scheme that enables vocationally registered GPs to claim slightly higher rebate payments composed of content- and time-based descriptors.

General practice reforms

By the early 1990s, the Commonwealth government was reviewing many aspects of the health system. In 1991–92, the Commonwealth introduced a number of initiatives that resulted in some structural changes to general practice. These changes focused on quality and the integration of general practice into the broader health care system. The General Practice Strategy Review Group had been established and started the reforms with vocational registration (Department of Health and Family Services 1998).

The Royal Australian College of General Practitioners (RACGP) has since 1996 provided mandatory vocational registration training (or its equivalent), which must be completed before a GP is permitted to practise and be issued with a Medicare provider number. More recently, the Howard government has restricted the number of medical school graduates who are offered vocational training. Those who do not complete vocational registration do not become eligible to practise with a Medicare number, and hence are not able to work in general practice. The requirements for vocational registration are

- completion of a formal general practice training program
- attainment of fellowship of the RACGP by examination
- demonstration of involvement in continuing education and quality assurance activities
- agreement to participate in peer review through an independent peer review organisation.

The four main themes identified for general practice in 1992 were gradually refined and developed in the following eight years. These themes were

- *quality of service*—initiatives including vocational training, registration, accreditation, an evaluation program, and continuing medical education
- *workforce*—which led to the development of controls for the number of overseas-trained doctors, 'provider number' registration, and the rural incentives program to redistribute doctors from the urban areas to rural areas
- *integration*—which is mainly addressed through the Divisions of General Practice
- *financing*—including the Coordinated Care Trials, incentive payments, alternative practice models trials, differential payments for vocationally registered and nonvocationally registered GPs, and the Relative Values Study.

After much negotiation between the government and the medical industry representatives (AMA and RACGP), the Commonwealth allocated $223.45 million to the General Practice Strategy in 1996–97 (Department of Health and Family Services 1998). In this instance, specific allocations were made to the Divisions and Projects Grants Program. Divisions of General Practice are funded local networks that enable GPs to come together as a group and that aim to provide closer integration of GPs with the rest of the health care system. In the twenty-first century, as part of this program, the role of GPs in population-based health and data collection has been enhanced.

The next scheme to be funded was the General Practice Rural Incentives Program. This program aims to attract GPs to rural practice and redress the oversupply of GPs in some urban areas. In addition, allocations were made to the Better Practice Program, now called the Practice Incentive Payments (PIP). The RACGP Training Programs evaluation projects and accreditation systems were also allocated recurrent funding resources. The Australian General Practice Accreditation of Practices program provides support to improve quality at the practice level. Specifically, it serves to improve programs such as information management, information technology, patient management systems, and infection control, and to encourage the use of evidence-based guidelines and decision support systems.

The Commonwealth government insisted on increased consumer input and representation on working, policy, and implementation groups. The Consumers' Health Forum received specific funding until 1999 to provide policy advice and to support consumer representatives on national GP committees. In the latter part of the decade, consumer policy advice began to challenge some of the assumptions about the role of GPs in the primary care system and the nature of the patient–GP relationship, particularly the saliency of expert knowledge. For consumers, issues such as communication and access became more important priorities. Consumers have consequently demanded a right to participate in the debates around GP reform; much of the rhetoric espoused in policy papers focuses on patient-focused practice. However, the project lost its funding although some individual projects, and consumer representatives are still maintained (Matthew Blackmore, Consumers' Health Forum, pers. comm., August 2001).

Not surprisingly, the implementation of the strategy has been complex and at times divisive, conflictual, and contentious (Cresswell 2001). The Relative Value Study has highlighted major differences in approaches to problems in general practice between the AMA, Australian Divisions of General Practice (ADGP), and the RACGP. In a review of the General Practice Strategy, the Department of Health and Family Services (1998) outlined a number of changes that had occurred since the strategy had been implemented. The strategy had been slow to promote the development of information technology (IT) and computer developments, and in the area of vocational training there had been considerable controversy. An additional change that resulted from the implementation of the strategy was increased conflict between government and the profession, as well as within the profession itself. Moreover, low morale was found among GPs who felt their remuneration was low, especially compared with that of specialists. In fact, the Department of Health and Family Services (1998) concluded that much of the blame for problems in general practice was attributable to the General Practice Strategy itself.

Those initiatives for alternative forms of remuneration for GPs that have been introduced to achieve particular goals in improving the quality of patient care include Divisions of General Practice and Practice Incentive Payments (PIP) (introduced in 1998–2000 and paid on a full-time GP basis when a practice gains accreditation). In order to achieve efficiencies of scale, small practices have been encouraged to amalgamate—physically or virtually—by sharing administrative infrastructure and bulk purchasing. In 2000–01, GPs were also paid additional funding for improving IT infrastructure and usage in their practices and clinical work. A third area of incentive payments is targeted towards encouraging GPs to increase levels of childhood immunisation (Department of Health and Aged Care 2000). The Department of Health and Family Services maintained that 'the remuneration aspect of the (General Practice) Strategy was considered a failure, with fee for service remaining inequitable and cumbersome and not rewarding quality' (Department of Health and Family Services 1998, p. 26). In addition, GPs were considered to be resentful since the 'level of indexation for recognised GP items in the Medicare Benefits Schedule was discounted in comparison with the indexation that applied to specialists' items' (Department of Health and Family Services 1998, p. 26).

It was also maintained that 'the lack of an agreed definition for "general practice" and the lack of baseline data further complicate attempts to evaluate the Strategy as a whole' (Department of Health and Family Services 1998, p. 25). Other factors to affect the evaluation and impact of the strategy have been casemix funding and the moves to primary health care, the increased influence of quality, and the coordinated care trials. In addition, the report referred to emerging structural changes that form the basis of concern for a wide section currently in health care: 'Some parts of the "industry" are becoming corporatised: this has implications for both the business and clinical aspects of service delivery' (p. 25).

Changing trends in the expectations of younger GPs and graduates fundamentally challenge traditional expectations of the nature of a career in general practice.

> Recent entrants to the GP workforce have differing expectations in relation to working conditions and remuneration. Many demand a more balanced lifestyle, which means shorter working hours and the ability to work part-time for extended periods (Department of Health and Family Services 1998, p. 25).

The 1998 report argues that many GPs are not willing to bear the responsibility and difficulty associated with running a small business. Overall, however, the strategy was considered to have had only a small effect on GPs, but it was considered to have had a negative financial impact because of the costs associated with having general practice engage to a greater degree with the rest of the health care system.

The development of corporatisation and its effects on general practice

Although the General Practice Strategy has had an effect on the way GPs do their work, a more dominant structural change has been taking place. Corporatisation has been having a significant effect on the structure of general practice in the health care system, which in turn has affected the status of GPs and the way they perform their services. With the increase of corporatisation and privatisation, there has been in Australia a substantial shift away from GPs being small business owners to becoming employees in a corporatised practice.

The wholesale purchase of practices by multinational corporations—a new phenomenon in Australia—has been an unexpected outcome of the incentive schemes. This differs from the entrepreneurial models of the 1980s and more clearly reflects the Health Maintenance Organisation (HMO) structures of the USA. These corporations are not so much concerned with providing extended services but with establishing medical monopolies. Corporatisation appeals to many GPs as there is a dwindling demand from newer GPs for buying stand-alone practices as overheads and other costs reduce their profitability. For many older GPs, corporatisation represents a windfall that enables them to retire. The major corporate bodies usually own pathology, radiology, and other diagnostic testing services. These services can be contained in a one-stop-shop approach to general practice within which GPs are encouraged or required to refer.

White and Collyer (1998) have observed that in New South Wales in 1989 the then Liberal government announced the sell-off of a substantial number of assets and the closure of numerous public hospitals and other facilities. In the 1990s, the Victorian Liberal government also announced public hospital closures and the building of a number of private facilities. It has been part of every Liberal government's platform to increase privatisation in the health care sector. White and Collyer outline a number of privatisation approaches (1998), which include offering private investment in the building of private hospitals and the leasing of public hospitals to private operators. In addition, there has been the offer of private company management contracts. Private companies have been allowed to build and operate public-status hospitals.

Importantly for general practice, entrepreneurial clinics in Australia represent another sign of privatisation. Entrepreneurial clinics were introduced first in the 1980s, and 'by 1985, Edelsten (financially backed by Abignano

Ltd) and competitors such as Viscount Holdings Ltd had introduced clinics into Victoria, New South Wales, Queensland and South Australia' (White & Collyer 1998, p. 494).

White and Collyer argue that this follows the trend in the USA where physicians have extensive interests in clinical and medical centres. They further argue that in the state's changing role, 'privatisation (albeit in the hospital sector) increases the power of corporations and contractors to pursue their own interests' (1998, p. 501). They suggest that the state's position to guide developments in health care nationally has been compromised, and that privatisation has limited its capacity to serve as an intermediary. In the past the state has acted as an arbitrator and regulator of general practice, legislating on how the profession can operate. It has also enabled general practice to become a powerful force in the medical community through activities such as the General Practice Strategy. With corporatisation, these roles of the state have diminished.

On the role of the state, White and Collyer maintain that

> the State does not just provide social and economic infrastructure (such as justice, the law, and a monetary system), but [it] has come to intervene in all social and economic practices, providing public services and benefits that shape class inequities and distribute wealth and resources (1998, p. 497).

One argument about the role of the state, which they maintain is losing favour, is that the state acts as 'an instrument of class interests' (1998, p. 497). The state has supported the dominance of medicine and at present supports the commercialisation and commodity approach towards health care. They refine this analysis of the state and show that the state is in a process of shaping and being shaped by a social struggle.

Discussing the effects of corporatisation, White (2000) presents a sustained argument on the development of general practice from the mid twentieth century, focusing on factors that have been important for the state as well as the profession. He maintains that, in Australia, the plethora of reports produced in the 1980s and 1990s

> discuss general practice in the absence of wider sociological changes in Australian society, focussing on the profession as if it were a self-contained occupation existing, by and large, independent of political and economic changes (White 2000, p. 286).

White also argues that much sociological literature is limited since, rather than focusing on structure and structural change, it has restricted the discussion of such issues as the relationship of general practice with alternative medicines and the power of general practice in defining states of illness and health.

White (2000) maintains that there have been some fundamental changes in the position of general practice in the community. These have been driven by the emergence of a number of factors, including increases in differentiation and specialisation in health care, the effects of feminism, and the consumer movement. The notion of a generalist practitioner has thus been weakened, which has led to deprofessionalisation as general practice faces the challenge that it is not the only custodian of legitimate knowledge about medicine.

The trend during the 1980s and 1990s to specialise has challenged the legitimate role for general practice. Consequently, GPs have been dealing with a number of encroachments upon their territory. The development of corporatised medicine and 24-hour clinics has meant that cost containment and efficiency approaches are used, and that practice management requires patient throughput rather than the utilisation of higher specialty skills by GPs. In this sense a de-skilling has also been taking place in the profession. The occupational analysis of territory was documented in the work of Willis (1983), in which he points out that medicine has carefully excluded other health professions from its territory. However, general practice, being seen as the poor cousin to specialties, has faced specialties increasingly taking over its territory. In addition, GPs—particularly in the USA but also in Britain—have had the threat of nursing practitioners taking over some of their bread-and-butter activities, such as prescribing and immunising. Even prior to corporatisation, GPs were facing important encroachments on their territory.

There is another trend that affects the relationship between capital, medicine, and the state. This has been through 'the dissolution of a male working class, and consequently of the latent social control function of general practice to discipline labour through control of the "sick certificate"' (White 2000, p. 286). White continues his structural analysis of general practice in relation to capital and the state by arguing the strong bonds that have existed in the past between general practice and the state in Australia. Further, White maintains that the changing relationship between state and general practice challenges the petit bourgeois basis of general practice, which, in Marxist terms, then becomes wage labour. In short, proletarianisation is occurring. GPs are moving from being small business people—a characteristic of middle and upper middle classes—to being people with only their labour to sell, a characteristic of the working class. This represents a fundamental structural change to the profession of general practice.

In Australia, general practice, while maintaining that it is an autonomous profession, has always depended quite heavily on state support (White 2000). For example, users of GP services have long been subsidised by the state, more recently through Medicare. In maintaining a close association between general practice and the state, White argues, social transformation in medicine has been central to health sector changes. 'Foremost among these are the interrelated changes in state policy, in the perception of the medical profession, and in labour and industry' (2000a, p. 288). Much of the recent development in corporatisation and entrepreneurial health care has been part of a changing trend in the organisation of labour and reliance on market forces, characterised by economic rationalist management and managerialism. In White's view, this has led to policies that emphasise individualism and 'the internalisation of medical norms of behavior' (2000, p. 289).

The diminished role of the state in general practice is part of a comprehensive move by conservative governments to lessen the role of government and to seek to outsource its services. The political and administrative climate over much of the past decade has been one of deregulation; the changes for general practice are paralleled in a number of spheres. Government rhetoric has been to let the market rule and this has produced many deregulated practices in health care. Apart from lowering government costs and thereby allowing the government of the day to appear to have a more balanced budget, policies not to invest in state provision or regulation have led to outsourcing traditional government roles to private industry. Privatisation and corporatisation have been part of a general trend established by economic rationalist management practices; however, for GPs this trend has resulted in the alteration of the structures of the profession. For nursing and some other health professions, the reduced role of the state as an arbiter and regulator has weakened their position in the health hierarchy, making them vulnerable to the business and budgetary guidelines of corporate managements. In this sense, the changing role of the state is an industry-wide phenomenon affecting the work practices of a number of health professions.

The phenomenon of corporatisation that has taken place has overtaken a policy and regulatory framework with unresolved issues regarding ownership of patient records, and GP accountability and autonomy. Some Divisions of General Practice are looking at developing a nonprofit-based corporate alternative for GPs, and policy rhetoric is beginning to embrace the notion of Divisions of Primary Care that could be fund holders.

Alternatives to the corporate model for organising general practice

Over the past few years there have been several models put forward on how to organise general practice under a more collective and corporatised model. Much of the debate has drawn on the USA-based managed competition and HMO models, as well as the British model of Fundholding. Duckett (1999a) has been one of the few authors to provide a carefully detailed analysis of the application of American health care models to Australia, and recommends that only some of the integration practices are appropriate to Australia. He has argued that much of the health policy formulation in the USA has had negative effects and resulted in costly services for consumers (Duckett 1999b). Yet many of the examples for developing the health care system in Australia have drawn uncritically on the managed care and HMO types of models. Whether these have worked particularly well in their home environments, or whether they are culturally appropriate for Australian general practice and consumers' expectations of care, are issues that tend to be overlooked.

A model that has not embraced the corporatised approach and that relies on regulation of general practice health services is the UK's Fundholding model, which includes purchasing allied health and hospital services, teaching employees to manage budgets, and medication purchases. Prichard and Beilby (1996) critically evaluated the application of the Fundholding model for Australian general practice and concluded that it has some application, but is limited by cultural constraints (Prichard & Beilby 1996). In their view, 'Fundholding is based on Enthoven's concept of managed competition and aims to transform general practices into purchasers and distributors of health care services … for enrolled patients within a regulatory framework' (1996, p. 215).

However, they are critical of its application to Australian general practice. Fundholding can control costs and be efficient in providing health care services, but under this system there might be a disincentive to service costly patients, though there could be a capitation formula that reflects practice operation and the needs of particular patient groups (Prichard & Beilby 1996).

GPs in the UK saw Fundholding as a way of addressing the small amount of control they had over factors related to the management of patients. However, in Australia, GPs have more control over patients, so the drivers for a regulated system might not be as strong. In fact, Scottish GPs have argued that Fundholding costs outweigh many of the benefits. The increased administration required of doctors has led to a reduction in clinical activities, which has potential for reducing the income derived from clinical activities. Further, due to fundamental differences in payment systems for clinical practice, the UK-based Fundholding system seems less appropriate to Australian general practice; there is little evidence of cost containment through Fundholding (Prichard & Beilby 1996).

Duckett (1999b) has also suggested that the UK system is not necessarily the most applicable for Australian conditions. There are a number of potential drawbacks of the Fundholding system for Australia, including

- the potential for discrimination against more costly patients
- possible neglect of the chronically ill and elderly
- a lack of funding additional to nonFundholding practices.

In addition, patient freedom to attend a number of practices might have to be preserved (Prichard & Beilby 1996).

In predicting changes in the GP role for the year 2025, Kilmartin (2000) argues that GPs will still have an important place; however, with the growth of competition with other health care providers and the growth of subspecialties, the GP 'will encroach on areas now regarded as specialties, since the knowledge base and skills needed to perform some specialist tasks will be readily available to the generalist' (Kilmartin 2000, p. 87). She maintains that there will mainly be large group practices and these will be integrated with other health care organisations. Salaried or shareholder GPs will predominate in group practices. The regulated Fundholding model and the corporatised model seem inappropriate to the cultural heritage of general practice as a profession in Australia and to meeting the needs of consumers. Even so, corporatisation has emerged as one of the major challenges to confront general practice in the past two decades.

Conclusion

Corporatisation is likely to continue in Australia, at least in the short term. In the UK, Fundholding was based on evaluating American HMOs and adapting the HMO model to the local cultural and political environment. Appropriate corporate models for Australia would need to be sensitive to cultural and political factors. Corporate models might need to be adapted to the needs of general practice to maintain doctors' occupational identity and territory, as well as the health care needs of consumers. Whether corporatisation delivers for consumers in meeting their needs is questionable; historically, the profit motive of corporations has tended not to be reflective of the needs of less powerful groups. The rhetoric of corporations promotes the benefits of the corporate model for health practitioners and consumers.

Apart from changing the way that general practice operates, the status of many GPs has changed as a result of corporatisation—they have moved from being small business people to being workers in a large corporation, which has implications for general practice in terms of the occupational hierarchy. In addition, it further limits the role that the state plays in regulating the profession as the profession becomes based on free-market forces. It also raises questions of medical autonomy—once the basis of the profession—and the increasing regulation by corporate interests in the market economy.

Corporatisation poses a policy problem for the federal government which, in reforming information management and information technology, is making it clear that it wants GPs and divisions to play a larger role in public health care than previously (Tongue 2001). Requirements for the provision of aggregated data about population health trends will be tied more firmly to practice incentive payments. If corporately owned practices in Australia follow the experiences of HMOs in the USA, these data will only be surrendered at a price, and not at all if this is deemed to be against commercial interests.

Corporatisation might be a manifestation of globalisation, and certain elements are sure to develop and remain. The corporatisation that developed in the USA was not a result of planned government policy, but took root in the last decade and quickly began to change the way that family medicine was delivered (Emmett, University of Pennsylvania, pers. comm., April 2001). However, sustained growth and development of corporatisation might well face critical opposition from general practice and the consumer movement. In that sense, it behoves Commonwealth, state, and territory governments to look a little beyond immediate cost containment approaches to the needs of consumers and health care professions. It might be that critical evaluation of the experiences of other countries with corporatised health care might save repeating some of the costly mistakes and lead to the evolution of a culturally and politically appropriate arrangement for general practice in Australia.

In the meantime, there are some significant threats to the occupational identity of GPs; it is these that might force some important rethinking about future directions and development.

References

Australian Institute of Health and Welfare 1998, *Australia's Health 1998*, AIHW, Canberra.

Bollen, M. & Saltman, D. 2000, 'A History of General Practice', in Commonwealth Department of Health and Aged Care (eds), *General Practice in Australia*, AGPS, Canberra.

Britt, H. et al. 2000, *General Practice Activity in Australia 1999–2000*, AIHW, Canberra.

Cresswell, A. 2001, 'GPs Strongly Oppose College over Values Study', *Australian Doctor*, 4 May.

Department of Health and Aged Care 2000, *General Practice in Australia*, AGPS, Canberra.

Department of Health and Family Services 1996, *General Practice in Australia*, AGPS, Canberra.

—— 1998, *General Practice: Changing the Future Through Partnerships*, General Practice Strategy Review Group, Department of Health and Family Services, Canberra.

Duckett, S. J. 1999a, *Health Care in the US: Lessons to be Learned by Australia*, Australian Centre for American Studies, University of Sydney, Sydney.

—— 1999b, 'Health Care in the US: Lessons to be Learned by Australia', Paper delivered to the School of Public Health Seminar Program, La Trobe University, Melbourne.

Goldman, S., Jasper, A., & Wellard, R. 2000, *A Study of Registrar Views to Evaluate Outcomes of the RACGP Training Program*, Royal Australian College of General Practitioners, Melbourne.

Kilmartin, M. R. 2000, 'General Practice in the Year 2025', *Medical Journal of Australia*, vol. 172, 17 January, pp. 97–8.

Peterson, C. 1996, 'Health Service Restructuring: Changes in the Roles of General Practitioners', *Australian Journal of Primary Health—Interchange*, vol. 2, no. 2, pp. 12–20.

Prichard, D. A. & Beilby, J. J. 1996, 'Issues for Fundholding in Australian General Practice', *Medical Journal of Australia*, vol 164, 19 February, pp. 215–19.

Tongue, A. 2001, Speech delivered to the General Practice Divisions of Victoria, Divisions Forum, April.

White, K. N. 2000, 'The State, Market and General Practice: The Australian Case', *International Journal of Health Services*, vol. 30, no. 2, pp. 285–308.

—— & Collyer, F. 1998, 'Health Care Markets in Australia: Ownership of the Private Hospital Sector', *International Journal of Health Services*, vol. 28, no. 3, pp. 487–510.

Willis, E. 1983, *Medical Dominance*, Allen & Unwin, Sydney.

12

Evidence–based Health: Three Cheers for Noncompliance

Jeanne Daly, Emma Hughes, and Corinne op't Hoog

There is a large and growing literature addressing the problem of noncompliance with health advice. This term refers mainly to patients who take little or no notice of the advice given them by their doctors. One estimate is that around 40 per cent of patients on medication fall prey to noncompliance, but when it comes to advice to make lifestyle changes the figure rises to 75 per cent (DiMatteo 1994). So common is this behaviour that it could be seen as the norm (Rapley 1997) were it not for the negative effects of large numbers of unnecessary deaths. McElduff et al. (2001) calculated that compliance with cardiac health promotion programs could reduce cardiac mortality by 40 per cent. Frazier et al. (2000) estimated that in a setting of 100 per cent compliance the incidence of colorectal cancer mortality could be reduced by half with a screening program using a single colonoscopy. In summary, there is mounting evidence in the medical literature that patients have much to gain from being compliant.

Noncompliance is also a problem for health policy makers. In the USA, the cost to the health care system of noncompliance has been estimated to be US$100 billion per year (Gerbino 1993). Smith (1985) aroused policy makers' interest by arguing that noncompliance accounts for 10 per cent of all hospital admissions. The colonoscopy screening program described by Frazier et al. (2000) could save the health industry US$92 000 per life-year saved. In times of budgetary constraint, such apparent wastage is not sustainable.

Based on these figures, an alternative to enlarging the health budget would be to increase the efficiency of the health system by improving patient compliance with health interventions. This is particularly important with drug treatment of infectious diseases. In the case of tuberculosis, for example, noncompliance creates a pool of cases in the community, putting both the infected individuals and the community at risk, which has the potential to escalate the costs of care. In instances where cases of tuberculosis spread into the community, this is serious enough for the World Health Organization to have devised an intervention in which patients were placed on a short course of therapy under direct clinical observation. Even this was not effective. Compliance rates with tuberculosis treatment turned out to be lower than in self-supervised regimens (Zwarenstein et al. 1998). The answer seems to be to try to understand this behaviour and then to fund interventions to rectify it. At last count the number of articles on the Internet on noncompliance in the health literature was slightly under 50 000—varying depending on which search engine was used—providing further evidence of the extent of the problem.

One strand of the research in this area quantified the extent of noncompliance by monitoring urine or blood levels, using pill dispensers, or by asking patients themselves (for an overview, see Cramer & Spilker 1991): the research established that patients were indeed noncompliant. Researchers then focused on trying to explain noncompliance in terms of patients' personalities or other individual characteristics and on devising appropriate interventions to increase compliance. Counselling was seen as appropriate for patients who had to be motivated to overcome complacency or who were simply negligent. Disturbed patients could be referred to a psychiatrist for extra help. Education programs were favoured for patients who would benefit from knowing why it was so important to comply with professional treatment regimes. It is important for doctors to be able to communicate their messages on the reasons for compliance so, where required, training in communications skills could be offered.

Considering the size of the research effort involved, carefully devised programs to improve compliance failed to show any real impact (Haynes & McKibbon 1996). Perhaps not surprisingly, some researchers decided that patients were irredeemably ignorant, recalcitrant, or both (Lerner 1997). Some researchers attempted to enlist the cooperation of patients in solving the problem. Noncompliance was recognised as being potentially stigmatising, so the preferred terms became 'adherence' or 'concordance'. One researcher objected that terms such as 'concordance' made the act of compliance seem a matter of personal choice, and suggested the use of 'fidelity' or the Dutch term 'therapie-trouw', translated roughly as 'therapy troth' (Urquhart 2001). Underlying these terms, the perception remains that patient behaviour needs to change by becoming more compliant with medical prescription.

The aim of this chapter is to put forward a different argument. Patients often do not follow medical advice. A narrow focus on what is to count as 'rational' in an evidence-based emphasis compared with what happens in the clinical setting has distorted our views of what can be expected of patients. Labelling patients as noncompliant can be seen in part as an outcome of evidence-based medicine. Some patients admit to being noncompliant through a lack of information, and this can of course be addressed. Leaving these patients aside—and they are the minority—we should perhaps celebrate the achievements of informed noncompliant patients in asserting their own values in the face of medical overprescription, if this is indeed what they are doing. After an overview of the origins of noncompliance research, we examine data from an ongoing study of patient noncompliance. The implications for policy makers are also suggested.

Noncompliance research

Traditionally, biomedicine, the laboratory-based scientific study of organs and tissues, was the basic science of medical practice. Among other benefits, biomedicine produced disease-specific drugs, safe anaesthetics, and vaccines against infectious diseases. In the 1970s, a new medical discipline arose in the USA and Canada: clinical epidemiology. The proponents of clinical epidemiology argued that clinical care needed a new set of skills, an additional basic science that focused on the way in which medical knowledge about diagnosis and treatment is applied at the bedside in clinical practice (Feinstein 1983; Sackett et al. 1985). Sackett at McMaster University was one of the founders of clinical epidemiology. He wrote a letter to the editor of the *International Journal of Epidemiology* in 1984 that appeared under the title 'Three cheers for clinical epidemiology'. In it, he extolled the virtues of the new discipline for training clinicians in the science of selecting the right diagnostic tests, interpreting the results accurately, choosing the right treatments, deciding on a plan of management, and evaluating the outcome. Clinical epidemiology was important for two reasons: it highlighted an under-researched area and proposed a research direction to fill the gaps in our knowledge about clinical practice.

Clinical epidemiology has as its central aim the production of scientific evidence of effective clinical practice based on the study of live patients instead of the study of laboratory animals. With evidence of what works and what does not work, it was argued, clinicians would rely less on clinical judgment and more on scientific evidence of benefit. Clinical epidemiology as a term never really caught the popular imagination. In contrast, its offspring, evidence-based medicine, had a self-evident appeal for both clinicians and policy makers. With growing evidence of what works and what does not work, organisations ranging from the World Health Organization to local health departments started devising guidelines for clinical practice to contain medicine within the limits set by what was known to be effective. This would also provide justification for health spending which, it could be argued, would be based on improved outcomes. Evidence-based practice has now earned a firm place in medical schools, and governments have a keen interest in evidence-based policy. Some clinicians find it useful, although there have been complaints about the way that evidence-based medicine distorts clinical decision making (see, for example, Benech et al. 1996; Feinstein & Horowitz 1997).

The problem of noncompliance appeared early in the history of clinical epidemiology. It has been recognised since the time of Hippocrates that patients ignore medical advice and then deny that they do so. If clinical epidemiologists were investing effort in producing scientific evidence of the benefit of or harm from medical interventions, then surely patients would see it as rational to comply with medical prescriptions based on such scientifically impeccable evidence? Unfortunately for the researchers trying to conduct scientifically rigorous studies of living patients, recalcitrance was a feature of study participants as well as patients (Roberts & Wurtele 1980). Unlike laboratory mice under observation, people participants went home, escaped observation, and a proportion did not conform to the requirements of study protocols. They subverted study designs by not doing what they were supposed to, by gaining access to new interventions that they were not supposed to have, or by dropping out of the study altogether. This introduced compliance bias into the trial, creating what Feinstein (1976, p. 165) referred to as 'major biostatistical delusions', leading to underestimation of the effectiveness of interventions, with the consequent risk of overmedication of future patients. The admission of problems with evidence did nothing to reassure noncompliant patients that there were real gains to be had by following medical prescription or, for that matter, to promote the aims of evidence-based medicine.

These problems gave a new impetus to the study of noncompliance (Sackett & Haynes 1976). Strategies that were developed for controlling study participants had the additional benefit of then being able to be tried with patients who were failing to fill their prescriptions or who were flushing pills down the toilet. Thus was born an expanding field of research into the nature, causes, and costs of noncompliance. Perhaps not surprisingly, given the context of rational decision making based on good evidence, noncompliant patients were targeted and demeaned. Strangely, taking into account the emphasis on studying real patients, much of this new field of study focused on the study of people while they were in the clinical setting and only on isolated aspects of their behaviour once they went home. What was much less popular was to ask why people did what they did. This is the gap in the literature that we decided to address.

We recognise that noncompliance with some therapies has serious direct health consequences for the individual and the community. The failure to treat an infectious disease can put the community at risk. The failure to comply with a therapeutic regimen for serious mental illness might put family members at risk. Our interest was not in cases where noncompliance puts a community at risk but in cases where compliance primarily benefited the individual and where there was an incentive for that individual to be compliant. We focused on heart attacks in the belief that a heart attack was extremely painful, amounted to a brush with death, and that the experience would predispose patients to follow medical advice on preventing a recurrence.

We devised a qualitative study of patients' responses to medical advice after a heart attack. Study participants were enrolled in the cardiac out-patient clinic of a large city hospital but were interviewed at home. The interview format was unstructured and based on their account of the advice they were given as patients and how they responded to that advice. In the analysis we categorised patients along a continuum based on their degree of compliance with both drug treatment and lifestyle changes.

The focus here is not on the minority of patients who followed medical advice with scrupulous attention to detail; instead, we focus on two noncompliant patients. Louise Craig in case study 1 (see box 12.1) is located towards the compliant end of the spectrum and we chose her for more detailed analysis because she epitomises the way in which patients are selective in deciding to follow some medical advice but not all. George Kominos in case study 2 (see box 12.2) comes from the noncompliant end of the spectrum and epitomises the kind of patient labelled as recalcitrant in the literature.

Box 12.1
Case study 1—Louise Craig

Louise Craig is 66 years old and married to a retired lawyer. The couple have seven children, most of whom live close to the family home. Ms Craig has been a devoted mother and takes care of grandchildren several times a week. She was interviewed a year after her heart attack.

We were struck by the stoic nature of Ms Craig's response to the heart attack, which she describes as 'an interesting exercise'. Giving birth seven times had acquainted her with pain; raising seven children has taught her to take everything in her stride. She went to her daughter's house to babysit a grandchild during the heart attack, at which stage her son-in-law called for an ambulance. She prides herself on being 'a good patient', who complies with her doctor's advice: 'If he said lie on a bed of nails, I'd do it.' After the heart attack, and following medical advice, she gave up smoking. 'I haven't smoked since. I was smoking a packet, maybe thirty a day ... I would love one, I miss it, but I just can't, I can't, that would be just ridiculous!' She has also complied 'absolutely' with the medication prescribed.

Ms Craig would seem to be the ideally compliant patient, but she has not followed all the advice she was given. After dealing with her various daily commitments, she tends to avoid doing the walking program her husband devised. When it comes to diet she points out that they eat a pretty healthy diet anyway, but in some areas she has 'let it slip'. Her life is very focused on her family and she would not like to deprive them of the sweet that they expect at the end of dinner. This is not because her family is unsupportive. On the contrary, in early convalescence when she considered dramatically changing her diet, her husband offered to cook the new 'fat-free' meals. This did not work out:

> He never cooked in his life. After two meals, I decided this wasn't acceptable ... I'd rather die than eat steamed vegies ... fat-free recipes, they should just put 'boring' on the top ... I love to cook in butter, so I've slipped back a bit ... Salads, sandwiches with just a scrape of butter, I couldn't eat a sandwich without butter. No bacon. I love bacon. I didn't think I could be bothered in doing all this, so I've sort of gone back to my old ways.

In addition, she is not convinced that weight loss is worth it.

> A friend was on a strict diet and we ate at another friend's house. He brought his own and it was a plate of steamed vegies that he brought. He was gaunt, and he had lost weight and [they] all thought that was marvellous. I thought he looked like a walking corpse, and I thought, No thanks, I'd rather not. If you've got to go, you've got to go.

The other area in which Ms Craig has been noncompliant is in not attending rehabilitation sessions at the local hospital:

> I've let that slip. They rang me and I said Yes, I'd be interested. Then they were trying to get a time, and then they didn't ring any

more and it's sort of slipped through. I've done nothing about the rehab, but then I thought, Well, what exactly will they tell me that I really don't already know? I'm not doing everything I should. I've chosen not to.

∎

Louise Craig has made changes to her lifestyle but has stopped short of making changes that would disrupt the quality of her and her family's life. If we take account of what Ms Craig values in her life, then her actions seem quite rational. Who would deny this woman a scrape of butter and the occasional slice of bacon? She has certainly not acted out of ignorance; nor does she hold any disrespect for the medical system. What she has done is to find an acceptable compromise between what she was prescribed and what she feels able to achieve.

Box 12.2
Case study 2—George Kominos

George Kominos has had a quite different response to his experience. At the age of 37, he has had two heart attacks, sixteen months and ten months before he was interviewed. He lacks personal and family resources. He did not complete high school but, as a first-generation Australian, aspires to something more than the life of his parents, who speak only a little English and 'grow vegetables in their back-yard'. Before his heart attacks George Kominos worked as a mechanic and fisherman and was established in his own house. At the time of the interview he had been forced to return to his parents' home as he was neither able to find work nor, even if he had found work, been well enough to work for long. The direct impact of heart disease on Mr Kominos's life chances, occurring as they did at an early age, has left him feeling alienated and angry. He feels he has been pushed aside. 'Society is telling you to get the hell out of the way.' His friends are young and do not understand why he is unable to go out with them. 'They cracked the shits ... "George, you can't keep doing this to us".' His view of life was not improved by learn-ing of the ways in which he was expected to restructure his life. After his first heart attack he made consistent changes, to no avail. He had another heart attack. He now presents as the epitome of a difficult, recalcitrant, and noncompliant patient. No longer employable, he is restricted in his social life. His body remains one area where George Kominos feels he can exercise some control, often in direct opposition to medical advice. In hospital, when he was given a bedpan, he jumped out of bed and started doing pushups.

> It makes me feel lower than an ant, when I'm quite capable of lifting up my legs, walking on my own two feet to the toilet ... They cracked up on me ... 'You idiot, you just had a heart attack two days ago!' ... I wasn't going to let anybody tell me to run my life the way they wanted to, for what suits them. Well, it's not their body, it's my body, and I'll do what suits me. They can advise me, but that's all they can do. They can't rule me on my own body.

After leaving hospital, he was told not to worry about the chest pain that he was still experiencing. This was a crucial episode for George. For him, these pains were evidence of further serious trouble and, having had two heart attacks, the fear of another was very real. Having denied the significance of his pain has made him angry and vengeful.

> When I do get pains in the chest ... I can still hear his voice telling me not to worry about it. 'Just ignore it' ... So that's what I do. But what happens if I just drop? Yeah, what happens then? ... Well, I'll tell you what I told him. I said, 'I won't worry about it, but if I drop, you're dropping with me!'

Lacking faith in the medical system has meant a reluctance to trust what doctors tell him and a greater emphasis on drawing his own conclusions about the evidence: 'It's not good enough. You want to see for yourself, read it for yourself, that's all there is to it.' This would seem to fit well with the aim of evidence-based medicine: if the evidence is there, it can be used both to sustain practice and persuade patients.

While still in hospital George asked for access to the medical library, but he was told it was just for the staff. The irony of this does not escape him: 'In other words if somebody wants to learn something, they'll have to get better first and get out of here and then go to the library.' He decided to refuse medication for pain as he felt it would mask the pain, which he needed to monitor for himself.

> I won't take the morphine. I refuse morphine, I refuse pethidine. [They are] trying to solve the problem by giving me something to kill the pain but that's not rectifying my problem. I want to know

my actual problem, what damage is in here. Don't just give me something for the pain and kill the pain, and let me lay in bed for four or five hours and then ask, 'Are you pain free?' And if you say 'Yes', 'OK, you can go home then.' I don't need that. I want to know my problem—if I can fix it or if I can't.

George Kominos's angry questioning of medical evidence undoubtedly has made him unpopular as a patient, but we were impressed by his determination to stand up for himself and others from a strong sense of social justice. In one memorable incident, visitors who came to the hospital to see him were turned away as they arrived out of visiting hours. They had travelled from the country town where they live, a journey of four hours. One of them was a 77-year-old neighbour who also had heart disease and whom Mr Kominos regarded as being 'three times as sick' as he was himself. When he found that they had been turned away, it was the last straw. 'I couldn't take it any more, so I just jumped out of bed, pulled all the monitors off, got dressed, discharged myself, [and] drove all the way to Mansfield.' He got there at half past three in the morning, apologised to his neighbour the next morning, gave her flowers, and drove back to the hospital. George Kominos's explanation was simple: he 'didn't want to die with a guilty conscience'.

■

George Kominos is angry and he is fighting the medical system. After his first heart attack he was compliant, which included giving up smoking, but his second heart attack made it seem a waste of time. However, he is still not smoking and it is not even clear that he is consistently noncompliant with other advice. This can be seen as evidence of his good sense.

Implications for policy

These two patients each experienced a life-threatening event. Each brought to it quite different capacities for responding to stress. Louise Craig is a person with a great respect for medical care but one whose limits to change were reached. She has a different perspective on the problem from that of a health policy maker who might quite reasonably focus on the potential saving to the health budget if thousands of cardiac patients followed medical advice to the last detail. The problem is that, while the benefit in the whole population may mean a considerable saving to the government, the benefit to each individual is small. In Louise Craig's case, the additional benefit of increasing her compliance with dietary and exercise recommendations and recommendations to attend rehabilitation classes would be smaller still. This small benefit is not justified in terms of her reduced quality of life as a result of disrupted food patterns, family obligations, and her clear recognition of the downside of compliance, or, as she put it, becoming a 'walking corpse'.

If we are to make sense of Louise Craig's decision, we need to recognise that there are two kinds of expertise and even two kinds of evidence. Health professionals are expert in the diagnosis and treatment of heart disease. They may well have at their fingertips the evidence for the cardiac benefits of a change in diet. Ms Craig, however, is expert in her own life. She is the only one who can judge the extent to which the advice she was given is relevant to her life, given that she already eats a healthy diet and expends plenty of energy looking after her grandchildren. She knows how the advice she was given articulates her particular circumstances and values and has made a considered judgment: her level of compliance is that which assures her the best quality of life for her. Certainly, it would be worth focusing on her real success in giving up smoking and taking medication instead of questioning her partial lack of success with diet and rehabilitation. Instead of calculating the cost of her noncompliance, we could quantify the contribution made to health savings by her compliance.

George Kominos presents quite a different challenge. He is confused. Who expects to have a heart attack at 37? He is angry that the changes he made after his first heart attack did not protect him from having another one only months later. He is proof that the evidence on secondary cardiac prevention is problematic. Again, the evidence that changes in lifestyle after a heart attack can prevent a second heart attack is derived from epidemiological evidence drawn from populations and does not reliably predict the effect on any one person. In a sense, patients are asked to wager a great deal of effort on the chance that the improvement in health will manifest in their particular case. George Kominos thought that he had made an agreement with his doctor; he had made the effort, but lost. Notions of risk and whole population health benefits are not as real as his anger at being let down, as he thought he had been, by his doctor. These notions of risk are implicit in much of the advice given to patients, but risk is a complex concept and is difficult to make explicit. The focus is on telling a patient what they can do to get well. The risk in this approach is the alienation of patients such as George Kominos.

Paradoxically, given the emphasis on education as a remedy for noncompliance, it appears that Mr Kominos was not encouraged to access and evaluate the evidence himself. Certainly, his view is that he is being denied access to professional material and this makes him suspicious of what health professionals might be hiding from him. When he acts in defence of his elderly friend he is taking a principled and compassionate path. Given how ill he was, he showed a commitment to moral principles over the risk to his own health. We should recognise the contribution he has made to health savings by complying with medical advice despite his level of frustration with and alienation from the health system.

Running through both these cases are troublesome issues. Health professionals have properly focused on trying to save the lives of these two patients. There is good evidence for their prescriptions from a population perspective. But from the perspective of the two patients, they might both have been treated in an unnecessarily intrusive way. Ms Craig takes a passive route in setting limits to the intrusion into her life; she stays away. Mr Kominos is confrontational, acting out his frustrations. The assumption that underlies much of the literature on noncompliance is that they both should in some way be made to comply. Given the good reasons (to them) why they are not doing so, further efforts at inducing compliance might well be counterproductive. Louise Craig might not go back to the hospital at all, and George Kominos might take some even more unfortunate direct action. Better by far to respect their judgments and accept that they are both, within the limits of their particular settings, making reasonable attempts at being 'good' patients.

Evidence-based policy

There is no question that biomedical science has been central to the development of effective medical care. Clinical epidemiology, too, has generated new methods for studying clinical care and is generating an everincreasing number of studies that demonstrate clearly what works and what does not work in the clinical setting. This is cause for celebration, as Sackett (1984) pointed out. Evidence-based medicine is quite reasonably seen as having the potential to change the way in which medical students are trained and it might change the way in which clinicians make treatment decisions. The evidence base has proved useful in devising guidelines for practice and for policy makers making funding decisions. The problem apparently lies with patients and their lack of compliance; however, this view can be questioned.

The laboratory is confined within four walls and is governed by standards of scientific rationality. Clinical epidemiology has extended its focus to the real-world clinical setting and concentrates on selected aspects of practice, typically answering the question 'Is treatment A more effective (or more cost-effective) than treatment B in treating disease X?' The answers produced are persuasive and the standards of scientific rationality have been retained. The problem arises when we attempt to extrapolate from this evidence to the social world of patients. Here, we encounter people who make their decisions in a manner that does not nearly approximate what happens in the laboratory or in a well-conducted trial of the cost-effectiveness of treatment. Instead, people live their lives by dealing with a confluence of influences and circumstances that constitute the social world. Scientific rationality has to be integrated into this world; it cannot govern it.

The popular appeal of the notion of patient noncompliance is based on its methodological origins. It would be rewarding if we could constrain the behaviour of participants in trials of therapy. Inspired by the promise of evidence-based medicine, it then seemed even more advantageous to constrain the behaviour of patients to fit the evidence. In thinking this way, we have defined a standard of rationality that excludes an understanding of the everyday social lives of human beings. Such a program cannot succeed.

The policy implications of these conclusions are complex and may well be unwelcome, as they appear to remove from the field the sense of certainty, which was one of the main attractions of evidence-based policy making. The promise that it holds in terms of cost constraints is that services only need to be provided to the extent that patients see them as necessary. This is in direct contrast with a health system governed by the lure of what medical science argues to be possible—with patients then being obliged to avail themselves of these treatments. We need to sound two important notes of caution here. We are neither arguing that noncompliant patients, however diagnosed, can simply be excluded from services that they are not going to use anyway, nor suggesting a health system responsive only to patient or consumer needs. Instead, our argument is that medical services might be prescribed to an extent that patients, in general, do not find useful or welcome. This is not a problem of noncompliant patients, but a problem of the expectation that patients will use services provided for them for their health advantage when these are services they do not wish to use. We should recognise that some patients will use these services, but others will choose not to do so. Where, especially, an intervention primarily stands to benefit the patient as individual, and where patients are well informed, there is little we can, or should, do to change this. Thus patients' nonuse or nonattendance can provide a filter for what is going to satisfy patient needs. The other necessary filter is that the intervention must meet professional standards of evidence of effectiveness. The health system could well be smaller but better used and more effective.

There are additional implications for health research. If our arguments are correct, we can call a moratorium on research programs that identify targets and devise interventions for bringing recalcitrant patients to (medical) heel. Rather, the research focus should be on the necessary next stage in our scientific understanding of the treatment of illness—studies of patients in their real, everyday lives outside of the medical setting. This requires us to gather evidence about noncompliant patients as they fulfil their roles as family members, with concerns for social justice, and with their own expertise in the way in which medical prescriptions articulate with their lives. The aim of these studies will be to explain how responsible citizens view the evidence from medicine in the light of the evidence about their own lives. Perhaps not surprisingly, we conclude that the social sciences stand to make a central contribution to the gathering of this new social evidence.

There is, however, a new role for epidemiologists in addressing one of the impediments that patients encounter in their efforts to get well—understanding the difficult and counterintuitive nature of conclusions based on the epidemiological study of risk. To select a first target for future research in this area, it might be necessary to devise effective ways of communicating notions of risk and evidence of benefit from a range of popular public health interventions, ranging from dietary change after a heart attack, to screening for cancer, or even to the debate on the evidence for risks versus benefits of immunisation programs.

We end this paper with three cheers for the people who came forward to share with us their thoughts on recovering from a heart attack.

Acknowledgment

This chapter draws on data from a research study, 'Patient non-compliance with health advice', funded by the National Health and Medical Research Council. The views expressed in the chapter are those of the authors alone.

References

Benech, I., Wilson, A. E., & Dowell, A. C. 1996, 'Evidence-based Practice in Primary Care: Past, Present and Future', *Journal of Evaluation in Clinical Practice*, vol. 2, no. 4, pp. 49–63.

Cramer, J. A. & Spilker, B. 1991, *Patient Compliance in Medical Practice and Clinical Trials*, Raven Press, New York.

DiMatteo, M. R. 1994, 'Enhancing Patient Adherence to Medical Recommendations', *Journal of the American Medical Association*, vol. 271, no. 1, pp. 79–83.

Feinstein, A. R. 1976, ' "Compliance Bias" and the Interpretation of Therapeutic Trials', in D. L. Sackett & R. B. Haynes (eds), *Compliance with Therapeutic Regimens*, Johns Hopkins University Press, Baltimore.

—— 1983, 'An Additional Basic Science for Clinical Medicine', Parts I–III, *Annals of Internal Medicine*, vol. 99, pp. 393–7, 544–50, 705–12.

—— & Horowitz, R. I. 1997, 'Problems in the "Evidence" of "Evidence-based" Medicine', *American Journal of Medicine*, vol. 103, no. 6, pp. 529–35.

Frazier, A. L. et al. 2000, 'Cost-effectiveness of Screening for Colorectal Cancer in the General Population', *Journal of the American Medical Association*, vol. 284, no. 15, pp. 1954–61.

Gerbino, P. P. 1993, 'Foreword', *Annals of Pharmacotherapy*, vol. 27, S3–4.

Haynes, R. B., Taylor, D. W., & Sackett, D. L. (eds) 1979, *Compliance in Health Care*, Johns Hopkins University Press, Baltimore.

—— & McKibbon, K. A. 1996, 'Systematic Review of Randomised Trials of Interventions to Assist Patients to Follow Prescriptions for Medications', *Lancet*, vol. 348, pp. 383–6.

Lerner, B. H. 1997, 'From Careless Consumptives to Recalcitrant Patients: The Historical Construction of Noncompliance', *Social Science and Medicine*, vol. 45, no. 9, pp. 1423–31.

McElduff, P. et al. 2001, 'Opportunities for Control of Coronary Heart Disease in Australia', *Australian and New Zealand Journal of Public Health*, vol. 25, pp. 24–30.

Rapley, P. 1997, 'Self-care: Re-thinking the Role of Compliance', *Australian Journal of Advanced Nursing*, vol. 15, pp. 20–4.

Roberts, M. C. & Wurtele, S. K. 1980, 'On the Noncompliant Research Subject in a Study of Medical Noncompliance', *Social Science and Medicine*, vol. 14A, no. 2, p. 171.

Sackett, D. L. 1984, 'Three Cheers for Clinical Epidemiology', Letter to the Editor, *International Journal of Epidemiology*, vol. 13, no. 1, p. 117.

—— & Haynes, R. B. (eds) 1976, *Compliance with Therapeutic Regimens*, Johns Hopkins University Press, Baltimore.

——, Haynes, R. B., & Tugwell, P. 1985, *Clinical Epidemiology: A Basic Science for Clinical Medicine*, Little, Brown, Boston.

Smith, M. 1985, 'The Cost of Noncompliance and the Capacity of Improved Compliance to Reduce Health Care Expenditures' in National Pharmaceutical Council, *Improving Medication Compliance: Proceedings of a Symposium*, Washington DC, 1 November, pp. 35–44.

Urquhart, J. 2001, 'E-Drug: The Terms Compliance and Patient', <http:www.healthnet.org/programs/e-drug-hma/e-drug.199909/msg00126.html>.

Zwarenstein, M. et al. 1998, 'Randomised Controlled Trial of Self Supervised and Directly Observed Treatment of Tuberculosis', *Lancet*, vol. 352, pp. 1340–3.

13

Carer Policy in Aged Care: A Structural Interests Perspective

Alice Creelman

Thursday, 2 April 1998. The 450 delegates assembling at the National Convention Centre in Canberra for the National Summit Conference of the Carers Association of Australia heard rumours that there was to be a last-minute change in the conference agenda. The previously circulated program stated that the keynote address would be given by the parliamentary secretary representing the Minister for Health and Family Services, but soon the rumours that a more senior politician would take her place were confirmed. In fact, none other than the Prime Minister himself was introduced to deliver the keynote address. Mr Howard spoke of 'our shared responsibility to provide for the care of older Australians' and 'the formulation of long-term policies in relation to community care'. He listed his Coalition government's achievements for older Australians and for carers, then proceeded to announce 'a major new package of initiatives worth $270 million over four years to help older Australians, their carers and carers generally' (Howard 1998, p. 9). But wait, there's more ... the Leader of the Labor Opposition was introduced as a keynote speaker on 'A Vision for Community and Health Care', and referred to the community care reforms undertaken by the previous Labor government, which had 'put a supportive architecture around carers in our community', and promised to do even more when Labor was next returned to government (Beazley 1998, p. 17). Then, in her keynote speech, the Leader of the Australian Democrats noted the importance of looking at 'the political context within which policies affecting Carers are being developed' and

---

The views expressed in this chapter are those of the author and should not be taken to represent the views of the Department of Health and Ageing.

expressed the opinion that 'the economic policies of both the major parties spell disaster for carers …' (Lees 1998, pp. 22, 23). Later, both the Minister for Family Services and the shadow minister articulated their respective carer policies (Carers Association of Australia 1998a). On Friday, 3 April, the Prime Minister's speech and policy announcement was the lead article on page 1 of the *Canberra Times* and featured prominently in all major Australian newspapers. The media coverage (including several editorials) continued over the weekend and into the following week.

Meanwhile, back at the conference, many delegates must have been remembering a time not so long before when the very notion of carer policy did not exist, let alone have the capacity to command the attendance of the leaders of political parties or draw national media attention. Carers as a client group of government community care services first appeared in Australian legislation in the *Home and Community Care Act 1985* (Cwlth), but it was to be another seven years before a first policy on assistance to carers appeared in a Commonwealth Budget (Department of Health, Housing and Community Services [DHHCS] 1992). Yet, less than six years later, no major political party in Australia could afford to be without an articulated carer policy.

What happened in so short a space of time to raise carer policy to national prominence? The emergence of carer policy as a distinct component of Australian aged care policy in the period between 1985 and 1998 is an interesting case for policy analysis. Most analysis of community-based aged care policy has focused on the development of policy in relation to services that support the aged and disabled to remain at home (Healy 1990; Sax 1993; Minichiello 1995). The chapter aims to take a different perspective and analyse the development of policy in relation to services that support carers. In doing so, Alford's structural interests thesis is used to assist in understanding why carer policy has emerged as an issue of national importance (Alford 1975). Recognising that the scope of carer policy is broad, the focus of the chapter is on carers of the aged in Commonwealth government community care policy from 1985 to 1998.

There are two reasons for choosing this focus. First, while carers of the aged have many needs in common with carers of younger adults and children with disabilities, the construction of ageing as a public policy issue differs in many respects from the construction of disability as an issue (Gibson 1998). Differences that impact on policy development include societal norms and expectations of the caring role and of the care recipient's participation in the community, the availability of family care at different life stages, and the history and patterns of government service provision. Second, while a comprehensive analysis of carer policy would also examine Commonwealth and state policy in relation to such areas as income support, housing, and transport (Bozic et al. 1993), the most integrated development of carer policy in Australia over the past fifteen years has occurred at the national level and within the context of the Commonwealth government's aged and community care programs.

Australia's aged and community care system

A wide range of health services and assistance is available to older Australians. The aged care system is generally taken to encompass those services that provide continuing support for frail and disabled older people, as well as support for those who care for them (Australian Institute of Health and Welfare 1999). With the nongovernment sector and private individuals, all levels of government have some role in the funding, administration, or provision of aged care services for older people. Of the three levels of government in Australia (national, state and territory, and local), the Commonwealth government is the major funder of aged care services.

The aged care system (Department of Health and Aged Care 1999) is structured around two main forms of care delivery—residential care and community care—each underpinned by a system of assessment and quality assurance. For most of the period under review, there were two tiers of residential care: nursing homes for higher-dependency residents needing access to ongoing nursing care, and hostels for lower-dependency residents requiring personal care services. From October 1997, the funding and administration of these care forms were restructured under one system of residential care, although the terms 'nursing home' and 'hostel' remain in common usage and many residential care facilities continue to specialise in either high- or low-level care. Residential care is financed and regulated by the Commonwealth government.

Community care is more diverse, and includes the jointly funded Commonwealth–state Home and Community Care Program, which provides a range of services including home nursing, delivered meals, home help, home maintenance, paramedical services, respite care, and transport. The Commonwealth also funds more intensive home-based personal care through brokerage arrangements known as Community Aged Care Packages.

Developments in the aged care system since 1985 have taken place within the policy context of a strategy to shift the balance of care provision gradually away from high-level residential care towards lower levels of residential care and community-based care (DHHCS 1991b). However, expenditure on residential care in 1997–98 ($2847 million) was still more than three times the combined expenditure ($895 million) on Home and Community Care (HACC) and Community Aged Care Packages (Australian Institute of Health and Welfare 1999).

The corollary of this shift in provision is that, proportionately, more highly dependent older people are remaining in the community, supported by home-based services and informal carers (Gibson 1998).

Who are the carers?

There is not a universally accepted definition of 'carer', and it is difficult to establish the number and characteristics of carers. Some definitions in current usage include:

> A carer is someone who provides care and support for a parent, partner, child or friend who has a disability, is frail aged, suffers from dementia or a chronic illness; or any former carer (Carers Association of Australia 1993b).

> A person such as a family member, friend or neighbour, who provides regular and sustained care and assistance to another person without payment other than a pension or benefit (HACC 1998).

> A person of any age who provides any informal assistance, in terms of help or supervision, to persons with disabilities or long-term conditions, or persons who are elderly (Australian Bureau of Statistics 1999).

The Australian Bureau of Statistics (ABS) conducts a five-yearly Survey of Disability, Ageing and Carers. Definitions and methodologies for identifying carers have varied somewhat between surveys. The 1998 survey distinguished between 'carers' and 'primary carers' (ABS 1999). The narrower category of 'primary carer' is defined as

> a person of any age who provides the most informal assistance, in terms of help or supervision, to a person with one or more disabilities. The assistance has to be ongoing, or likely to be ongoing, for at least six months and be provided for one or more of the core activities (communication, mobility and self care) (ABS 1999, p. 71).

Most of the analysis of carer data published by the ABS relates to primary carers. However, the target population of a particular carer support program may well be broader (or, in some cases, narrower) than the population of primary carers.

According to the ABS survey (ABS 1999), in 1998 there were more than 2.3 million carers in Australia, of whom about 450 000 were primary carers. Of the latter, 45 per cent were caring for aged people (65 years and older). The largest group of primary carers (43 per cent) was providing care to a partner, with a high proportion of partners being aged. A further 22 per cent were providing care to a parent, with a large proportion of parents also being aged. About 70 per cent of principal carers are women, and about 22 per cent are themselves older than 65 years.

It has been noted that caring is 'a more common than uncommon experience' (Howe et al. 1997, p. 1028), taking into account the duration of caring, the spread of caring across age groups, and the extent of inter-generational exchange in caregiving. One large population-based survey conducted in Victoria found that more than 40 per cent of carers had been caring for more than five years (Howe et al. 1997).

The caring role has been shown to have a major impact on carers' incomes, expenses, workforce participation, family relationships, social life, health, and wellbeing (Braithwaite 1990; Office of Women's Affairs Victoria 1994; ABS 1995; Carers Association of Australia 1997, 1998b, 2000). As a predominantly female activity, caring can have a particular impact on women who may be maintaining multiple roles including those of carers of elderly parents, mothers of dependent children, and employees in the workforce (Murphy et al. 1997).

The Australian Institute of Health and Welfare (AIHW) analysed the earlier 1993 ABS survey data in terms of carers' expressed need for assistance in their caring role. Of principal carers providing care to people 65 years and older, 16 per cent expressed an unmet need for help (Australian Institute of Health and Welfare 1997). The AIHW analysis also noted that 'the vast majority of assistance required by persons with a profound or severe handi-cap' was provided by informal carers, not formal services (Australian Institute of Health and Welfare 1997, p. 252).

It should be noted that the ABS survey is based on self-reported data and probably underestimates the number of carers. Many people view caring as an extension of their family role and do not self-identify as carers. It may also be the case that the invisibility of carers is based on the stereotype of women's roles (DHHCS 1991a). Women undertake most informal caring. It is unpaid and generally not valued as work; it also tends to be taken for granted in public discourse (Hancock & Moore 1999). The emergence of caring as a policy issue may be an indicator of (as well as a contributor to) a greater tendency for people to self-identify as carers.

Major milestones in national carer policy

The development of Australian community care policy in relation to carers of the aged can be divided into three periods, each beginning with a major mile-stone. The first of these milestones was legislative, the second was budgetary, and the third was political.

1985-91

The Commonwealth Home and Community Care Act was passed in 1985. This was the major community care achievement of the Hawke Labor government. It subsumed four smaller Acts in an expanded and integrated program of domiciliary and community-based support services for frail aged people and younger people with disabilities who were at risk of premature or inappropriate institutionalisation. It was the first piece of community care legislation to identify specifically carers of these people as part of the client group. The main service targeting carers' needs was respite care, which had not been funded under the previous four Acts.

The Home and Community Care Act was a key element of the Commonwealth's Aged Care Reform Strategy, which aimed to shift the balance of aged care service provision away from residential care and towards community care (DHHCS 1991b). During the next six years, funding under the Home and Community Care Act was increased substantially.

In 1988, the ABS conducted its second Survey of Disabled and Aged Persons, which also surveyed carers. Publications from this survey increased policy makers' knowledge about carers and started to provide a database for policy development (ABS 1990).

In 1991, the *Report of the Mid Term Review of the Commonwealth's Aged Care Reform Strategy* was published. It included a major discussion paper on *The Role of Carers in Aged Care: Policies and Programs for Support*, which highlighted the need to take account of carers in policy development (DHHCS 1991a).

1992-95

In August 1992, the first carer policy appeared in a Commonwealth Budget. The aged and community care budget initiatives included a package of assistance for carers worth $93 million over four years. The money was used to establish the Commonwealth Respite for Carers Program, increase the level of the Domiciliary Nursing Care Benefit, provide information and support to carers through the development of a carers' kit, and to the funding of a National Carers' Week (DHHCS 1992).

The Budget was followed in September by the launch of the Keating Labor government's 'Commitment to Carers' national policy statement, which proclaimed that 'commitment to carers is a cornerstone of the Australian Government's Community Care Policy' (Australian Government 1992). In 1993, the Carers Association of Australia was established with funding from the Commonwealth government. The Association saw its 'initial and primary role' as being 'to lobby the government on issues related to carers' (Carers Association 1993a).

Also in 1993, the Australian Bureau of Statistics conducted an expanded Survey of Disability, Ageing and Carers. Publications from this survey, particularly the widely distributed *Focus on Families: Caring in Families—Support for Persons who are Older or have Disabilities*, were influential in creating a 'language around caring' and placing carers on the public agenda (ABS 1995).

The 1993, 1994, and 1995 Commonwealth Budgets contained various changes in relation to services for carers, including the establishment of a National Respite Review to evaluate provision, analyse needs, and identify the scope for improved effectiveness (Department of Human Services and Health 1995). In 1995, the Commonwealth Department of Human Services and Health (DHSH) sponsored a workshop titled 'Towards a National Agenda for Carers' to stimulate thinking about carer issues and consider principles for the development of carer support strategies (DHSH 1996a, 1996b).

1996–98

In the leadup to the March 1996 federal election, the Carers Association ran its first election-related political campaign, which involved mailing a campaign kit to every candidate from every major party. For the first time, all major political parties launched a carer policy (Carers Association of Australia 1996). The Liberal and National Parties' policy document, *National Carer Action Plan*, promised to implement a carer policy (Liberal Party and National Party 1996).

The first Budget of the newly elected Howard Coalition government was widely recognised as a cost-cutting Budget. One area where this did not apply was in relation to support for carers, where the government moved to implement its election promise by providing $36.7 million over four years to establish a National Respite for Carers Program and Carer Resource Centres in every capital city (Department of Health and Family Services [DHFS] 1996a). The 1997 Coalition Budget further extended support for carers as part of the National Carer Action Plan, with particular emphasis on income support and needs assessment, information and advice, and targeted support for people with dementia and their carers (DHFS 1997).

Then, in April 1998, the Prime Minister attended the Carers Association National Summit Conference to announce the $270 million *Staying at Home—Care and Support for Older Australians* package. In the words of Warwick Smith, then Minister for Family Services, 'The Government has delivered on its words of support for carers. We are serious about supporting the carers in our community' (Smith 1998).

The role of interest groups in carer policy

In reviewing the influences on the development of carer policy since 1985, the role of the Carers Association of Australia stands out. Carers' advocacy and support groups are well advanced in Australia compared with other countries (Gibson 1998). Indeed, the first carers' association in the world was established in New South Wales in 1975, and the forerunner to the Carers Association of Australia was active at the national level from the late 1980s. From the time it was formally established with Commonwealth funding in 1993, the Carers Association has lobbied intensively on behalf of carers and appears to have achieved many notable policy successes (Carers Association of Australia 1996). Throughout this period, it has been the main group attempting to influence public policy in favour of carers.

There was also the Victorian Carers Program, which functioned from 1991 to 1996 (Schofield 1998). This was primarily a research and health promotion program based in just one state. Nevertheless, research centres can also function as interest groups, including in the aged care arena (Howe 1990), and the findings of the program's research were brought into the national policy process through publications and consultations (Bozic et al. 1993; DHSH 1996b).

According to pluralist theory, power is widely distributed among different groups. Groups participate in the policy process in order to defend their interests and values and secure resources for their policies (Ham & Hill 1984). An interest group such as the Carers Association attempts to mobilise its resources in order to influence public policy in favour of the interests of its members (Gardner 1995a). Groups that are organised, articulate, motivated, and wealthy are more likely to be effective in achieving their goals.

The difficulty with relying solely on pluralist theory to account for the development of carer policy is that it does not answer a number of pertinent questions. Why should carer policy come to prominence during this period, when families have always been the main carers of aged relatives? Why should the Commonwealth government have chosen 1993 to fund a carers' lobby group, when a group had been in existence a long time previously? Why has the Carers Association, which, despite its government funding, has always operated on a small budget, apparently been so successful in achieving its policy objectives in the 1990s? Why were such significant advances achieved in the 1996–98 period, when researchers were asserting in 1996 that 'Currently, there are significant impediments to effective policy development and service provision' (Schofield et al. 1996, p. 167)?

To explore these questions, this chapter now turns to an alternative model, which looks more broadly at the interaction of social, economic, and political factors in determining why particular interests prevail in policy development.

A structural interests perspective

Alford (1975) has put forward a structural interests perspective as a model for analysing why policy decisions that serve particular interests are taken. He does not adopt the pluralist focus on the organised activities of interest groups in attempting to gain benefits. Instead, his view is that interests are 'served or not served by the way they "fit" into the basic logic and principles by which the institutions of society operate' (Alford 1975, p. 14). He classifies these structural interests into three categories:

- *Dominant*: these are served by the structure of social, economic, and political institutions as they exist at any given time, so these interests do not have to organise and act to defend themselves.
- *Challenging*: these are created by the changing structure of society, and they act to challenge the dominant interests.
- *Repressed*: these interests are the opposite of dominant ones and the structure of societal institutions means that these interests will not be served except in special political circumstances.

Alford's thesis is that health policy needs to be understood in terms of a continuing struggle for control of health care resources between these three structural interests, which he identifies with, respectively,

- *professional monopolists*, principally medical practitioners and some other health care professionals who seek to maintain the status quo by preserving a professional monopoly over health care production
- *corporate rationalisers*, who may be bureaucrats, administrators, some health professionals, academics, and politicians whose interests are served by the promotion of greater efficiency, effectiveness, and equity in health provision
- *the community structural interest or equal health advocates*, whose interests lie in improving the health care available to the community population.

This framework was used to analyse changes in Australian health policy between 1965 and 1983 (Duckett 1984) and health system reform in Victoria in 1992–93 (Lin & Duckett 1997).

Structural interests in aged care policy

The structural interests perspective can usefully be applied—with some adaptation—to aged care policy. The dominant structural interest in Australian aged care is represented by the residential aged care sector, particularly the nursing home industry. The technology of aged care differs from the mainstream health care sector because the needs of the clients are related to dependency, disability, and chronic illness, not to the need for acute medical or surgical intervention. A range of health professionals is involved in controlling access to and provision of nursing home care, and the medical profession's position is not as dominant as in the health care sector. However, the main group with an interest in maintaining the aged care status quo is service providers, many of whom are private for-profit companies. The sector's industry organisations and lobby groups have a powerful voice and exert considerable political influence (Minichiello 1995). The threat of a nursing home closure tends to attract adverse political publicity. Despite many modifications to funding systems (Gibson 1998), the Commonwealth government has provided recurrent nursing home funding since 1962. The nursing home sector continues to benefit from a secure income stream, a high occupancy rate, and the prestige of being a health service. The sector's interests lie in preserving acceptance by government of the residential mode of care as the norm in aged care service provision.

The corporate rationalisers are also a challenging structural interest in aged care. These include bureaucrats from what is now the Department of Health and Ageing, and the departments that preceded it, various academic researchers, and some health care professionals involved in community care services. Over the years, the corporate rationalisers have drawn on data about the ageing of the population and other demographic changes, the increasing costs of residential care, and the substitutability of less intensive forms of care, to challenge the dominant role of nursing homes by proposing alternative models of service provision (DCS 1986; Howe 1990; EPAC 1994). This activity benefits the corporate rationalisers by enlarging their role in the planning and administration of aged care.

The repressed structural interest in aged care can broadly be identified with the aged themselves, their carers and families, and volunteer-based community groups. For the most part, this group is not seeking access to nursing home care. It is broadly accepted that, given the choice, most aged people would choose to stay at home (Gibson 1998). However, this group does have an interest in having ageing and caring viewed as public issues and as legitimate areas for government funding of service provision, even when they take place at home. Until the period we are considering, these interests had effectively been kept off the political agenda. The dependent aged who are consumers of aged care services do not speak with an organised or powerful political voice. The Carers Association of Australia and the various state carers' associations are the only groups specifically established to lobby for carers and care recipients. Perhaps the term 'equitable care advocates' would appropriately describe their focus.

Social, economic, and political circumstances

Alford (1975) asserts that it is the particular combination of prevailing social, economic, and political circumstances that determines which interests are served. This section highlights some of the broad trends relevant to carer policy between 1985 and 1998.

The structure of Australian society has been changing in a number of ways that impact on aged care policy (EPAC 1994; Gibson 1998). The population is ageing, so that the old old (who are more likely to be disabled) are forming an increasing proportion. Family patterns are changing, with women having fewer children and at a later age, reducing the supply of family carers and increasing the likelihood of competing care responsibilities. Female workforce participation rates have increased markedly, again with the effect of reducing the supply of family carers.

Analysis of the impact of population ageing and changing demographics has been largely undertaken by social scientists and policy makers who form part of the baby boom generation, which will move into old age in coming decades. This group has exhibited increasing levels of awareness of 'the twin problems of how to pay for the support of burgeoning numbers of older people in the present and yet have sufficient resources available to ensure that they are themselves appropriately cared for in the future' (Gibson 1998, p. 5).

From an economic perspective, the attention paid by the bureaucracy to the need to constrain rising aged care costs, largely driven by changing demographics, was a feature of this period. To an increasing extent, methods were being explored that would shift costs from government expenditure to private expenditure. At the same time, there was recognition that to sustain some cost savings in residential care it would be necessary to increase expenditure in community care (Minichiello 1995).

Australia's federal system sets up opportunities for cost shifting between the levels of government, and arguments over cost shifting have been a feature of Commonwealth–state health financing negotiations (Swerissen & Duckett 1997; Duckett 2000). The opportunity for cost shifting in aged care derives from the fact that residential care is the responsibility of the Commonwealth, whereas community care is partly cost shared with the states and territories. Expanding residential costs during this period thus increased the incentive to shift the focus to community care and also provided the rationale for a national approach to carer policy to sustain this focus.

Economic rationalism was the prevailing economic ideology and political orthodoxy shared by both political parties during this period. Economic rationalism advocates the use of strategic policy methods and the introduction of market mechanisms in the public sector (Gardner 1997). It can be viewed as an attempt to introduce more coherence and rationality into public policy, and it relies on putting appropriate financial incentives in place so that the most cost-effective policies are chosen. It is an approach that is consistent with the bureaucratic drive for more efficient service delivery.

Political ideology was also an important factor (Gardner 1995b). The Hawke Labor government was in power from 1983 to the end of 1991, when Keating replaced Hawke as Labor leader. The Labor government throughout this period was committed to a social justice ideology. The Howard Coalition government was elected in March 1996, and was committed to a family ideology. Paradoxically, both these ideologies were consistent with calls for increased government involvement in supporting family carers.

The shifting balance of structural interests 1985–98

We can now draw some of these strands together and explore the three periods, outlined earlier, of carer policy development.

1985–91

The first challenge to the dominance of the nursing home industry came with the passage of the *Home and Community Care Act 1985* (Cwlth). The conditions that facilitated this were an awareness of the changing demographics of the population and the increasing costs to the government of residential aged care. Politically, the Hawke Labor government was embracing the principles of economic rationalism while also being committed to a social justice ideology. This enabled the corporate rationalisers to successfully challenge the dominant interests of the nursing home industry, while also giving some recognition to the interests of informal family carers.

In the first few years after 1985, carer policy was not identified separately from community care policy. The emphasis was on the provision of community care services to support the aged in their homes, and carers were viewed as one of the resources contributing to that objective. However, as the policy changes introduced under the Aged Care Reform Strategy began to take effect, the reduction in residential care provision combined with the continued ageing of the population to produce a situation in which a larger proportion of highly dependent aged people were remaining in the community. More research about the role played by carers was becoming available, and carers were beginning to organise and put to bureaucrats and politicians the view that they shared common interests.

In particular, during this period recognition of the social and economic value of caring was brought into the public arena (Rosenman 1991; Tilse et al. 1991), which can, in part, be attributed to greater societal acceptance of women as income earners, leading to recognition of the opportunity costs of caring.

1992–95

By 1992, the Keating Labor government had been persuaded of the need to articulate a separate carer policy and to emphasise the provision of services to carers as clients in their own right. Behind this approach was an awareness that 'without the continued support of their carers, many more frail aged people or people with disabilities would require residential care' (Keating 1992, p. 34). It was therefore economically rational to provide support to carers if this could be done at a lesser cost to government than the cost of residential care. Equally, however, the government's public statements emphasised that 'carers deserve and must have respect and recognition, financial assistance and support … Their contributions enrich the lives of many thousands of Australians by … enabling them to remain at home among family and friends' (Australian Government 1992).

This period also saw the funding of the Carers Association and the effective incorporation of the group into government policy making processes, marking recognition that the interests of the corporate rationalisers and the equitable care advocates had become aligned. The remaining years of the Keating government was a period when economic and social factors continued to serve the interests of both these groups. Economic rationalism was ascendant and there was a continuing drive for efficiency in government expenditure, while the ABS 1993 survey and other research highlighted that the overwhelming majority of care needs of aged people at home were met by informal carers (ABS 1995).

In a paper presented in August 1995 at a major workshop on carer issues, Shaver and Fine (1996, p. 19) noted that 'private households have now become the preferred site for the exercise of public responsibility for many of the most vulnerable and dependent citizens'.

1996–98

With the election of the Howard Coalition government in 1996, the political context changed in ways that again served the interests of carers and facilitated the influence of the Carers Association.

First, the new government was committed to an ideology of the family. The Department of Human Services and Health was renamed the Department of Health and Family Services (DHFS 1996b). The new Minister for Family Services, Judi Moylan, started her Budget statement with these words:

> The family is the core social unit in our society. For generations the family has endured as the primary and most effective provider of assistance and support for people of all ages and from all backgrounds. The Coalition is absolutely committed to ensuring that the needs of families remain at the centre of public policy' (Moylan 1996, p. 1).

This political ideology was consistent with the social values articulated over many years by carers—that older people want to stay at home, cared for by their family—and which had been powerfully placed on the political agenda by the Carers Association's mailout campaign before the election. However, it was also consistent with economic rationalism. The Coalition election document noted that 'Carers make an untold contribution to the life of our community, saving billions of dollars in residential and hospital care. They ask for very little in return' (Liberal Party and National Party 1992, p. 3).

Second, in 1997, a major political crisis arose over the government's attempts to restructure the financing of the nursing home industry (announced in the cost-cutting 1996 Budget). In a major furore over proposed nursing home accommodation bonds, the government suffered considerable political damage when it appeared that aged people might need to sell the family home in order to fund entry to a nursing home; on 5 November the Prime Minister personally intervened to reverse the policy (Short 1997). In this context, the political largesse distributed at the Carers Association Conference in April 1998 could be interpreted as an attempt to win back the trust of the older constituency in what was widely expected to be an election year, and to shift the focus away from nursing homes and towards staying at home. Political commentators interpreted the funding package in that light (Contractor 1998).

The period of the first Howard government was thus interesting for the way in which political factors reinforced economic and social trends to favour particularly the interests of family carers of the aged, to the point where carer policy became an issue of national importance.

Conclusion

This chapter has charted the changes in government policy between 1985 and 1998, which came to favour the previously repressed structural interest group, and has explored the social, economic, and political circumstances that combined to produce these changes.

The notable trend was for an increasing alignment of the interests of the corporate rationalisers and the equitable care advocates in the development of carer support policies. Corporate rationalisers recognised the efficiency arguments for putting in place service supports that would sustain the capacity of unpaid, informal carers to provide care that would substitute for more expensive residential care. The equitable care advocates sought service supports that would legitimise the value of caring, be responsive to the desire of older people to remain at home, and provide much-needed practical support for the often arduous tasks of caring. Sustaining the process of carer policy development throughout this period were powerful political ideologies, which, in different ways, were consistent with a role for the state in supporting family carers.

The dominant structural interest in aged care—the nursing home industry—has had to cede some ground. Nevertheless, it cannot be said to have lost its dominant position. Residential aged care still attracts far more Commonwealth funding than community care and carer support services. Community care continues to be presented in policy documents as a substitute for residential care rather than as the norm. An interesting development since the mid 1990s has seen residential aged care providers increasingly moving to provide the equivalent of residential care in the home, including through a pilot Commonwealth program of nursing home care packages (Gibson 1998). While this may represent a growing alignment with the interests of both corporate rationalisers and equitable care advocates, it may also be viewed as a move to reappropriate control of aged care resources.

The development of policy inevitably involves competing interests and competing values. There is a dilemma to be faced in considering the effects of the increasing importance accorded to carer policy. While developments in carer support programs appear to be an enlightened response to the expressed claims of carers and older people, might it also be asserted, as some observers have, that the real interests of carers are being ignored by programs that facilitate the state's reliance on their unpaid work (Shaver & Fine 1996; Hancock & Moore 1999)?

Caring will continue to be a key component of aged care policy. The issue for the future will be to determine whose interests are being served in the further development of carer policy.

References

Alford, R. R. 1975, *Health Care Politics: Ideological and Interest Group Barriers to Reform*, University of Chicago Press, Chicago.

Australian Bureau of Statistics 1990, *Carers of the Handicapped at Home*, Cat. no. 4122.0, ABS, Canberra.

—— 1995, *Focus on Families: Caring in Families—Support for Persons who are Older or have Disabilities*, Cat. no. 4423.0, ABS, Canberra.

—— 1999, *Disability, Ageing and Carers: Summary of Findings*, Cat. No. 4430.0, ABS, Canberra.

Australian Government 1992, *A National Policy Statement: 'Commitment to Carers'*, Canberra.

Australian Institute of Health and Welfare 1997, *Australia's Welfare 1997: Services and Assistance*, AIHW, Canberra.

—— 1999, Australia's Welfare 1999: Services and Assistance, AIHW,. Canberra.

Beazley, K. 1998, 'Forging New Directions: A Vision for Community and Health Care', in *Community, State or Family: A Question of Responsibility*, Proceedings of National Summit Conference, 2 and 3 April, Carers Association of Australia, Canberra, pp. 16–21.

Bozic, S., Herrman, H., & Schofield, H. 1993, *Government Policy and Unpaid Family Carers: An Overview of Federal and Victorian Government Policy in Relation to Unpaid Family Caregivers—The Case of the Invisible and the Invaluable*, University of Melbourne, Melbourne.

Braithwaite, V. A. 1990, *Bound to Care*, Allen & Unwin, Sydney.

Carers Association of Australia 1993a, *First Annual Report 1992–93*, Carers Association of Australia, Canberra.

—— 1993b, *Strategic Plan*, Carers Association of Australia, Canberra.

—— 1996, *Annual Report 1995–96*, Carers Association of Australia, Canberra.

—— 1997, *Caring Enough to be Poor: A Survey of Carers' Incomes and Income Needs*, Carers Association of Australia, Canberra.

—— 1998a, *Community, State or Family: A Question of Responsibility*, Proceedings of National Summit Conference, 2 and 3 April, Carers Association of Australia, Canberra.

—— 1998b, *Caring Costs: A Survey of Tax Issues and Health and Disability Related Costs for Carer Families*, Carers Association of Australia, Canberra.

—— 2000, *Warning—Caring is a Health Hazard: Results of the 1999 National Survey of Carer Health and Wellbeing*, Carers Association of Australia, Canberra.

Contractor, A. 1998, '$270m Grey Pitch: PM Under Fire', *Canberra Times*, 3 April, pp. 1–2.

Department of Community Services 1986, *Nursing Homes and Hostels Review*, AGPS, Canberra.

Department of Health and Aged Care 1999, *Aged Care in Australia—August 1999* <http://www.health.gov.au/acc/about/agedaust/agedaust.htm>, 16 February 2001.

Department of Health and Family Services 1996a, *Budget Papers 1996–97*, AGPS, Canberra.

—— 1996b, *Annual Report 1995–96*, AGPS, Canberra.

—— 1997, *Budget Papers 1997–98*, AGPS, Canberra.

Department of Health, Housing and Community Services 1991a, 'The Role of Carers in Aged Care: Policies and Programs for Support', Discussion Paper no. 1, *Aged Care Reform Strategy Mid-Term Review 1990–91: Discussion Papers*, AGPS, Canberra.

—— 1991b, *Aged Care Reform Strategy Mid-Term Review 1990–91: Report*, AGPS, Canberra.

—— 1992, *Budget Papers 1992–93*, AGPS, Canberra.

Department of Human Services and Health 1995, *Budget Papers 1995–96*, AGPS, Canberra.

—— 1996a, *Towards a National Agenda for Carers: Report on the Workshop*, Aged and Community Care Service Development and Evaluation Reports no. 21, AGPS, Canberra.

—— 1996b, *Towards a National Agenda for Carers: Workshop Papers*, Aged and Community Care Service Development and Evaluation Reports no. 22, AGPS, Canberra.

Duckett, S. J. 1984, 'Structural Interests and Australian Health Policy', *Social Science and Medicine*, vol. 18, no. 11, pp. 959–66.

—— 2000, *The Australian Health Care System*, Oxford University Press, Melbourne.

Economic Planning Advisory Council 1994, *Australia's Ageing Society*, Background Paper no. 37, AGPS, Canberra.

Gardner, H. 1995a, 'Interest Groups and the Political Process', in H. Gardner, (ed.), *The Politics of Health: The Australian Experience*, 2nd edn, Churchill Livingstone, Melbourne.

—— 1995b, 'Political Parties and Health Policies', in H. Gardner, (ed.), *The Politics of Health: The Australian Experience*, 2nd edn, Churchill Livingstone, Melbourne.

—— (ed.) 1997, *Health Policy in Australia*, Oxford University Press, Melbourne.

Gibson, D. 1998, *Aged Care: Old Policies, New Problems*, Cambridge University Press, Melbourne.

Ham, C. & Hill, M. 1984, *The Policy Process in the Modern Capitalist State*, Harvester Wheatsheaf, Hemel Hempstead.

Hancock, L. and Moore, S. 1999, 'Caring and the State', in L. Hancock (ed.), *Health Policy in the Market State*, Allen & Unwin, Sydney.

Healy, J. 1990, 'Community Services: Long-term Care at Home?', in H. L. Kendig & J. McCallum (eds), *Grey Policy: Australian Policies for an Ageing Society*, Allen & Unwin, Sydney.

Home and Community Care Program 1998, *National Minimum Data Set: HACC Data Dictionary, version 1.0*, AusInfo, Canberra.

Howard, J. 1998, 'Keynote Address', in *Community, State or Family: A Question of Responsibility*, Proceedings of the National Summit Conference, 2 and 3 April, Carers Association of Australia, Canberra, pp. 9–13.

Howe, A. 1990, 'Nursing Home Care Policy: From Laissez Faire to Restructuring', in H. L. Kendig & J. McCallum (eds), *Grey Policy: Australian Policies for an Ageing Society*, Allen & Unwin, Sydney.

——, Schofield, H., & Herrman, H. 1997, 'Caregiving: A Common or Uncommon Experience?', *Social Science and Medicine*, vol. 45, no. 7, pp. 1017–29.

Keating, P. J. 1992, *Towards a Fairer Australia: Social Justice Strategy 1992–93*, AGPS, Canberra.

Lees, M. 1998, 'Forging New Directions: A Vision for Community and Health Care', in *Community, State or Family: A Question of Responsibility*, Proceedings of the National Summit Conference, 2 and 3 April, Carers Association of Australia, Canberra, pp. 22–5.

Liberal Party & National Party 1996, *National Carer Action Plan*, Election policy document.

Lin, V. & Duckett, S. 1997, 'Structural Interests and Organisational Dimensions of Health System Reform', in H. Gardner (ed.), *Health Policy in Australia*, Oxford University Press, Melbourne.

Minichiello, V. 1995, 'Community Care: Economic Policy Dressed as Social Concern?', in H. Gardner (ed.), *The Politics of Health: The Australian Experience*, 2nd edn, Churchill Livingstone, Melbourne.

Moylan, J. 1996, *Strengthening Families*, AGPS, Canberra.

Murphy, B. et al. 1997, 'Women with Multiple Roles: The Emotional Impact of Caring for Ageing Parents', *Ageing and Society*, vol. 17, pp. 277–91.

Office of Women's Affairs 1994, 'The Price of Care: A Progress Report on Women as Carers', Conference of Commonwealth and State Ministers for the Status of Women, Melbourne.

Rosenman, L. 1991, 'Community Care: Social or Economic Policy?', in P. Saunders & D. Encel (eds), *Social Policy in Australia: Options for the 1990s*, Proceedings of National Social Policy Conference, Sydney, 3–5 July, vol. 1, Plenary Sessions, Social Policy Research Centre Reports and Proceedings, no. 96, University of New South Wales, Sydney.

Sax, S. 1993, *Ageing and Public Policy in Australia*, Allen & Unwin, Sydney.

Schofield, H. (ed.) 1998, *Family Caregivers: Disability, Illness and Ageing*, Allen & Unwin, Sydney.

—— et al. 1996, 'Family Carers: Some Impediments to Effective Policy and Service Development', *Australian Journal of Social Issues*, vol. 31, no. 2, pp. 157–72.

Shaver, S. & Fine, M. 1996, 'Social Policy and Personal Life: Changes in State, Family and Community in the Support of Informal Care', in Department of Human Services and Health, *Towards a National Agenda for Carers: Workshop Papers*, Aged and Community Care Service Development and Evaluation Reports no. 22, AGPS, Canberra.

Short, J. 1997, 'I Was Wrong: PM's Aged Care Retreat', *Australian*, 6 November, pp. 1–2.

Smith, W. 1998, 'What Older Australians Want', Media release, WS 19/98, 2 April, Canberra.

Swerissen, H. & Duckett, S. J. 1997, 'Health Policy and Financing', in H. Gardner (ed.), *Health Policy in Australia*, Oxford University Press, Melbourne.

Tilse, C., Rosenman, L., & Le Brocque, R. 1991, 'Who Pays for Community Care? Income Support and Caring', in P. Saunders & D. Encel (eds), *Social Policy in Australia: Options for the 1990s*, Proceedings of National Social Policy Conference, Sydney, 3–5 July, vol. 1, Plenary Sessions, Social Policy Research Centre Reports and Proceedings, no. 96, University of New South Wales, Sydney.

14

Promoting Australian Health Industry Exports: The Role of Public Policy

Simon Barraclough and Amanda Neil

The purpose of this chapter is to chronicle the efforts by Commonwealth, state, and territory governments to foster Australian health industry exports and to explore the policy tools used in that process. We are also concerned to analyse the domestic and international issues raised and to highlight policy problems that need to be dealt with in order to improve the promotion of exports by the health industry. Exports include the provision of goods and services that earn foreign currency whether provided inside or outside Australia. They do not include the provision of goods and services through Australia's foreign assistance programs since these constitute part of the Australian domestic economy. In broad terms, the export potential of the Australian health industry can be divided into the categories listed in box 14.1.

For more than a decade, both national and state governments in Australia have sought to promote the export potential of the health industry. This endeavour has been in keeping with the wider agenda of identifying and fostering value-added, 'clever-country' exports, which exploit Australia's comparative advantage in health care and certain health technologies. Moreover, these exports are congruent with future trends of increasing international trade in services and the liberalisation of tariffs on therapeutic goods by the world's major industrial nations. Such an export orientation also attracts and retains the financial capital—as well as the managerial and technological knowhow—of transnational corporations for whom Australia can serve as a springboard into the Asia-Pacific region.

Public policy for the promotion of Australian health industry exports has faced a range of formidable obstacles; some are rooted in the very

Box 14.1
A typology of Australian health industry exports

Health care services
- The provision of health care to foreign patients in Australia, as well as services provided by individuals and corporations overseas.

Therapeutic goods
- Medicinal drugs, natural therapies, and therapeutic equipment and devices.
- Medical and hospital equipment, and infrastructure construction.
- Nontherapeutic equipment, and design and construction services for health facilities.

Education and training
- Services offered by public and private sectors encompassing formal and informal courses delivered within Australia or overseas, and fellowships and training placements conducted in Australia.

Health information technology
- Includes data processing, hardware, software, and telemedicine (also known as telehealth and e-health).

Health systems policy, planning and management
- Consultancy services, including such areas as health insurance, casemix funding, waste management, and aged care.

Research and development
- Private and public sector activities in universities, research centres, and corporations generating export earnings.

nature of the industry, while others are a function of tensions within Australia's federal system of governance.

In terms of marketing, a prime concern in the promotion of any brand is the nature of the product. Although the term 'health industry' might slip easily off the tongue, the heterogeneous nature of the industry means that it cannot easily be encapsulated and promoted as a single entity. The health industry encompasses producers of both goods and services (see box 14.1). Some producers, such as medical equipment and pharmaceutical manufacturers, are highly specialised and operate only within the health sector, while others, such as architects, educational institutions, financial consultants, and information technology suppliers, regard the health sector as merely one of their diverse markets. Moreover, as one of the most specialised sectors of the economy, the health sector is characterised by identities and organisations centred on professional and technical specialisation, often with a history of independent action. Appeals to such diverse interests to identify and take concerted action as 'the health industry' are therefore problematic.

Accurate data on the value of health industry exports are not available. While general trade data are available through the Australian Bureau of Statistics (ABS) on certain categories of commodity exports, such as pharmaceuticals and medical goods, and some information is available on services supplied to foreign patients (figure 14.1), it is not possible to identify most health-related services. Moreover, private corporations and even public institutions often seek to keep details of their exports confidential for fear of alerting competitors to potential markets.

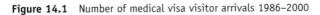

Figure 14.1 Number of medical visa visitor arrivals 1986–2000

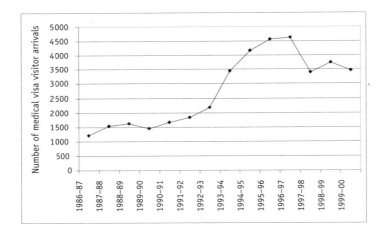

The Australian health industry is also characterised by huge variations in the relative size of its constituents and the nature of their ownership. Some companies are small operators with limited capital and staff, and seek to exploit market niches; a few others are major domestic or multinational corporations. Although most companies are privately owned, a number of listed public companies also participate strongly in the health sector.

Further, in terms of health care services, many of the leading providers are in the public sector, adding an additional complexity to the industry's profile. The public health care sector has, historically, been domestic in focus, and has not had a strong commercial culture, let alone one that has incorporated a commitment to exports of health services. Governments have also been sensitive to the danger of health exports being perceived as favouring foreign above local patients. There are also limitations on government departments and agencies exporting their services, which may be done in support of the national interest or when an improvement to services can be demonstrated as a result of the activity. Such export activity can only be pursued if a private sector or other provider cannot perform the task more effectively. In addition, competitive neutrality must be observed so that government agencies do not obtain an unfair commercial advantage over their private sector rivals. Not surprisingly, such restraints leave only limited scope for government departments and agencies for exporting their services.

Crosscutting lines of authority and moral responsibility also complicate the task of public policy in promoting the export activities of such a disparate industry. The federal government plays a leadership role in foreign trade. The Australian Trade Commission (Austrade) maintains an international network of offices, offers advice to exporters, and provides market intelligence and some financial assistance. For example, the Export Market Development Grants scheme subsidises eligible organisations to offset some of the cost of export marketing. In the case of health industry exports, Austrade has assisted in the staging of trade fairs and has provided financial support for exhibitors.

Individual states and territories also conduct their own trade promotion activities, including the establishment of representative offices in foreign countries. Not surprisingly, there is strong competition between states and territories for domestic and foreign investment, as well as for export markets. Such competition may be counterproductive from a national perspective. Added to these centripetal forces is the difficulty for governments to get competitive private sector interests to share information and work together for the national common good.

A further issue in public policy on export promotion in general, and in health industry exports in particular, has been the ambivalence of governments about their appropriate role. At times, governments have regarded export promotion as largely the responsibility of particular industries. In the case of the federal government this has led to an insistence upon attempts at cost recovery for services provided by Austrade and the removal of subsidies to industry export groups. At other times, both federal and state governments have sanctioned subsidies for health industry trade fairs and export promotion activities. In one rare case, discussed in the next section, the New South Wales government even invested capital to further international connections in health care services.

Federal government involvement in promoting health industry export potential

It is during the 1980s and 1990s that efforts to foster health industry exports can be identified as a substantial element of the export policy agenda, although evidence of an interest in promoting pharmaceutical products can be found as early as 1960 (Industries Division, Department of Trade 1960, p. 1). The promotion of health industry exports was intensified in the wake of the balance of payments pressures of the mid 1980s and the then Labor administration's policy of greater global economic engagement. Such exports also served Labor's drive to foster Australia as the clever country, in which technologically sophisticated products and services would underpin Australia's prosperity in a growing global market. As Paul Keating, the federal Treasurer for most of the Labor incumbency, has observed in his memoirs, 'Australia had a rich legacy of innovation in pure and scientific research upon which to draw and services that could compete with any in the world' (Keating 2000, p. 16).

The Liberal–National Coalition government, which succeeded Labor in 1996, continued a commitment to health industry export promotion, albeit with reduced funding and a degree of policy inconsistency. An array of policy tools can be employed in export development and promotion. Most of these tools, which can be categorised in the ways described in box 14.2, have been employed in health industry export promotion at the federal level. The application of these tools is detailed below.

Box 14.2
Policy tools for health industry export promotion

Consciousness raising
Ministerial speeches, government sponsorship of conferences, and workshops.

Strategic planning
Development of industry export plans and strategies, commissioning of reports on special markets.

Industry Commission
Enquiries.

Diplomatic and promotional
Ministerial visits, trade missions, memoranda of understanding, hosting delegations and official visits, and sponsoring international conferences.

Agencies
The provision of support through government export and industry development agencies and units in the form of advice, introductions, intelligence, clearinghouse activities, and websites.

Fostering industry groups
Encouraging industry support groups, and providing secretarial and financial assistance.

Subsidies
Subsidies for export activities, such as trade fairs, publications, and trade delegations.

Fiscal measures
Tariff policies.

Commercial ventures
Establishing trading corporations, capital investment in strategic projects.

Regulatory
International harmonisation of regulations and standards, simplification of medical visa requirements.

■

The Australian Labor government (1983–96)

Pre-current-account crisis (1983 to March 1985)

The Australian Labor Party recognised the economic potential of the health industry when in opposition in the early 1980s and included biotechnology and medical technologies in the sixteen 'sunrise industries' within the party's science and technology policy for the 1983 federal election. In May 1983, priorities to encourage the growth of these industries and the establishment of the National Biotechnology Program were announced (Jones 1983). The aim of this program was to bridge the gap between research in the laboratory and its industrial implementation (Australian Industrial Research and Development Incentives Board 1985, p. 71).

During 1984, the hospital and medical equipment industry was identified as having the potential for rapid export growth, and was included in the interim Global Marketing Plan developed by the Department of Trade (Department of Trade 1984, pp. 12, 15). Throughout Labor's tenure the department was to provide continuous support to export development within the medical equipment industry.

The potential for the development of the pharmaceutical and acute health services sectors was also raised during Labor's first term. In

1984, a reference was sent to the Industries Assistance Commission (IAC) acknowledging problems with pricing and the need for an industry development strategy in the pharmaceutical industry (Button 1984a). The IAC, subsequently renamed the Industry Commission (IC) and then the Productivity Commission (PC), has been the Commonwealth government's principal advisory body on all aspects of structural reform, involving all levels of government. This has included encouraging the development of internationally competitive industries, facilitating structural adjustment, and reducing unnecessary business regulation.

In 1984, the government also recognised that more could be done to promote tradable services in education and medicine (Button 1984b, p. 879). In the case of medical services, this represented a marked policy reversal, since the export of acute health services had hitherto been actively discouraged. Indeed, patients wishing to undergo treatment in Australia were required to provide evidence that the service was unobtainable in their countries of origin and that Australia was the closest provider, in order to obtain a medical visa (IAC 1989, p. 31).

Post-current-account crisis (March 1985 to 1996)

In the period 1985–86, wider economic factors in the form of a current-account-deficit crisis and the government's response to an economic downturn were a major impetus for the promotion of health industry exports. In March 1985, following poor balance of payment figures, a 20 per cent devaluation of the Australian dollar occurred. According to the government, this was partly the result of structural weaknesses within the Australian economy characterised by a narrow export base and the failure to exploit the fast-growing world demand for manufactured goods and services (Keating 1985, p. 563; Dawkins 1986, p. 1825).

The marked decline in Australia's terms of trade (which fell by 14 per cent between March 1985 and March 1987) led Treasurer Keating to seek to jolt the consciousness of Australians by warning of the risk of the country becoming a 'banana republic' (Keating 2000, pp. 15–16). In mid 1986, a two-year national export drive was initiated under which export strategies were to be developed for each industry with export potential. By 1988, four export strategies had been inaugurated, including one for the medical and scientific equipment industry and another for acute health services (Austrade 1988).

Medical equipment industries

As growth through exports became the catchcry of industry policy there was a shift towards high technology industries (Department of Industry Technology and Commerce [DITAC] 1988, p. 5). The medical equipment industry was presented as an exemplar of the sort of 'clever-country' industry that the government wished to see develop. This industry operated with low levels of assistance and exports were 40 per cent of turnover, compared with 6 per cent for manufacturing as a whole (Button 1986). Moreover, medical equipment had been responsible for six of Australia's top ten leading high technology product groups in 1985 (Jones 1985).

A reference on the development potential of the medical equipment and appliances industry was forwarded to the Industries Assistance Commission. During the course of its inquiry the government also set about encouraging an internationally competitive hearing aid manufacturing industry through a positive procurement strategy; the federal government being the second largest government distributor of hearing aids in the world (Button & Blewett 1986).

Early into Labor's third term, in December 1987, Industry Minister John Button released the government's response to the *IAC Report into the Medical and Scientific Equipment Industries*. The commission's recommendation that the industries needed be involved in greater international marketing efforts was accepted (DITAC 1987, p. 31). Significantly, the industries' calls for specific assistance were not heeded, although both sides subsequently cooperated in implementing an export strategy.

Pharmaceutical industry

In the case of the pharmaceutical industry, the government was willing to provide assistance. In September 1987 the ministers for Industry, Technology and Commerce, and Community Services and Health jointly announced policies for the development of the pharmaceutical industry (see page 299). This followed the release of the IAC report into the industry. The initiative—the Pharmaceutical Industry Development Program (or Factor 'f' Scheme as it came to be known) in reference to one of the factors the Pharmaceutical Benefits Pricing Authority (PBPA) had to consider in pricing decisions—aimed to encourage the growth of the pharmaceutical products industry in Australia. Among the objectives was that of creating an environment that would lead to improved exports (Button & Blewett 1987). In effect the program involved the government agreeing to pay higher prices for products listed on the PBS to manufacturers who undertook approved development programs. This was to be effected by the PBPA through consideration of Factor 'f', which took into consideration:

> the level of activity being undertaken by the company in Australia, including new investment, production and research and development where the activity is orientated towards international competitiveness (Button & Blewett 1987, Attachment).

The scheme was initially implemented for five years, but in 1992 was liberalised and extended until 1999. In extending the program, the government believed that this action would 'send a positive message to multinational companies' at a time when many were rationalising their research and manufacturing facilities on a global basis (Button 1992, p. 5867). The government wanted Australia to be 'firmly established as a strategic location in the Asian region for research and development and manufacturing activity by the world's major pharmaceutical companies' (Button 1992, p. 5876). The scheme also aimed to reverse the trend of disinvestment by multinational pharmaceutical companies.

During the operation of the Factor 'f' scheme, participating companies generated $387.3 million in export value added in the first phase, and $1.5 billion in export value added in the second phase (IC 1996a, pp. 107, 121). The scheme also encouraged a number of alliances between multinational pharmaceutical corporations and Australian pharmaceutical and biotechnology companies. This was considered essential to the viability of the biotechnology industry, which largely comprised small indigenous research-orientated firms.

Acute health services
In addition to medical equipment and pharmaceutical products, interest in the export potential of acute health services had also intensified in the wake of the current account crisis. The Export Market Development Grant scheme was expanded to include education, and hospital and medical service exporters; however, incongruously, health services provided in Australia were excluded. Under the premise that minor excess capacity existed among private health hospitals and that it made good economic sense to export services that would otherwise be underutilised, medical visa requirements were eased in December 1986 (Hurford 1986).

In 1987, health and medical export services were specifically identified as a key area with export potential by the newly established Trade in Services Advisory Group to the Trade Development Council (Hayden 1988, p. 94). The credentials of the Australian health industry were extolled by the government, as was the country's potential as a regional centre of excellence in health care goods and services.

A Health and Medical Services Exports Task Group, comprising representatives of four major federal government departments, was established in June 1989. Australia was held to command 'the broadest range of technical capabilities in the Southern Asian region spanning resource extraction, manufacturing, services, space, health and environment' and was also claimed as a world leader in biotechnology, agriculture, and medical research (Button 1988). In 1994, Industry Minister Peter Cook claimed that, since Australia had the second largest services sector in Asia, it was by default a regional services centre, a position he reaffirmed the subsequent year when he referred to Australia as a 'regional medical and health node' (Cook 1994, p. 3746).

The growing interest in acute health services found recognition in Labor's fourth-term industry and exports strategy, which included the export of services (including health services) and extended the Export Market Development Grant scheme to health services provided to foreign patients in Australia. In addition, the IC was specifically asked to investigate the export of health services (Hawke 1990, pp. 5596–7).

On the trade promotion front, health and medical services were included under the auspices of the Health Business Development Unit, or health cluster, within Austrade. The cluster, which also covered pharmaceuticals, and scientific and medical instruments and equipment, was established as part of Austrade's reorganisation in 1991 (Austrade 1991, p. 15). The objective of this move was to develop more broadly based sectoral networks with an enhanced capacity to capture a wider range of international business opportunities (Austrade 1991, p. 54). This is the first known instance of the health industry being treated as a single entity in national export promotion.

Ironically, interest in the export potential of acute health services was not noticeably assisted by the Industry Commission report *Exports of Health Services*, released in December 1991. The report, requested as part of the government's industry and export strategy, focused narrowly upon the treatment of foreign patients in Australia and used this discussion as a platform for a critique of Australia's health care system. It was not received favourably by the government. The reforms canvassed by the Commission were not considered to be worth the limited foreign earnings that might come from health service exports (Howe 1992).

In December 1992, the then deputy Prime Minister, Brian Howe, formally responded to the IC's report (Howe 1992), and called for the development of a new export strategy for health and medical services focusing on services other than the treatment of overseas patients in Australia, a field that was seen as likely to offer reduced financial returns in the future. Health services identified as having export potential profitability included health management and training systems, hospital construction, health-related computer software and hardware systems, and technology-intensive services such as remote diagnostic and telemedicine services (Howe 1992).

In contrast to the government's reservation about the potential of foreign patients coming to Australia, the federal parliament's Joint Committee on Foreign Affairs, Defence and Trade considered that Australia's capabilities in this area should be actively pursued. In its report into services exports to Indonesia and Hong Kong, the Joint Committee recommended that Austrade and the Department of Health and Family Services consider ways to improve awareness of the availability of high-quality medical services in Australia, in markets such as Indonesia (Australia, Joint Committee on Foreign Affairs, Defence and Trade 1996, p. 137).

Telemedicine

Telemedicine, with its application of computer and electronic communication technologies to diagnostics, education, and health information, also attracted attention as a potential export revenue earner. An analysis of the effectiveness of employing telemedicine 'as a basis for the development of a competitive advantage strategy' for the export of Australian medical services to the Asia-Pacific region was prepared for the Service Industries Research Program (Steidl 1993). This was followed by the announcement in January 1995 of a feasibility study into establishing a National ASEAN Telemedicine Centre in Perth, jointly funded by the Department of Industry, Science and Tourism (DIST), the Western Australian government, and a private company (Cook 1995).

Aged care

Another specialised export niche identified by policy makers was aged care. In 1993, a trade delegation was sent to Japan in the course of developing a Health Export Strategy framework (Department of Health, Local Government and Community Services 1993, p. 228). Howe's report, *Exporting Aged Care Services to Asia*, was published in February the following year (Howe 1994). Immediate and long-term commercial opportunities in the aged care sector were posited, with Japan identified as the most immediate short-term market for Australian services (Howe 1994, p. 4467). However, aged care export opportunities were considered to be dependent upon immediate action from government and industry, as well as long-term commitment, including the formation of export consortia drawing on a range of expertise and services.

A small unit was established within the Department of Human Services and Health to implement some of the report's recommendations. Initially, the aim was to 'identify opportunities for the export to overseas markets of both Government and private sector aged care programs, systems and services' (Department of Human Services and Health 1994, p. 226). This involved making contacts with regional government officials to encourage cooperation in aged care issues, and hosting officials and professional delegations from Japan, Thailand, and New Zealand. The department also advised Austrade on Australia's expertise in aged care services. In 1994–95, the unit established contacts with government departments in Japan, Hong Kong, Singapore, and Indonesia, supported the development of an aged care exporters' network, and provided a secretariat for the first twelve months' operation (Department of Human Services and Health 1995). The Australian Aged Care Exporters (AACE) network, which is still in operation, consists of public and private participants in the aged care industry; its aim is to service the needs of clients in the Asia–Pacific region.

Industry support groups

A major organisational initiative of the Labor government to encourage health industry exports was the Australian Health Industry Development Forum (AHIDF) convened in 1994 under the auspices of the ministers of industry, science and technology, and human services and health (Cook & Lawrence 1994). The AHIDF's brief was to recommend policies that would maximise health exports and enable the Australian health industry to capitalise on its international competitive advantage (AHIDF 1995).

Health service exports were considered to have virtually unlimited prospects, particularly through partnership between the private and public sectors, and the joint provision of goods and services for particular projects (Cook & Lawrence 1994). Establishment of the AHIDF was also intended to overcome industry fragmentation—including interstate rivalries—and generally to assist networking and clustering within the health industry. A number of countries were to be targeted through special interest groups established to develop links with Indonesia, India, Malaysia, and China. This policy initiative was consistent with the wider Asian engagement being pursued as public policy by the Labor government.

Other initiatives

Engagement with Asia in the health field was also furthered through the establishment of memoranda of understanding on health cooperation with Indonesia (1992), China (1993), and Thailand (1993). Efforts to promote or assist exports to Indonesia were pursued through the health industry trade promotions in Indonesia and the commissioning of a report, *Maximising Australia's Health Industry Export Potential to Indonesia*, in November 1994. In addition, the Joint Committee on Foreign Affairs, Defence and Trade reported on services exports to Indonesia and Hong Kong (Joint Committee on Foreign Affairs Defence and Trade 1996).

A concern with health industry exports was also articulated in Australia's official foreign aid policy. A special health initiative to strengthen the health component of Australia's official foreign aid program was announced in the 1994–95 Budget. This was part of the government's response to the recommendations of the House of Representatives Standing Committee on Community Affairs Inquiry into Australia's international health programs. According to the government, the initiative would 'help to expand the access of Australian firms to the growing regional health market, reinforcing the domestic push for increased service sector exports' (Bilney 1994, p. 24).

The government had also sought to encourage the health industry to secure exports through multilateral procurement programs, such as those conducted by United Nations agencies. Multilateral procurement was considered to be an export market with considerable potential. An examination of Australia's procurement performance undertaken in 1991 had indicated a low level of success (Blewett 1991, p. 1486). A second study was commissioned to investigate impediments and to recommend practical measures for improving performance in the area (Blewett 1991, pp. 1486, 1490).

In the final years of the Labor administration, the role of the Internet as a promotional avenue was actively pursued. The Department of Industry, Science and Tourism, in association with the New South Wales Department of Health, the South Australia Health Commission and the AHIDF, supported the development of the HealthNet Australia site, as well as supporting a feasibility study into a National Health Industry Clearing House (Department of Industry, Science and Tourism 1996, p. 43). As a result of this study the government entered into a strategic alliance with Australian Business Limited to develop Australian Health Online, an Internet-based industry directory and source of trade opportunities (Department of Industry, Science and Tourism 1996, p. 43; Australian Business 1998).

In October 1995, the Australian Health Ministers Advisory Council recognised the dysfunctions of poor coordination, as well as negative rivalries between states and territories, and commissioned Coopers and Lybrand to undertake a 'study into the options for the structure, function, financing of a nationally based organisation which would facilitate commercial participation in international health projects' (Coopers and Lybrand 1996, p. 1). *Review of Options: Mechanism for Government Participation in Health Exports* was released in November 1996, after the change in government. Despite the obvious need for a national approach to health industry exports, the report did not lead to any policy action.

Developments during the final term of the Labor government were associated with a general shift in government policy away from large enterprises towards small- and medium-sized enterprises (SMEs) and niche markets. This was of particular relevance to the medical equipment industry. To further assist the development of the medical and scientific equipment industry, a new reference was forwarded to the IC in January 1996 to examine 'the development potential of the Australian medical and scientific equipment industries in domestic and export markets; and to identify barriers to that potential being realized, and where appropriate to suggest measures to remove them' (IC 1996b, p. 1).

A reference into the pharmaceutical industry was also forwarded to the IC.

The Liberal–National Coalition government (1996–)

The Coalition continued its predecessor's encouragement of health industry export efforts. Shortly after the change in government, the new Minister for Health and Family Services, Dr Michael Wooldridge, wrote of 'the commitment of Australia's government and private enterprises [producing] an ever-expanding range of health-related products and services that are highly competitive in international markets' (Wooldridge 1996, p. 1).

The government also identified the health industry as one of four sectors with scope for expanding value-added exports in the inaugural *Trade Outcomes and Objectives Statement* released in February 1997. Areas of greatest potential were identified as research and development; professional and community education; planning, design, and construction of health facilities; medical products and services; patient care; caring for older people; and telemedicine (Department of Foreign Affairs and Trade 1997). The statement also noted that the government was identifying and supporting market opportunities for the Australian health sector through bilateral agreements and the development of specific programs of mutual activity; and by showcasing Australian health competencies in regional markets (p. 170).

However, despite such encouragement, direct financial support for health industry export promotion was reduced within the general context of the government's efforts to restrain public expenditure. The health business unit within Austrade was disbanded and formal sponsorship of the AHIDF was discontinued in the 1996–97 Budget. The AHIDF continued to function under the auspices of Australian Business Limited, supported by a year's funding from the federal government as well as membership subscriptions (Grezl 2000, p. 58).

Despite financial constraints, several government departments initiated export promotion activities that included the health industry. For example, in early 1997, the Department of Industry, Science and Tourism entered into a major eighteen-month project with Australian Business Limited aimed at building domestic and international consortia of health equipment companies (Department of Industry, Science and Tourism 1997, p. 28). This was followed by the development of a package entitled Australian Health to promote Australia's health industry and expand opportunities for export during 1997–98 (Department of Industry, Science and Tourism 1997, p. 55).

Pharmaceutical and medical equipment industries

During its first term the Coalition responded to the IC reports arising from the inquiries into the pharmaceutical and medical and scientific equipment industries commissioned by the previous government. It was announced that a review of the Pharmaceutical Benefits Scheme (PBS), as recommended by the IC, would not be undertaken and, as such, the need and appropriate options for industry policy measures post-Factor 'f' would be considered (IC 1996c, p. 283). In April 1997 it was decided that, in view of the likely suppression of prices arising from the price setting arrangements under the PBS; a Factor 'f' replacement program would be introduced (Moore 1997a). The intention was to maintain an internationally competitive operating environment for the industry into the twenty-first century. The Pharmaceutical Industry Investment Program was confirmed in the

1997 Budget. The major initiative under the program was the provision of $300 million over five years (Moore 1997b). This amounted to a partial renewal of the Factor 'f' scheme.

In May 2001, it was announced that an Action Agenda for the pharmaceutical industry was to be prepared in conjunction with industry in order to maximise future growth of the pharmaceutical industry in Australia. This was seen as ascertaining 'ways to increase the rate of commercialisation of Australian research, lift the levels of manufacturing and export, and raise Australia's profile as an attractive investment location' (Minchin 2001a). In general, action agendas are promoted as powerful mechanisms for building partnerships between industry to improve the operating environment for business and to encourage a more globally competitive and strategic focus to business activities (Minchin 2001b).

The final response to the report on the medical and scientific equipment industry was released in July 1998, 18 months after its submission. The government agreed to reduce tariffs on all medical and scientific equipment to zero and announced that the regulation of medical devices was to be harmonised with the European Union (Moore 1998). The latter was partially achieved through the implementation of the Mutual Recognition Agreement with the European Union (initiated by the previous Labor government), which had been signed in June 1998. In September 1999, the government committed itself to enacting legislation in order to adopt the internationally accepted classification and essential requirements from the European Union (Tambling 1999). An Action Agenda was also considered for elements of the medical equipment industry in the most recent Budget (2001–02), but no decision was made.

Telemedicine

Another major area of interest to the Coalition government during its first term was the information economy, including telemedicine. Three reports of relevance to the industry were released in 1997 (House of Representatives Standing Committee on Family and Community Affairs 1997; Information Industries Taskforce (Goldsworthy Report) 1997; Information Policy Advisory Council 1997). These were followed by the release of a National Scoping Study in March 1998 (Mitchell 1998, p. 2), and a preliminary strategy for the information economy in July 1998.

Within the National Scoping Strategy (Mitchell 1998, p. 52) it was held that

> Australia does not seem to have progressed from the position outlined in the 1993 strategic analysis, which had suggested that Australia:
> * has a competitive 'product' as well as a natural geographic advantage in terms of location in relation to developing Asia-Pacific markets;

- has failed to develop and implement a well-focussed Telemedicine market strategy, particularly in terms of building relationships with overseas specialists and institutions;
- has a fragmented approach to the export of medical services; and
- may again end up as a follower, rather than a leader, with Singapore (and possibly others) establishing and operating a domestic and export orientated Telemedicine network before Australia.

The National Scoping Strategy proposed that an Australian telemedicine centre be established; however, the conclusions of the earlier Steidl study were also reiterated. Steidl had maintained that before telemedicine could become a viable export product a number of perceived barriers needed to be addressed, including the following.

- The current lack of cooperation and coordination between states and individual institutions and specialists involved in telemedicine applications. If this issue is not addressed, it will result in a fragmented domestic telemedicine infrastructure, causing inefficiencies and providing a rather weak platform for export activities.
- There needs to be consensus between all relevant government agencies if Australia wants to participate alongside Canada, the USA, and others in the application of telemedicine projects in developing countries.
- Telemedicine has to be considered as a national challenge, not an opportunity by any particular state to outdo other states (Steidl 1993, pp. 6–7).

In its preliminary statement, *Australian Strategy for the Information Economy*, also released in July 1998, the government identified the creation of online health and education services as one of its objectives. In part, this was to 'enable Australia to benefit from the online export of these services' (Ministerial Council for the Information Economy 1998, p. 17).

In April 1999, the Australian health ministers established the National Health Information Management Advisory Council (NHIMAC). One of several roles of the council is to encourage the development of a market for Australian health information technology and services. In November 1999, NHIMAC released a health information action plan. Within this plan, endorsed by Australian health ministers, the development of online health services for export was identified as a primary objective (National Health Information Management Advisory Council 1999, pp. 2, 6).

Biotechnology

From the end of the Coalition's first term, biotechnology also became a major focus of government interest, reflecting the position that innovation will be a key driver of the competitiveness of firms and economies into the twenty-first century. Indeed, it has been held that the Coalition wanted biotechnology to be Australia's answer to Silicon Valley (Pheasant 2000). The development of a Biotechnology Action Agenda was announced in the 1998 election policy statement, followed by the announcement of Biotechnology Australia in the 1999 Budget.

Industry support groups

Having divested its responsibilities for the AHIDF to Australian Business Ltd (ABL) in 1996, the federal government was obliged in 1998 to resume its sponsorship role in the wake of ABL's withdrawal. The secretariat of AHIDF was provided by the Department of Health and Family Services (Davidson 1998; Juurma 1998). One of the major initiatives of the department was to organise the Health Industry Outlook Conference 1999. Due to poor industry response, the conference was cancelled and, in late 1999, official support for the AHIDF was discontinued. The first-ever attempt to foster a national forum for promoting health industry exports had ended in failure.

Aged care services

Aged care services exports continued to receive attention under the Coalition. Senator Bronwyn Bishop, Minister for Aged Care, led a trade mission to Hong Kong and Japan in 1999 and to Malaysia and Singapore a year later. Prominent representatives of both the public and private sectors of Australian aged care services accompanied her on these missions. The missions emphasised Australian expertise in community and residential care, the design of facilities, support services, and retirement living.

Other health services

During the Coalition's second term there was also renewed interest in the potential of health care services exports in general (Department of Industry, Science and Resources 1999, p. 21), although this interest was not sustained. The initial interest was reflected in the reorganisation of the Department of Industry, Sciences and Resources in March 1999, with the establishment of the Services and Emerging Industries Division, and the Services Industries Section within that division. The objective of the Services Industries Section was to provide a focus and coordination for service industries in the department, since service industries were becoming integral to many manufacturing industries and new technologies, and their importance was expected to grow with the move towards a knowledge-based economy (Department of Industry, Science and Resources 1999, p. 34). The health industry was a major focus. After the first year, however, support for the Services Industries Section was reduced, the most recent Budget resulting in a loss of 50 per cent of the section's funding and a third of its human resources funding. This was seemingly incongruous given that, in this country, services account for more than 70 per cent of gross domestic product (GDP) and more than 20 per cent of exports.

There were some positive developments from 1999 to 2000. Three studies were commissioned to identify initiatives for promoting export market development in the health services and products field (Department of Industry, Science and Resources 2000). The first, *AustMed: Export Wealth from Australia's Health* (Grezl 2000), arose out of the Emerging Industries and Technologies Forum and sought to investigate various export models for the Australian medical and health industry. The intent was to ascertain whether a new national networking initiative would help Australia better realise the export potential of its health and medical technology. The report concluded, in part, that a major initiative should be explored, but that adequate resources and bipartisan support was essential to its success (Grezl 2000, pp. v, 7). Another conclusion was that an action agenda should be prepared for the industry. Partly in consequence of this study, a proposal for an action agenda for the medical equipment industry was put forward during the 2001–02 Budget round (Services Industries Section, Department of Industry, Science and Resources, pers. comm., July 2001), but as previously noted no decision was made.

The second report, *The Health Product and Services System in Australia* (AEGIS 2000), was a major analysis of the dynamics of innovation within the health product and services system, and included an examination of health industry exports. The study concluded, in part, that the health system was not realising its potential in terms of innovation and growth because of incoherence within, and the complexity of, the system. A subsequent study extending the findings of this research was to be undertaken, but due to the withdrawal of funding from the Services Industries Section this could not be pursued.

The third study focused on public health in relation to water quality and was aiming to assist such activities in India (Services Industries Section, Department of Industry, Science and Resources, pers. comm., July 2000).

State and territory government promotion of health industry exports

Victoria

The Cain and Kirner Labor governments had sought to exploit international commercial opportunities in the health industry, especially for foreign aid projects, through a generic state agency, the Overseas Projects Corporation of Victoria (OPCV). The Liberal–National Coalition, elected in 1992 under the leadership of Jeff Kennett, decided that a specific policy for Victorian health industry exports was required. Of all Australian governments, Victoria adopted the most formal approach to the promotion of health industry exports. This involved the convening of a ministerial advisory group on health exports, the promulgation of a written policy, and the creation of an export unit within the Victorian Department of Human Services (DHS).

In December 1994, a formal health export policy for Victoria was published (Health and Community Services 1994). This document lucidly defined what constituted health exports, described potential exports and markets, identified strengths and weaknesses in Victoria's export capacity, and made a number of recommendations, including the establishment of a ministerial advisory committee. This document was the first attempt by any Australian government to develop a comprehensive published policy document dealing with health industry exports. The aims and objectives of the policy (see box 14.3) represented a generic template for health industry exports.

Box 14.3
Victoria's strategy for the export of health services

Aims
- To position the health sector to recognise, develop, and access export opportunities.
- To package products successfully for overseas markets.
- To use collaborative relationships to add value to products and services in existing distribution networks.

Objectives
- To identify key markets, products, and services.
- To develop a coordinated approach from the Victorian health sector in order to better respond to export opportunities.
- To develop a supportive network for public and private sector exporters.
- To establish an information base to identify health industry capabilities.

Source: Health and Community Services 1994, p. 1

■

The strategy listed specific areas for further action, including identifying target markets in the Asia–Pacific region, potential products for export, and four primary export segments (import of patients, health projects under aid programs, commercial contracts, and education and training). In addition, the strengths, weaknesses, opportunities, and threats to the Victorian industry would be analysed and the capabilities of the Victorian health export sector assessed. The strategy also recognised the need for the development of information sharing networks among health industry exporters in different market segments in order to encourage collaboration and a coordination of effort (Health and Community Services 1994, p. 1).

The bipartisan Victorian Ministerial Advisory Committee on Health Exports was established in April 1995. This committee originally included former Labor Party Senator John Button and former Liberal–National Party Opposition leader Andrew Peacock—two one-time federal parliamentarians with considerable ministerial experience in international trade. John Button had been responsible for a development plan for the Australian medical goods industry, while Andrew Peacock had served as Australia's foreign minister. The committee's brief was to facilitate the development of the health export industry in Victoria and enable the state's health industry to benefit from opportunities in the Asia-Pacific region.

In 1996, the then Department of Health and Community Services convened a workshop under the auspices of the Ministerial Advisory Committee on Health Exports to identify the export potential for Victorian health education and training courses and the level of interest in develop-ing a coordinating mechanism for such endeavours. A year later the Corporate Strategies Division of the Victorian DHS established the Export Development Office.

The Victorian government was an active participant in health trade fairs in Malaysia and Indonesia and sponsored the visits of a number of health industry officials to Victoria to enable them to gain firsthand experience of Victoria's health industry. Business Victoria published a medical equipment directory, which was directed at export markets in the southern hemisphere.

The Victorian government also cooperated with the Commonwealth to establish the Australian Medical Solutions Network, a specialised group of Victorian commercial companies and nonprofit agencies. The network offered medical equipment, medical consumables, and training and consultancy support to overseas hospitals and health care organisations.

With the change to a Labor government in Victoria in 1999, institutional support for health industry exports within the Victorian DHS waned. The Export Development Office was abolished and the accumulated expertise and corporate memory of its staff were lost.

New South Wales

The government of New South Wales adopted a model of health services export promotion that combines the international protocol functions of a health department, the coordinating capacity of an industry umbrella organisation, and the operational imperatives of a commercial corporation. This was achieved through the establishment of a limited company fully owned by the government.

Aus Health International Pty Ltd (AHI) was established in 1996 by the government of New South Wales with the minister for health and the treasurer as shareholders. The management of AHI is responsible to the board of directors. The company's brief is to facilitate export and other commercial activities in the health field, including overseas development assistance projects. AHI is commercially orientated and is not subsidised by the Department of Health. Significantly, AHI also has a mandate to represent the New South Wales Department of Health in international affairs, as a result of which it has been able to build upon existing government relationships when seeking to develop commercial partnerships and new markets.

Although AHI is a creation of the New South Wales government and purports to represent the New South Wales health system, it also claims to provide 'a one point, coordinated access to Australia's health care industry' since it has developed a 'wide network of health professionals around Australia' (Aus Health International 1999). Although AHI is based in New South Wales and owned by that state's government, it seeks to recruit partners and individuals from throughout Australia when putting together tenders or responding to business opportunities.

Aus Health International has not restricted its activities to tendering for contracts and the provision of services. It has also invested equity in a joint venture to establish an oncology centre in a private hospital in Kuala Lumpur. The New South Wales Cabinet approved A$1.5 million capital for the project through the mechanism of the issue of redeemable preference shares by AHI to the Department of Health. A joint venture company was registered in Malaysia and the first chemotherapy offered in 1997; radiotherapy services commenced in 1999.

The joint venture was more than just a profit-seeking enterprise. For Aus Health International, this project represented an 'important flagship' for future growth by the company in Malaysia, as well as providing opportunities for 'leveraging', whereby other goods and services could be provided by the Australian health industry.

South Australia

For some years the government of South Australia has been active in seeking to foster health industry exports as part of an overall policy of encouraging exports. Health industry export promotion has been undertaken through commercial encouragement and advice from government and financial assistance to a locally based health industry development organisation. Until its privatisation in 2000, a state-owned corporation provided a third policy element for health industry export promotion.

The initial period of policy interest in health industry exports was characterised by a rational, comprehensive approach. In 1995, the state government, through the South Australian Centre for Manufacturing (SACFM) funded a major pioneering mapping exercise of the export potential of organisations that had their head offices in South Australia, that had at least half of their turnover generated from health industry activities, and that were engaged in export activities (or that planned to be). This exercise resulted in a publication listing the export capabilities of South Australian health organisations (South Australian Centre for Manufacturing 1995). The SACFM established a health industry research and development team, pledged that it would collect and collate new survey data annually, and articulated a three-stage plan to assist the South Australian health industry to integrate with global trade (South Australian Centre for Manufacturing 1995).

The South Australian Department of Human Services was originally given a role in export promotion and established the Health Development and Export Unit; however, this was discontinued in 1998 and responsibility for the promotion of health industry exports was transferred to the Department of Industry and Trade's Business Centre. The Department maintains offices in China, Singapore, Indonesia, Japan, and the United Kingdom.

The centre maintains a web page to provide details of the South Australian health industry. Local organisations can obtain a listing free of charge. In addition, the centre subsidises the production, by a commercial publisher, of an export guide of South Australian health and medical exports, *South Australian Health and Medical Exports*, as well as sponsoring advertisements in the national version of this guide (Kompass 1998). In the 1999–2000 edition of the national guide, the entire cover was sponsored by the South Australian government and carried the slogan, 'Adelaide—intellectual capital for health'. This publication illustrates the endemic rivalry between states in seeking to promote their health industries and the potentially confusing message given to prospective international customers.

As is the practice of government export promotion agencies in other states, the centre offers advice, export readiness training, marketing training, and limited financial assistance (up to a maximum of $5000) to South Australian enterprises wishing to commence or intensify their export activities. Such subsidies may be used for such things as participation in trade exhibitions, visits to potential markets, negotiations with potential customers, and the cost of producing advertising material. In the spirit of intergovernmental rivalry, any business receiving support from another state or federal government agency is not eligible for such assistance.

Until 2000, the government of South Australia made use of a state-owned corporation, SAGRIC International, to foster its state's participation in both domestic and international projects. SAGRIC promoted itself as being 'at the forefront of exporting Australia's health care capability and extensive expertise', and regards its key services in the health fields as health promotion, HIV/AIDS and STD prevention and care, maternal and childcare, epidemiology, hospital management, and community health system development (SAGRIC International n.d.b, p. 4). The privatisation of SAGRIC in March 2000 reduced the range of policy tools available to the state government in promoting health industry (and other) exports.

A further element of public policy to promote South Australian health industry exports involves the subvention of locally based industry umbrella group Australian Health Industry Incorporated (AHII). This organisation was formed in 1996 in the wake of the state government's mapping exercise of the local health industry. The state government contributed seeding funds, and the Department of Industry and Trade provided office space and some support services.

According to its mission statement, the organisation exists 'to promote economic growth and international trade in the Australian health industry'. Each year AHII presents an award to a local enterprise that has distinguished itself in export or import substitution activities.

Despite the identification of international trade in its objectives, the AHII has undertaken only limited activities in this sphere. Links have been developed with the Australian Institute of Export and Intelligence, and information about export opportunities is disseminated to members. AHII has considered conducting export-ready workshops to prepare health industry companies for the tasks associated with becoming exporters. The organisation is also ready to arrange trade missions and specialised fairs in order to promote the health industry. A link has also been established with the Industrial Supplies Office in South Australia to identify possibilities for import substitution. AHII also cooperates with other export-oriented organisations in Australia.

In its operations, AHII must face the perception that, although it has members from other states, it is essentially a South Australian organisation, partly financed by the government of that state and colocated in offices used by the state government's Business Centre. The organisation also faces reduced government funding, with the expectation that it will become self-funding through membership subscriptions.

Western Australia

For some years, the government of Western Australia adopted a different approach from other states and sought to develop a coalition of service providers from the public and private sectors in order to project the export potential of the state. Originally, a health export unit was established within the Health Department, but a wider health industry-based body subsequently replaced it. The Australia Clinic was launched in 1996 as a consortium of the

Health Department and a number of Perth's public and private hospitals. Participants financed the establishment and running of the body and the chief executive officers of participating entities sat on the clinic's board. A modest secretariat consisting of a director and two support staff was established under the auspices of the Western Australian government. In addition, some hospitals were affiliated to the clinic as alliance partners rather than formally belonging to the consortium.

The Australia Clinic was intended to play both a marketing and brokerage role in promoting the export of Western Australian health products and services. As its name suggested, the consortium emphasised the provision of health care services, either in Perth or overseas, although project consultancies and education and training programs were also an element of the services marketed. The Australia Clinic offered international services to patients coming to Perth and claimed a leading role for Western Australian hospitals in the fields of cardiac surgery, neurosurgery, the treatment of cancer, and trauma rehabilitation (Kompass 1998, p. 26).

In marketing its services the clinic emphasised Western Australia's proximity by air travel to most of Southeast Asia and to the Indian Ocean region, the fact that its time zone facilitates communications with these regions, and the multicultural nature of the state's population. Prior to the Asian financial crisis, the perceived principal market for the clinic was Indonesia, but Malaysia and Thailand were also promising markets. However, in the wake of the financial crisis of 1997, which had serious consequences for these countries, the clinic diversified its marketing to the Indian subcontinent, China, and some African countries (Australia Clinic 2000).

Western Australia's consortium model differed from health industry policy in other states in that it sought to provide government-instigated coordination in the context of a flexible coalition of interests spanning both the public and private sectors. The model offered the attraction of the integrity of service provision under the auspices of the state government, while allowing for private sector participation in the context of a corporate umbrella organisation. At the same time, this model could be readily integrated into the state government's international trade promotion activities. Participants were expected to demonstrate their continuing commitment to the coalition both financially and through membership of the board of directors. The consortium model had the potential not only to provide an export identity for Western Australian health services as it sought to compete with other Australian states, but also allowed for considerable flexibility, since members could leave and new members could be recruited at any time.

By 2000, the Australia Clinic model had proved unworkable. The legal status of the entity in terms of its ability to participate in joint ventures and consortia was unclear, and the organisation reverted to functioning as a health export agency within the Department of Health. In this role—and despite limited funding—it successfully attracted more than 200 foreign patients to Western Australia, overseeing their travel and accommodation requirements for which it charged a handling fee to generate revenue.

In December 2000, the Western Australian government moved to establish the Australia Clinic as an agency under the state's Health Services Act. It also decided to obtain legal advice on any legislative authority necessary to legitimise commercial participation in joint ventures and bids for international multilateral projects.

Queensland

The Department of State Development actively promotes health industry exports as part of the 'Smart State' image and maintains a Website containing information about the Queensland health industry and state and national export networks. The Department is able to make use of its own offices in several countries, as well as working with Austrade. Queensland treats hospital patients from Papua New Guinea, the Middle East, and Southeast Asia.

Although no comprehensive plan for health exports has been developed, the Queensland government has identified a number of areas of competitive advantage for strategic alliances and joint ventures as part of its encouragement of health industry exports. These include telemedicine, clinical trials and cancer research, and genomics; in addition, health systems consultancies for rural and public health systems and medical training have been highlighted (Department of State Development 2000a).

The Queensland government has identified three emerging export priorities in the health sector:
- health information technology services to China
- aged care facilities construction and gerontology educational services to Japan
- joint ventures in the Indian hospital sector (Department of State Development 2000b).

In addition, the Health and Aged Care Trade Action Plan has been developed to focus on Queensland enterprises and aims to make that state the lead supplier of a range of health industry goods and services to the Asia–Pacific region.

Queensland's plan contains the familiar elements:
- development of a database of private sector capabilities
- the assessment of international markets
- raising the export consciousness of the local health industry
- providing intelligence on export opportunities
- promoting the local health industry's goods and services internationally (Queensland Health and Aged Care Trade Action Plan 1999).

Northern Territory

The health industry of the Northern Territory is of limited size in comparison with the states. Nevertheless, the government of the Northern Territory has sought to develop links with Indonesia with a longer-term view to the provision of health services to this market. The Territory's sole private hospital provides air retrieval services to offshore oil and gas rigs in Indonesian waters and caters for international patients. In 1994, a Charter of Cooperation Concerning Development of Community Health Services was signed by the Minister for Health and Community Services of the Northern Territory and the Governor of the Indonesian Province of East Nusa Tenggara. The agreement committed the parties to cooperate in the interests of community health and to jointly seek external funding for various projects. Among the activities identified in the agreement were discussions to develop a joint clinic and various training and management matters.

Approaches to health industry export promotion policy at state and territory level

The brief exploration of health industry export promotion at the state level has not only revealed considerable activity, but has also shown that markedly different models have been used by different states. Health export promotion has been undertaken with almost no attempt at national coordination and with little cooperation between states; indeed, much of the activity has been unashamedly based upon interstate competition. Although such export promotion has been centred upon state jurisdictions, the New South Wales and Western Australian governments have appropriated an Australian identity for their export bodies (Aus Health International and the Australia Clinic), while South Australia's government-subsidised industry organisation has assumed the title of Australian Health Industry Incorporated, notwithstanding its limited operational area. Aus Health International regards New South Wales as the gateway to the Australian health system, whereas—as we have seen—the South Australian government promotes the catchcry of Adelaide as the intellectual health capital of Australia.

The survey also reveals tensions in some states between the health and the industry portfolios in the organisation of health industry export promotion. Three states (Victoria, South Australia, and Western Australia) originally set up export units within their respective health departments, but all three were subsequently dissolved. New South Wales alone seems to have avoided these tensions through the agency of a commercial organisation with organic links to its department of health. It should be noted, however, that different kinds of tensions can be generated by such an arrangement, since private sector corporations might resent what they see as an unfair advantage gained by a competitor with such close ties to government.

In the case of New South Wales, public policy has taken a line at variance with the retreat from state-owned commercial enterprises, which has characterised the era of privatisation, since the government has sought to promote health exports through a fully owned state corporation and has also invested capital in an overseas venture. By contrast, the government of Western Australia attempted the device of a consortium linking the private and public sectors and to which participants were required to make a financial contribution. Victoria sought to develop a comprehensive policy for health exports and even appointed an advisory committee to assist in its development. As with South Australia, Victoria has abandoned the promotion of health exports from within its health department, preferring to make use of its business ministry for such activities and providing occasional financial subsidies to assist with networks and strategic projects likely to generate export opportunities. Queensland has also invested health export promotion within its state development department and has sought to develop export strategies for the sectors of its health industry, which it regards as having a comparative advantage.

Conclusion

This chapter has documented the recognition by federal, state, and territory governments—irrespective of political party—of the potential of health industry exports, and their willingness to support the promotion of such exports through public policy. To this end, various mechanisms and strategies have been employed, ranging from (in one case) direct capital investment in projects and the establishment of government-owned corporations, to relatively minor sponsorship.

Yet our exploration has also identified a number of problems. State, territory, and federal governments have waxed and waned in their degree of commitment to health exports promotion. Specialised export units have been formed and then disbanded; at times even modest financial support has been withheld from promotional and coordination activities that promised to create a greater consciousness of export potential and a degree of practical cooperation. Domestic health policy concerns have often prevailed over an interest in health exports on the part of health ministers. A longer-term view of development has been lacking.

Although the issue of effective national coordination of promotional activities has been repeatedly raised, it has proved impossible to achieve.

Responsibilities in this policy area are divided between state and federal jurisdictions and between various government departments within single jurisdictions. While there has been cooperation between states on some projects, there has also been a degree of unhealthy competition, with states vying to demonstrate their preeminence in the health field. A national brand for Australian health exports has not been established, even though several state promotional agencies have appropriated an Australian national identity for their activities.

Several priorities are evident in the public policy agenda for promoting health industry exports. Governments need to maintain a longer-term commitment to fostering export consciousness among the disparate elements of the Australian health industry. The Australian Health Industry Development Forum foundered because of its inability to deliver short-term commercial benefits to participants and the reluctance of the federal government to fund its activities adequately.

Strategic support is also required for particular sections of the industry with more immediate export potential. It is, therefore, disappointing to note that support for service industries—let alone the health service industry—has been reduced within the Department of Industry, Science and Resources, and that the proposed Action Agenda for the Medical Equipment industry was not supported in the 2000 Budget.

There is an obvious need for the federal government to exercise both symbolic and substantial leadership in the field of health industry export promotion. Such leadership needs to be negotiated with the state and territory governments in such a way that existing state agencies are included in a national network and that promotional programs recognise the legitimate interests of each state. Potential foreign customers should be able to identify a national agency with permanent staff who can assist with matching their needs to an appropriate supplier. A national clearinghouse for intelligence on export opportunities would be more efficient and cost-effective than the duplication of this function on the part of state governments. Moreover, there is a need for a corporate memory of networks and contacts in the health industry in order to allow a rapid response to commercial opportunities.

Any national health export agency should be ready to broker cooperative tenders from Australian suppliers for large health projects from national or transnational customers (such as the various agencies and programs of the United Nations). The failure of the Australian Health Industry Development Forum suggests that a vague blanket appeal for components of the industry to network and cooperate for the national export cause has not worked. A more promising approach is to appeal to enlightened self-interest through project-based cooperation in which the individual and collective rewards are self-evident and the purpose of cooperation is clear.

Problems in coordinating the respective export promotion roles of health, trade, and industry departments require attention. In many cases the legitimacy bestowed upon an export provider by an association with a government health department is most valuable. This can be seen in the *modus operandi* of Aus Health in New South Wales and the model of an industry delegation accompanying the Minister for Aged Care on international export promotion visits. Yet health departments do not have sufficient staff or the necessary expertise to handle export promotion activities without the participation of trade and industry specialists. The coordination of these two branches of the health industry export enterprise will require greater creativity on the part of policy makers. Perhaps a specialised agency, combining both health and trade expertise, is a solution to this problem, rather than merely having officers in the health portfolio with some export responsibilities and officers in the trade and industry portfolios who include health in their wider work allocations.

The ever-expanding potential of the Worldwide Web must be further capitalised upon as a mechanism to further Australian health exports. The Web has the potential to provide a relatively inexpensive vehicle for a virtual health industry forum to replace the defunct one. It would allow the registration of interested corporations and organisations, facilitate their communication, and, most importantly, provide a window for the world on Australian health industry exports. This will require existing websites dealing with the Australian health industry to be enhanced and appropriately linked. Enhanced use of the Web for health industry export promotion will require both national coordination and a financial commitment to fund the creation and maintenance of the network.

References

AEGIS 2000, *The Health Product and Service System in Australia*, Report, AEGIS, Canberra.

Aus Health International 1999, *About AHI*, <http://www.ahi.com.au/aboutbody.htm> 13 December.

Australia Clinic 2000, Homepage, <http://www.australiaclinic.health.wa.gov.au>, 10 February.

Australian Business 1998, *Australian Business Health*, Australian Business Limited, Sydney.

Australian Health Industry Development Forum 1995, *Newsletter*, no. 1, AHIDF, Canberra.

Australian Industrial Research and Development Incentives Board 1985, *Annual Report* 1983–84, AGPS, Canberra.

Austrade 1988, *Australian Trade Commission Annual Report 1987–88*, Australian Trade Commission, Canberra.

—— 1991, *Annual Report 1990–91*, Australian Trade Commission, Canberra.

Bilney, G. 1994, *Australia's Development Cooperation Program 1994–95*, Budget Related Paper no. 2, AGPS, Canberra.

Blewett, N. 1991, 'Doing Business with the United Nations, Address to the National Conference of the United Nations Association of Australia', Canberra, 13 September, *Ministerial Document Service*, vol. 91–2, no. 51, pp. 1478–91.

Button, J. 1984a, Media statement, 17 October, *Commonwealth Record*, vol. 9 no. 42, p. 2066.

—— 1984b, Speech to an ASEAN, Australia, and Japan Economic Symposium, Kuala Lumpur, 7 May, *Commonwealth Record*, vol. 9, no. 20, pp. 877–9.

—— 1986, Speech to Australian Medical and Diagnostic Association, 7 May, *Commonwealth Record*, vol. 11, no. 18, pp. 758–60.

—— 1987, 'Government Decision on Medical and Scientific Equipment Industry', Media statement 174/87, 9 December.

—— 1987, 'Policies for the Development of the Pharmaceutical Products Industry', Joint media statement 115/87, 13 September.

—— 1988, Media statement, 24 October, *Ministerial Document Service*, vol. 88–9, no. 80, pp. 2885–8.

—— 1992, Statement on the Pharmaceutical Industry, 31 March, *Ministerial Document Service*, vol. 91–2, no. 169, pp. 5868–77.

—— & Blewett, N. 1986, Media statement, 21 October, *Commonwealth Record*, vol. 11, no. 41, pp. 1884.

Cook, P. 1994, 'Tapping into Opportunities: Australia and APEC Post-Bogor', Keynote address to the Business Potential of the Asia-Pacific Community Congress, Sydney, 4 December, *Ministerial Document Service*, vol. 94–5, no. 101, pp. 3740–52.

—— 1995, Media release, 23 January, <http://www.isr.gov.au/media/1995/january/nr760.doc>.

—— & Lawrence, C. 1994, Media statement, 9 September, *Ministerial Document Service*, vol. 94–5, no. 48, p. 1695.

Coopers and Lybrand Consultants 1996, *Review of Options: Mechanism for Government Participation in Health Exports*, Australian Health Ministers' Advisory Council, Canberra.

Davidson, J. 1998, *Future of the Australian Health Industry Development Forum*, Department of Health and Family Services, Canberra.

Dawkins, J. 1986, Speech at the National Export Drive Launch, Canberra, 8 October, *Commonwealth Record*, vol. 11, no. 40, pp. 1825–6.

Department of Foreign Affairs and Trade 1997, 'Trade Outcomes and Objective Statement', Commonwealth of Australia, Canberra, <http://www.dfat.gov.au/toos/archive/1997/index_toos97.html>.

Department of Health, Local Government and Community Services 1993, *Annual Report 1992–93*, AGPS, Canberra.

Department of Human Services and Health 1994, *Annual Report 1993–94*, AGPS, Canberra.

—— 1995, *Annual Report 1994–95*, AGPS, Canberra.

Department of Immigration and Multicultural Affairs 2000, *Temporary Entrants 1998–99*, Statistical Report no. 29, Department of Immigration and Multicultural Affairs, Statistics Section, Canberra.

—— 2001, *Temporary Entrants 1999–00*, Statistical Report no. 31, Department of Immigration and Multicultural Affairs, Statistics Section, Canberra.

Department of Industry, Science and Resources 1999, *Annual Report 1998–99*, AusInfo, Canberra.

—— 2000, *Annual Report 1999–2000: Output 1.1 Strategic Industry Leadership*, <http://www.isr.gov.au/department/annualreport99_00/html/output_1_1/output_1.1.html>.

Department of Industry, Science and Tourism 1996, *Annual Report 1995–96*, AGPS, Canberra.

—— 1997, *Annual Report 1996–97*, AGPS, Canberra.

Department of Industry, Technology and Commerce 1987, *Annual Report 1986–87*, AGPS, Canberra.

—— 1988, *Annual Report 1987–88*, AGPS, Canberra.

Department of State Development 2000a, *Export Capacity*, <http://www.statedevelopment.qld.gov.au/export/industry/health/capacity>, 7 November 2000.

—— 2000b, *Queensland Government Emerging Export Priorities*, <http://www.statedevelopment.qld.gov.au/export/industry/health/priorities>, 7 November 2000.

Department of Trade 1984, *Annual Report 1983–84*, AGPS, Canberra.

Government of Western Australia n.d., *The Australia Clinic*, Government of Western Australia, Perth.

Grezl, K. 2000, *AUSTMED: Export Wealth from Australia's Health*, Final report, Environmental Industries Development Network, Newcastle.

Hawke, R. J. L. 1990, 'Labor's Export Plan for the 1990s', 28 February, *Ministerial Document Service*, vol. 89–90, no. 152, pp. 5594–610.

Hayden, B. 1988, 'Transforming Australia's Trade', Address to the Business Council of Australia, Melbourne, 11 March, *Australian Foreign Affairs Record*, vol. 59, no. 3, pp. 90–4.

Health and Community Services 1994, *Victorian Strategy for the Export of Health Services 1994–96*, Health and Community Services, Acute Health Services Division, Melbourne.

House of Representatives Standing Committee on Family and Community Affairs 1997, *Health on Line, Report into Health Information Management and Telemedicine*, AGPS, Canberra.

Howe, B. 1992, Media statement, 10 December, *Ministerial Document Service*, vol. 92–3, no. 116, pp. 4779–80.

—— 1994, Speech at launching of 'Exporting Aged Care Services to Asia', 14 February, *Ministerial Document Service*, vol. 93–4, no. 127, pp. 4465–9.

Howells, J. 2000, *The Nature of Innovation in Services*, Report presented to the OECD Workshop on Innovation and Productivity in Services, 31 October–3 November 2000, Sydney; online version available at <http://www.isr.gov.au/industry/services/oecdworkshop.html>.

Hurford, C. 1986, Media statement, 12 December, *Commonwealth Record*, vol. 11, no. 48, p. 2274.

Industries Assistance Commission 1989, *Exporting Health and Education Services, Inquiry into International Trade in Services*, AGPS, Canberra.

Industry Commission 1993, *Annual Report 1992–93*, AGPS, Canberra.

—— 1996a, *Annual Report 1995–96*, AGPS, Canberra.

—— 1996b, *Medical and Scientific Equipment Industries*, AGPS, Canberra.

—— 1996c, *The Pharmaceutical Industry*, vol. 1, AGPS, Canberra.

Industries Division Department of Trade 1960, *The Australian Pharmaceutical Products Industry*, AGPS, Canberra.

Information Industries Taskforce 1997, *The Global Information Economy: The Way Ahead, The Goldsworthy Report*, Information Industries Taskforce, Canberra.

Information Policy Advisory Council 1997, *A National Policy Framework for Structural Adjustment within the new Commonwealth of Information*, Policy Advisory Council report to the Commonwealth Minister of Communications and the Arts, Information, Canberra.

Joint Committee on Foreign Affairs, Defence and Trade 1996, *The Implications of Australia's Services Exports to Indonesia and Hong Kong*, Parliament of the Commonwealth of Australia, Canberra.

Jones, B. 1983, 'Sunrise Industries', Speech to Management Technology Education Conference, Sydney, 31 May, *Commonwealth Record*, vol. 8, no. 22, pp. 744–8.

—— 1985, Media statement, 7 June, *Commonwealth Record*, vol. 10, no. 22, p. 864.

Juurma, E. 1998, Open Letter to Australian Health Industry Development Forum Members, *Australian Business*, Sydney.

Keating, P. J. 1985, Speech to Asia Society (USA), 22 April, *Commonwealth Record*, vol. 10, no. 16, pp. 563–7.

—— 2000, *Engagement: Australia Faces the Asia-Pacific*, Macmillan, Sydney.

Kompass Australia 1998, *Australian Health and Medical Exports 1999–2000*, Kompass Australia, Melbourne.

Minchin, N. 2001, 'Industry Ministers to Continue to Cooperate to Promote Australian Industry', Media release 01/166, 27 April.

—— 2001, 'Action Agenda for the Pharmaceutical Industry', Media release 01/232, 29 May.

Ministerial Council for the Information Economy 1998, *Towards an Australian Strategy for the Information Economy*, Preliminary Statement of the Government's Policy Approach and a Basis for Business and Community Consultation, Ministerial Council for the Information Economy, Canberra.

Mitchell, J. 1998, 'The Telemedicine Industry: Fragmentation to Integration', in *The Telemedicine Industry in Australia*, National Scoping Study, Department of Industry, Science and Tourism, Canberra.

Moore, J. 1997a, 'New Policies Promote Investment in Australia's Pharmaceutical Industry', Media release 87/7, 8 April, Department of Foreign Affairs, Defence and Trade, Canberra.

—— 1997b, 'New Measures for the Pharmaceutical Industry', Media release 142/7, 13 May, Department of Foreign Affairs, Defence, and Trade, Canberra.

—— 1998, 'Government Responds to IC Report on Medical and Scientific Equipment Industries', Media release 198/98, 24 July, Department of Foreign Affairs, Defence, and Trade, Canberra.

National Health Information Management Advisory Council 1999, *Health Online: A Health Information Action Plan for Australia*, National Health Information Management Advisory Council, Canberra.

Pheasant, B. 2000, 'The Value of Pure Thought', *Australian Financial Review*, 12 August, p. 26.

Queensland Health and Aged Care n.d., *Draft Trade Action Plan*, Queensland Health, Brisbane.

SAGRIC International n.d. a, *Health Service Delivery*, SAGRIC International, Adelaide.

—— n.d. b, *Technology to the World*, SAGRIC International, Adelaide.

South Australian Centre for Manufacturing 1995, *Health Contacts*, South Australian Centre for Manufacturing, Adelaide.

Steidl, P. 1993, *Exporting Medical Services to Asia Pacific: The Potential of Telemedicine*, Australian Coalition of Service Industries, Canberra.

Tambling, G. 1999, 'Medical Devices Reforms', Meeting of Key Stakeholders, Parliament House, Canberra, 17 September.

Wooldridge, M. 1996, *The Australian Health Care Industry: Supplier of Choice to International Markets*, Australian Health Industry Development Forum and Department of Foreign Affairs and Trade, Canberra.

15

Towards a National Food Safety Policy

James C. Smith

The quality and safety of the commercial food supply has been a public health policy issue since the advent of the sanitary reform movement of the nineteenth century. This movement was significant for many reasons; however, one important aspect was the recognition of the direct links between health or illness status, poverty, and the physical environment. The local production and commercial supply of food, being part of the immediate physical environment, consequently became an important focus for governmental intervention primarily through regulation of the food industry.

The regulation of the food industry by government for the purpose of ensuring adequate standards of food safety and the associated policy issues is the focus of this chapter. Apart from the public health importance of the safety of the food supply, the economic importance of the food industry and the subsequent tension between public health and economic policy priorities, and the changes this has brought about in Australian food safety regulation as attempts are made to develop a national food safety administration, are also discussed.

The public health features of food

In the mid nineteenth century, the links between food and health were concerned with the supply of adequate amounts of safe food. As Gordon explains: 'Hence even local famines caused much loss of life in centuries gone by. Yet probably more prolific of mortality than actual famine was the constantly recurring malnutrition often due to lack of vitamin C. This meant that children so affected succumbed readily to infection'

(Gordon 1976, p. 160). The lack of proper food was also a feature of the early white settlement of Sydney (Cumpston 1989, p. 46); however, over time, improvements occurred in health status due to improved sanitation and nutrition. In due course the notion that food of itself is a potential medium for the transmission of infectious disease through contamination (Cumpston 1989; Hedberg et al. 1994)—and that food or its byproducts, or the premises from which food is produced, could pose a 'nuisance'—led to the development of food controls (Cumpston 1989).

Over the past 150 years, food production has changed from a purely subsistence economy to a food industry, and has changed from serving primarily local needs to serving export demands (Davis et al. 1988). This in turn has impacted upon food technology, which has had to develop from preservation methods for short-term food storage to the development of technology that supports the demands from huge farming, processing, packaging, retailing, and marketing sectors that make up the current food industry, which competes on the world food market.

Outside the naturally occurring health hazards in certain foods, the number of complex food processes that occur from paddock to plate provide increased chances for the contamination of foods from various environments. Examples include pesticide residues from the agricultural environment, additives such as colouring and flavouring agents from the food processing environment, and the increased potential for microbiological contamination of foods from food handling associated with specialised manufacturing and retailing processes. Not only is the increased public health risk associated with what are perceived to be hazardous foods such as meats, poultry, and so on, but it is also associated with mass production in general.

> Fresh fruits, vegetables, and other cold food items are now being mass-produced and distributed through large and complex networks of distribution. The size and complexity of these operations can greatly magnify the public health significance of food-borne contamination (Hedberg et al. 1994, p. 675).

This statement is significant given the thrust of recent health promotion campaigns pertaining to health, healthy foods, and diet generally, and to concerns about misrepresentation of foods. Indeed, it is the principal function of the Australia New Zealand Food Authority (formerly the National Food Authority [NFA]) to develop safety standards for Australian food prescribing 'the use of food additives, as well as production, storage, labelling and packaging, and maximum levels of pesticide residues and contaminants in food, including heavy metals' (National Food Authority 1992, p. 7).

As advances in food technology have been a feature of food safety, so too have the changes in consumer behaviour and expectations in regard to food, and this has, in turn, further increased the potential health risks from food. Examples of these changes include the following.

- Food products are increasingly being produced at one location for national distribution (food was once predominantly grown locally and then prepared and consumed at home).
- Food is increasingly consumed away from home.
- A larger proportion of food is now being sold in a form that is either partially prepared, or is ready to be eaten without further preparation.
- Self-service at retail level as well as within eating establishments is becoming more widespread.
- There has been a rapid expansion in the food service industry, which includes licensed clubs and small family restaurants.
- Food retailing increasingly involves national networks including, for example, supermarkets and family restaurant chains.
- Manufacturing, packaging, and transportation methods have been developed to increase durability and shelf life.
- New technologies are now available for preparation and preservation of foods—for example, vacuum packaging and cook–chill food service system techniques (National Food Authority 1994, p. 10).

Although the use and misuse of food additives over many years has impacted negatively on consumer confidence (Abbot 1994), including the presence of agricultural and veterinary chemicals in foods (National Food Authority 1993), the potential for food to act as a vehicle for the transmission of pathogenic microorganisms has more recently attracted the attention of policy makers and consumers. This is particularly so when episodes of food contamination occur, such as those associated with *mettwurst* in South Australia (February 1995) and peanut butter in Victoria (June 1996).

At the international level, the sheer magnitude of the results of poor microbiological food safety are probably best demonstrated by the following statistics.

> Foodborne diseases remain one of the major health problems and an important cause of reduced economic productivity… It is estimated that of the 1500 million episodes of diarrhoea which occur in children under the age of five, and the more than 3.2 million children who die as a result, 70 per cent of cases are due to contaminated food (including drinking water) (Kaferstein et al. 1994, p. 15).

The World Health Organization (WHO) has acknowledged the importance of food to health by identifying food as one of the prerequisites for health in the *Ottawa Charter* and as an essential element of primary health care as articulated within the *Declaration of Alma Ata* (WHO 1978, 1986). In terms of food safety, the joint Food and Agriculture Organization of the United Nations (FAO) and WHO International Conference on Nutrition in Rome (1992) was the first international event that focused explicitly on food safety. The conference stated that a high priority must be given to 'establishing food safety and quality control infrastructures, including food inspection, sampling, and laboratory facilities to enforce the law and regulations, to ensure that food products

comply with applicable requirements for domestic consumption or export'
(Kaferstein et al. 1994, pp. 15–16).

As a result of this attention many countries, including Australia, are
participants in efforts to develop international standard food safety programs
and processes. Perhaps the most significant of these has been the signing of
the General Agreement on Tariffs and Trade (GATT) in 1994, by which
trade barriers, in this case food standards, would be changed by Australia so as
to conform as far as possible with the food standards of the Codex Alimentarius Commission. Similar trade-orientated concerns have seen moves towards
a proposed uniform food standard system between Australia and New
Zealand (Wright 1994, p. 450). Subsequently, closer economic relations
(Edwards 1988, p. 371) have been referred to as 'harmonisation of food standards' by New Zealand, and as 'the development of a joint food standards-
setting system with New Zealand based on New Zealand entering the
Australian system' by Australia (Codex Alimentarius Commission 1994, pp.
4–5). Significantly, the Australian statement clearly signifies that there is some
expectation, if not agreement, that New Zealand would enter formally into
an Australian policy and legislation-setting process and comply with the outcomes of the process, as do the Australian states and territories, so that uniform food standards between the two countries would be achieved.

In Australia, foodborne illness is defined as a notifiable disease in all
states and territories, and notifications of foodborne illness to the respective
health authorities are compiled by the National Notifiable Diseases Surveillance System (NNDSS). The main notifiable foodborne illnesses are
Salmonellosis, Campylobacteriosis, Listeriosis, Shigellosis, and Yersiniosis.
Notifications for Salmonellosis since 1991 are provided in table 15.1. The
notification of Salmonellosis seem to have increased steadily over the
period, with significant increases in notification in 1998 and 1999.

In 1994 there were 10 117 cases of Campylobacteriosis, which constituted one of the highest annual adjusted rates of notification—that is, 85.8
per 100 000 population (table 15.2). It was also observed that there were
large swings in notification rates between jurisdictions—for example, the
Northern Territory (189.3 per 100 000 population) and in Western
Australia (63.2 per 100 000 population). Notification rates in Aboriginal
people were much higher than the respective jurisdictional notification
rate. In the Northern Territory the rate was 280.0 per 100 000 population
and in Western Australia it was 97.2 per 100 000 population (Department
of Human Services and Health 1995, pp. 546, 551).

Although there is an increasing notification rate of Campylobacteriosis
it is uncertain whether this is due to improved reporting or improved
diagnostic capability, or whether there is a real increase in incidence, or a
combination of all of these. Significantly, WHO reported that foodborne
illness cases could be underestimated by a factor of 10 (NFA 1994).

Table 15.1 Notifications of Salmonellosis (NEC) received by state and territory health authorities (1991–2000, and to August for 2001)

Year	Jan	Feb	Mar	Apr	May	Jun	Jul	Aug	Sep	Oct	Nov	Dec	Total
1991	366	569	575	763	626	336	474	394	255	344	372	366	5440
1992	482	501	642	511	423	326	299	262	272	283	311	302	4614
1993	494	517	546	448	462	322	255	286	228	331	411	431	4731
1994	456	684	711	523	452	381	337	299	278	353	424	429	5327
1995	556	839	864	472	493	471	328	315	299	388	469	401	5895
1996	677	701	567	451	608	369	415	292	289	404	516	530	5819
1997	724	638	803	1323	480	393	350	292	386	477	604	536	7006
1998	820	814	900	794	653	609	541	338	483	567	638	543	7700
1999	739	827	1444	802	533	614	328	350	370	380	511	432	7330
2000	624	644	759	518	742	397	312	314	299	383	493	539	6024
2001	714	789	810	631	602	500	425	349	2	0	0	0	4822

Source: Communicable Diseases Network Australia National Notifiable Diseases Surveillance System, pers. comm., 7 September 2001

Table 15.2 Notifications of Campylobacteriosis received by state and territory health authorities (1991–2000, and to August for 2001)

Year	Jan	Feb	Mar	Apr	May	Jun	Jul	Aug	Sept	Oct	Nov	Dec	Total
1991	456	514	602	864	715	610	813	821	628	959	894	796	8 672
1992	722	711	681	669	584	632	650	620	842	1 036	995	994	9 136
1993	835	673	739	553	637	512	585	638	607	760	820	752	8 111
1994	728	811	832	673	801	796	767	871	777	981	1 213	867	10 117
1995	816	939	909	709	837	809	795	984	944	1 041	1 217	933	10 933
1996	1 251	1 032	951	828	992	731	1153	961	879	1 137	1 155	1 088	12 158
1997	1 213	980	823	947	939	903	891	875	884	1 080	1 174	1 142	11 851
1998	1 109	1 086	904	819	759	970	976	1 170	1 158	1 416	1 672	1 410	13 449
1999	1 065	1 015	1 254	826	957	1 001	1 061	1 190	954	1 008	1 291	1 022	12 644
2000	1 012	1 019	1 103	897	1 187	1 127	1 149	1 247	1 000	1 325	1 355	1 059	13 480
2001	1 154	1 067	1 145	1 099	1 298	1 335	1 263	1 319	20	0	0	0	9 700

Source: Communicable Diseases Network Australia National Notifiable Diseases Surveillance System, pers. comm., 7 September 2001

It would appear then that food safety, and particularly those aspects that relate to food hygiene, cleanliness, and foodborne illness, are not public health issues of the past, but continue to pose actual and potential threats to public health today. Perhaps it might be said that this public health issue is even more important today because of the increasing development in the size of the food industry, increasing technology, and higher consumer expectations for the safety of their food.

The economic features of food and the food industry

As well as being a critical public health issue, food and the food industry also can be seen as a critical economic resource. It is this dual importance—at least from the policy development viewpoint—that has brought about a long history of political conflict between public health and economic interests. The economic importance of food and associated industries to Australia can be appreciated by examining table 15.3.

Almost half of all retail turnover is related to food (47.8 per cent) and over half the number of employees in the retail industry are employed in the food retail sector. Significantly, the large number of business locations,

Table 15.3   Statistical data on food retail and food manufacturing in Australia during 1991–92

Category	No. of locations	People employed	Employees per location	Annual turnover ($m)
Food retail				
Specialised food				
fresh meat, fish, poultry,	7 349	28 459	4	2 787
fruit, and vegetables	3 670	18 189	5	1 893
liquor retailing	1 847	8 593	5	2 094
bread and cake retailing	4 771	30 066	6	1 174
takeaway food	20 324	118 212	6	4 885
other	5 719	21 954	4	1 876
Supermarkets and groceries	9 486	180 826	19	26 102
Cafes and restaurants	14 740	136 894	9	5 167
Total of all food retail	67 906	543 193		45 978
Food retail as a proportion of all retailing activities (%)	39.3	50.8		47.8
Food manufacturing				
Meat products	590	43 721	74	8 236
Milk products	210	15 667	75	5 031
Fruit and vegetable products	183	10 224	56	2 417
Margarine, oils, and fats	33	2 188	66	721
Grain and flour products	145	8 583	59	2 570
Bread, cakes, and biscuits	1 920	34 506	18	3 238
Beverages and malt	386	17 104	44	5 489
Other food products	756	31 108	41	7 100
Total of all food manufacturing	4 223	163 101		34 802
Food manufacturing as a proportion of all manufacturing industry	10.2	18.0		20.7
Sum of all food retail and manufacturing	72 129	706 294		80 780

Source: National Food Authority, *Safe Food Handling Australia*, 1994, p. 8

together with the average number of employees per location of around eight, indicates one important feature of the industry—the importance of small businesses. The food manufacturing sector is also of some importance as it represents the largest subdivision of total Australian manufacturing turnover (18 per cent) and some 17 per cent of total manufacturing employment (NFA 1994, p. 9).

The implication here is that any public health interventions utilising the development of business regulatory strategies will have an economic impact on the food industry in terms of both employment and, importantly, export earnings. At the national and individual state and territory levels food exports have become an increasingly significant part of Australia's engagement in the world market. This significance has been realised by the food industry and its representatives.

> Its [the Food Industry Council of Australia's] efforts in recent times have been particularly designed to allow Australian companies to refocus their priorities from predominantly domestic issues to thinking outwardly and of opportunities presented by international markets. This change of focus, we believed, was critical to securing a long-term future for the industry (Gittus 1994, p. 2).

To achieve this change, industry believes that Australian management must be able to focus on this task and, not surprisingly, '... without distractions caused by intervention from governments and groups whose priorities and agenda for change are very different from the industry's' (Gittus 1994, p. 2).

The federal government's Agri-Food Strategy, announced in July 1992 by the Ministers for Industry and Technology and Commerce and Primary Industries and Energy, sought to increase food exports from $2.3 billion in 1992 to $7 billion by the year 2000. Part of the strategy was to remove impediments to industry at the government level so that this target could be achieved. The NFA saw that this would include prescriptive food hygiene regulation (NFA 1994). Indeed, the food industry has been successful in influencing government public health policy through the important economic portfolio of industry.

Food safety administration and its complexity

Historically, food safety policies were determined by each state government through Acts of parliament, which addressed public health and food safety within that context, or addressed food safety directly through specific Acts. The various state Public Health Acts and their frequent amendments tended to address the prevention of adulteration of foodstuffs or ensuring the selling and preparation of food in sanitary conditions. This generic approach was supplanted by a more specific approach heralded by the passing of the Victorian Pure Food Act in 1905. The passing of this Act was significant in that it 'made provision for the perpetuation of those general provisions designed to secure the cleanliness and purity of food' (Cumpston 1989, p. 403). Importantly, the Pure Food Act provided for the establishment of an expert committee, the Food Standards Committee, the major role of which was to advise the health authority on the compositional standards of foods, with the first regulations prescribing such standards coming into effect as from October 1906 (Cumpston 1989).

Other state governments followed a similar course of action; by 1912 there was legislation covering food across the whole of Australia (Business Regulation Review Unit 1988a). The aspects of food safety covered were primarily those relating to the prevention of adulteration and contamination, requirements for clean and sanitary food premises, and some requirements for the accurate labelling and compositional standards of certain classes of foods. Today, the various state Food Standards Committees still perform an advisory function regarding, *inter alia*, compositional standards of food. Of particular significance, however, the administration of food safety laws was and still is the responsibility of the individual state governments.

Despite the best intentions, food safety policy—and particularly its implementation—has been a highly problematic and dynamic area of public policy, probably best explained by the following three features of food safety administration. First, each Australian state and territory has sovereignty over food safety. Second is the complexity of state and territory government administration of food safety legislation. Third is the rationalisation of the administration of food safety legislation.

State sovereignty over food safety

As has been stated, the Commonwealth does not have powers under the Constitution in relation to food safety policy, which was confirmed by the 1929 Royal Commission on the Constitution. Consequently, since 1908 there have been regular, frequent, and in the main unsuccessful discussions between the Commonwealth and state governments to achieve an agreed uniform approach to food policy. Two significant events did assist in the facilitation of a uniform approach to food safety. The first of these was the establishment in 1955 of the National Health and Medical Research Council's (NHMRC) Food Standards Committee, which had the role of developing and recommending food safety standards to the Commonwealth and states for adoption (Business Regulation Review Unit 1988a). Although a useful strategy for policy development, there were still underlying policy implementation issues, which the establishment of the Food Standards Council could not address.

Governments were not obliged to adopt the advice or the standards developed by the NHMRC and, in a number of cases, the standards were adopted and then modified to meet the perceived demands of the local state or territory situation, which was the usual justification for modifications. The location of the administration of food policy often changed or was shared between various Commonwealth departments, agencies, and portfolios, including Health, Consumer Affairs under the Attorney-General, and Primary Industry (Business Regulation Review Unit 1988a).

The second event was that after 5 years of development, a Model Food Act was endorsed by health ministers in 1980 and, in the following year, a National Food Standards Council Agreement was signed by the prime minister, all state premiers, and the chief minister of the Northern Territory. This Agreement established the National Food Standards Council, which comprised all ministers responsible for food standards legislation (Business Regulation Review Unit 1988a). As with other national issues, an extra-constitutional mechanism had to be developed to facilitate the achievement of a national objective—in this case, uniform food standards.

Although progress had been made towards uniformity, there still existed—according to the 1988 Inquiry into Food Regulation in Australia by the Commonwealth Business Regulation Review Unit—many constraints to the uniform application or implementation of food legislation:

> … a significant impediment to the development of an efficient and competitive export industry, and the current administrative mechanisms were costly in terms of time and resources … these mechanisms have reduced the efficiency and competitiveness of the Australian food industry through increased costs and impediments to product innovation and adoption of new technologies (National Food Authority 1992, p. 6).

In response to these criticisms a special premiers' conference in 1990 agreed to the establishment of an independent statutory authority, the National Food Authority, which had the role of maintaining and developing uniform national food standards (National Food Authority 1992, p. 6). The authority was under the jurisdiction of the Human Services and Health portfolio and, from February 1994, reported directly to the Parliamentary Secretary to the Minister for Human Services and Health (National Food Authority 1994a, p. 5).

The establishment of the NFA, and its successor the Australia New Zealand Food Authority (ANZFA), provided a central focus for food safety policy. Subsequently, in July 2000 all health ministers, meeting as the Australia New Zealand Food Standards Council (ANZFSC), agreed to adopt the first three of four proposed national food safety standards (ANZFA 2001a). These standards, the first national standards for Australia, become legally enforceable as they are adopted by each state and territory. Of interest is the decision not to include the standard requiring food safety programs for food businesses. This requirement has been given the status of a model standard should any individual state or territory wish to introduce the requirement. Certainly, this seems paradoxical: on one hand there is a step to uniform standards, but on the other, potential is introduced for undermining uniformity.

On 3 November 2000, the Council of Australian Governments (COAG) agreed to major changes for the administration of food regulation (Department of Health and Aged Care 2001, p. 8). These changes included the establishment of the Australia New Zealand Food Standards Council and development of an intergovernmental agreement between the states and territories. Of importance is clause 26 of this agreement, which states that 'No State or Territory shall, by legislation or other means, establish or amend a food standard other than in accordance with this Agreement' (ANZFA 2001b). According to ANZFA, under this Agreement the states and territories have agreed to adopt without variation food standards approved by the ANZFSC (ANZFA 2001c). The latest initiatives, which are an outcome of many years of development, have been most significant steps in achieving uniformity.

The complexity of state government administration of food safety legislation

Generally speaking, state governments, through the agency of their health authorities, made the food safety laws and regulations; local government authorities, except in New South Wales, were charged with the responsibility of enforcing the food safety legislation as part of their public health role. Clearly, the formulation of food safety policy was the responsibility of the state government through the health department and its predecessors, and food safety policy implementation was the responsibility of each local government authority. In 1992 there were 210 municipalities administering food safety legislation in Victoria alone—thus, together with the division of responsibilities between state and local governments—increasing the potential for nonuniform approaches and implementation of the legislation.

For the purposes of illustration, Victoria is taken as a case study of food safety administration within a state jurisdiction. Even though each individual local government authority had—and has—delegated legislative responsibilities for the administration of the *Food Act 1984* (Cwlth), the actual administration is performed by Environmental Health Officers (EHOs). On a day-to-day basis, EHOs are called upon to inspect, investigate, and take action in regard to a wide variety of issues that occur at the community level with food premises, food production, and food selling. The action taken is often reactive and influenced by a number of factors:

- the experience and knowledge of the individual EHO
- the culture of EHOs as an organised unit of the council and as a professional group generally
- the service policies and priorities of the local council
- the relationships between local industry and council, and between local industry and EHOs
- the food policies and priorities of the state health department and state government
- local consumer and resident expectations regarding food safety
- current interpretations of food safety policy and legislation and its intent.

Apart from cultural aspects, the above factors reflect the same stakeholders in food safety at the local level as there are at the state and national levels: consumers, elected representatives, local and state public health administrators, and industry. The lack of uniform interpretation by local administrators was a criticism levelled by the food industry and the Inquiry into Food Regulation in Australia (Business Regulation Review Unit 1988b). Given the factors affecting local food safety administration it should not come as a surprise that there are, and will be, variations while local government continues to have responsibility for the administration of food safety legislation.

This is not to say that uniform approaches cannot or should not be achieved. The Inquiry into Food Regulation in Australia recommended a number of initiatives to achieve uniformity, including the establishment of a food unit with the role of giving authoritative advice, the development of standardised food inspection reports, and mandatory reporting of food safety data by local government (Business Regulation Review Unit 1988b). As with the later establishment of the NFA by the federal government, the proposal for a food unit in the health department appeared to be an appropriate and meritorious strategy, as this would then have created a focus for food safety policy making. However, it appeared that the review members assumed that the creation of a food unit in the state health department was the same as establishing a state government food unit. In this way, they were in error and, further, did not fully comprehend the very criticisms that they had identified about the need for rationalised state food legislation.

The review members also did not appreciate and consider the complete context for food safety administration, in that the whole of Victorian local government was under review as part of the state Coalition government's reform agenda. Specifically, public health legislation and the role that state and local governments fulfilled in public health were also under review. With regard to the appropriate relationship between the Victorian health department and local government, the *Local Government Review Report* tentatively concluded that care had to be exercised in not imposing rigid regulatory controls on local government that would limit its ability to respond to changing needs in each municipality. It was also acknowledged that consultation would need to occur with local government regarding its capacity to undertake any new functions. Importantly, there was recognition that a new relationship between the state health department and local government had to be forged if there was to be a change from purely mandated activities to public health outputs at the local level. This third conclusion of the review of local government was concerned with a joint public health planning process between the Health Department and local government (Health Department Victoria 1986).

Apart from the establishment of a food unit, the other recommendations from the Inquiry into Food Regulation in Australia—that is, the standardisation of food inspection reports and reporting requirements related to food safety—was a move towards increased central control by the state health department over local government authorities. This was inconsistent with the policy directions of the broader intergovernmental and public health review. Interestingly, each review failed to acknowledge the other, which perhaps indicates the rather disjointed approach to policy making, particularly in the appreciation of the context for policy implementation between levels of government in a federal system.

Rationalisation of the administration of food safety legislation

Prior to the establishment of the NFA, there were some concerns relating to the shared responsibilities for food safety administration at the national level. These concerns appeared to have been addressed, as the NFA had been established as the new national agency responsible for a streamlined food standards system (NFA 1994). This is not necessarily the case in the states and territories. Historically, states and territories have created two features of state food safety administration—delegation to local government authorities (except for New South Wales), and sharing food safety responsibilities between state departments. Prior even to the development of Pure Food Acts in the nineteenth century, separate food safety control systems were developed for the meat and milk industries because the veterinary aspects were thought to be so important as to require a change in the method of control (Cumpston 1989). It was recognised that to achieve acceptable food safety standards, appropriate animal health controls had to be put in place at the point of slaughter in the case of meat and, in the dairy shed, in the case of milk supply. As a consequence, the primary responsibility for control of these two food systems rested in most states with the Department of Agriculture.

Although on the surface the division of control seems quite appropriate, the demarcation of jurisdictions is not at all clear, particularly in the enforcement of legislation. Then there is the issue of potential duplication of controls and implementation that results from these two features of food safety administration. Generic administration of food safety standards occurs through local government authorities, as discussed above, but overlap of control occurs at the industry and municipal levels with specific controls and administration from the meat and dairy authorities. Further complexity is introduced with recent trends for specific foods (for example, icecream) to be removed from generic administration to the meat authority in Victoria.

In essence, the problem lies around where and at what specific point of the paddock-to-plate process do the respective jurisdictions and responsibilities begin and end, given that in this instance the motivation for all state and territory government departments and local government is about the protection of public health. When an episode or incident of food poisoning or food contamination does occur, which authority, agency, or level of government is willing to take responsibility for the control measures they have put in place to prevent such an incident from occurring? Who has been collecting the licensing or registration fees?

Conclusion

Food safety has been an important policy area for government for the past 150 years and is still so today. Food is a prerequisite for health and at the same time is also a potential source of health problems; food and food standards are always of interest to almost all the population.

As with other health policy areas, food safety policy is complex and involves the interests of many stakeholders who often have mutually exclusive policy expectations. Governments find themselves in the almost traditional conflict between the interests of industry and the interests of public health. However, governments who want to determine a food policy and who are willing to pay the cost for such a determination do not seem to make policy implementation easy. Often, implementation and administrative responsibilities are shared between departments that may have quite different *modus operandi,* cultural norms, and policy interpretations. Often, policy formulation and implementation roles are divided and shared between all three spheres of government, and it has been shown just how exceedingly complex policy implementation can become. When policy reviews are undertaken, the complete context for the review is often not understood—for example, that food is a public health issue as well as an economic issue, and these reviews are not integrated with other broader policy reviews, particularly those that have role implications for levels of government.

It would seem that the establishment of an Australia New Zealand Food Authority has provided a focus for food safety policy and has eliminated divided responsibility for its administration; however, in the states and territories there still exists a complex set of implementation responsibilities between state departments and between state and local governments. If the establishment of a food safety authority was a way of overcoming constitutional constraints to national food safety policy, perhaps a similar authority established in each state and responsible to the respective health ministers might overcome the constraining features of the current state food safety administration. Further, the establishment of state food authorities responsible both for policy and standards development and their implementation would not only overcome (from the viewpoint of the states) some of the intergovernmental issues encountered at local and federal levels, but would also clearly define responsibilities pertaining to food safety.

References

Abbot, P. 1994, *Proceedings of the Second Asian Conference on Food Safety*, Text and Journal Publication Company, Bangkok.

Australia New Zealand Food Authority 2001a, *Food Standards News 26, Special Edition: Food Safety Standards Update*, ANZFA, Canberra.

—— 2001b, <http://www.anzfa.gov.au/about anzfa>.

—— 2001c, <http://www.anzfa.gov.au/about anzfa/intergovernmentalagr780.cfm>.

Business Regulation Review Unit & Commonwealth of Australia and Regulation Review Unit, Government of Victoria 1988a, *Report of an Inquiry into Food Regulation in Australia, Part 1: National Issues*, BRRU, Canberra.

—— 1988b, *Report of an Inquiry into Food Regulation in Australia, Part 11: Victorian Issues*, Business Regulation Review Unit, Canberra.

Codex Alimentarius Commission 1994, *Report of the Third Session of the Codex Coordinating Committee for North America and the South-West Pacific*, FAO and WHO, Rome.

Communicable Diseases Network Australia, National Notifiable Diseases Surveillance System, 7 September 2001, Personal communication.

Cumpston, J. H. L. 1989, *Health and Disease in Australia: A History*, AGPS, Canberra.

Davis, A. & George, J. 1988, *States of Health, Health and Illness in Australia*, Harper & Row, Sydney.

Department of Health and Aged Care 2001, *Working Together, Discussion Paper: Review of Administrative Arrangements of Public Health and Safety Regulation for*

Chemical Safety Assessment, Medicines, Medical Devices, Gene Technology and Food, Regulatory Reform Taskforce DHAC, Canberra.

Department of Human Services and Health 1995, *Annual Report of the National Notifiable Diseases Surveillance System 1994*, vol. 19, no. 22, DHSH, Canberra.

Edwards, R. A. 1988, 'Food Legislation in Australia: The Last Twenty Years', *Food Australia*, September, pp. 369–75.

Gittus, I. 1994, 'Food Law: An Industry Perspective', Paper delivered at Food Industry Forum 1994, Moorabbin Industry Training Centre, Melbourne.

Gordon, D. 1976, *Health, Sickness and Society*, University of Queensland Press, St Lucia.

Health Department Victoria 1986, *Review of Health Legislation, Discussion Paper, Series No. 1: Public Health Legislation in Victoria: An Overview*, Government Printer, Melbourne.

Hedberg, C. W., MacDonald, K. L., & Osterholm, M. T. 1994, 'Changing Epidemiology of Food-borne Disease: A Minnesota Perspective', *Clinical Infectious Diseases*, vol. 18, pp. 671–82.

Kaferstein, F. K. & Motarjemi, Y. 1994, *Proceedings of the Second Asian Conference on Food Safety*, Text and Journal Publication Company, Bangkok.

National Food Authority 1992, *First Annual Report*, AGPS, Canberra.

—— 1994a, *Annual Report 1993–94*, AGPS, Canberra.

—— 1994, *Safe Food Handling Australia: A Discussion Paper on the Future Direction of Food Hygiene Regulation*, AGPS, Canberra.

World Health Organization 1978, 'Primary Health Care', *Health for All*, Series 1, WHO, Geneva.

—— 1986, *Ottawa Charter for Health Promotion*, WHO, Ottawa.

Wright, E. J. 1994, 'Australian Food Standards and the GATT', *Food Australia*, vol. 46, no. 10, pp. 450–1.

Acronyms

AACE	Australian Aged Care Exporters	CHF	Consumers' Health Forum
ABS	Australian Bureau of Statistics	CM	complementary medicine
		CMEC	Complementary Medicines Evaluation Committee
ACCC	Australian Competition and Consumer Commission	COAG	Council of Australian Governments
ACHA	Australian Complementary Health Association	CPI	Consumer Price Index
		DCS	Department of Community Services
ACSQHC	Australian Council for Safety and Quality in Healthcare	DHAC	Department of Health and Aged Care
ADGP	Australian Divisions of General Practice	DHFS	Department of Health and Family Services
AHA	Australian Hospital Association	DHHCS	Department of Health, Housing and Community Services
AHC	Australian Hospital Care		
AHI	Aus Health International	DHS	Department of Human Services
AHIDF	Australian Health Industry Development Forum		
AHII	Australian Health Industry Incorporated	DHSH	Department of Human Services and Health
AHIMA	American Health Information Management Association	DIMA	Department of Immigration and Multicultural Affairs
AHMAC	Australian Health Ministers' Advisory Council	DRGs	Diagnosis Related Groups
		DIST	Department of Industy, Science and Tourism
AIHW	Australian Institute of Health and Welfare	DITAC	Department of Industry, Technology and Commerce
AIRC	Australian Industrial Relations Commission	EHOs	Environmental Health Officers
AIRDIB	Australian Industrial Research and Development Incentives Board	EPAC	Economic Planning Advisory Council
AMA	Australian Medical Association	ESD	Ecological sustainable development
ANF	Australian Nursing Federation		
ANZFA	Australia New Zealand Food Authority	FAGs	Financial Assistance Grants
		FAO	Food and Agriculture Organization of the United Nations
ANZFSC	Australia New Zealand Food Standards Council		
BRRU	Business Regulation Review Unit	GATT	General Agreement on Tariffs and Trade
BOOT	build, own, operate, and transfer	GDP	gross domestic product
		GSP	gross state product
CDCP	Centers for Disease Control and Prevention (USA)	GST	goods and services tax
		GP(s)	general practitioner(s)
CGC	Commonwealth Grants Commission	GPPs	General Purpose Payments
		HACC	Home and Community Care

HCoA	Health Care of Australia	NHS	National Health Service
HFG	Hospital Funding Grant	NIMBY	not in my back yard
HIC	Health Insurance Commission	NNDSS	National Notifiable Diseases Surveillance System
HMO	Health Maintenance Organisation	NPHP	National Public Health Partnership
HR	human resources		
IAC	Industries Assistance Commission	NRCCH	National Reference Centre for Classification in Health
IC	Industry Commission	OECD	Organization for Economic Cooperation and Development
ICLEI	International Council for Local Environmental Initiatives		
		OPCV	Overseas Projects Corporation of Victoria
IMA	Integrative Medicine Association	OTC	over the counter
IMIR	Institute for Magnetic Imaging Research	PAHO	Pan American Health Organization
IOMR	Institute of Medicine Reporting	PBAC	Pharmaceutical Benefits Advisory Committee
IOS	International Organization for Standardization	PBPA	Pharmaceutical Benefits Pricing Authority
MBS	Medical Benefits Schedule	PBS	Pharmaceutical Benefits Scheme
MoU	memorandum/memoranda of understanding	PC	Productivity Commission
MSAV	Medical Scientists' Association of Victoria	PIP	Practice Incentive Payments
		POPs	persistent organic pollutants
NCC	National Coding Centre	PHLI	Public Health Leadership Institute
NCCH	National Centre for Classification in Health	RACGP	Royal Australian College of General Practitioners
NEHCN	North East Health Care Network	SACFM	South Australian Centre for Manufacturing
NEHPC	North East Health Promotion Centre	SMEs	small- and medium-sized enterprises
NEHRT	National Electronic Health Records Taskforce	SPPs	Specific Purpose Payments
NEHS	National Environmental Health Strategy	SSROC	Southern Sydney Regional Organisation of Councils
NFA	National Food Authority	TCM	traditional Chinese medicine
NHDD	National Health Data Dictionary	TGA	Therapeutic Goods Administration
NHIA	National Health Information Agreement	UNCED	United Nations Conference on Environment and Development
NHIM	National Health Information Model	VDPs	voluntary departure packages
NHIMAC	National Health Information Management Advisory Council	VHA	Victorian Hospitals' Association
NHIMG	National Health Information Management Group	WFPHA	World Federation of Public Health Associations
NHMRC	National Health and Medical Research Council	WHO	World Health Organization

Notes

Introduction

1   The Australian Commonwealth comprises six states (Victoria, New South Wales, Queensland, Western Australia, South Australia, Tasmania) and two territories (the Northern Territory and the Australian Capital Territory). In subsequent discussion, wherever the reference is to states, it can be taken to include the territories.

2 Australian Federalism, Politics, and Health

1   The main payments in this category relate to nongovernment schools and local government general-purpose assistance. Funds paid to the states (a small number of Special Purpose Payments made direct to local government) relate to childcare programs administered by local governments on behalf of the Commonwealth, and funding for aged and disabled people's homes and hostels. In terms of federal–state funding, grants to local government constitute only a small proportion of total Commonwealth assistance (4.3 per cent) and are not discussed separately.

2   Local government has no formal recognition in the Commonwealth Constitution; however, since 1996 the Council of Australian Governments (COAG) has recognised the significant role played by local government in areas of health and community services. Local government typically encompasses cities, towns, shires, boroughs, municipalities, and district councils, with a focus on road and bridge construction and maintenance, water sewerage and drainage systems, health and sanitation services, building supervision, and administration of regulations, along with some service provision in recreation, culture, and community services. Its revenue source comprises direct grants from the Commonwealth (about 20 per cent of revenue) and local government revenue, which comes mainly from property rates along with fines and service charges.

3   For a summary of the background to federation in its earlier years, see Summers (1994); and for later periods, see Fletcher (1991).

4   Several High Court decisions have expanded the scope of Commonwealth powers (Summers 1994), including the Mabo (1992) and Wik (1996) cases relating to Native Title. Among the most controversial for changing the federal–state balance are section 51 (xxix) cases, which deal with the Commonwealth's power over external affairs. These cases concern the Commonwealth overriding the states in areas affected by Australia being a signatory to international agreements.

5 The federal government raises about 73 per cent of combined Commonwealth–state general government revenue but its outlays for its own expenditure are only 58 per cent of total general government outlays (Commonwealth of Australia 1999, Budget paper No. 1, table 1, and Budget paper No. 3, chart 3).

6 The new system of Commonwealth–state financial relations provides the states with that GST revenue raised by those states (minus collection costs) to be spent according to their own budget priorities, and replaces abolished state taxes such as accommodation tax and financial institutions duty, as well as stamp duties on quoted marketable securities, which were abolished from 1 July 2001.

7 These grants increased during the Whitlam Labor government from 25.8 per cent of Commonwealth transfers to the states in 1972–73 to 48.5 per cent in 1975–76. Under the Fraser Liberal government, they fell to 41.5 per cent in 1980–81 and to 32.7 per cent in 1981–82, then grew again under the Hawke and Keating Labor governments to a peak of 52.8 per cent in 1995–96. SPPs were reduced under the Howard Coalition to 50 per cent in 1998–99 and fell to around 49 per cent of total payment to states and territories in 1999–2000 (James 1997, pp. 15–29; Commonwealth of Australia 1999, Budget paper 3, ch. 3, p. 17).

8 This organisation emerged out of the joint review of Commonwealth–state financial arrangements conducted by the Special Premiers' Conference in 1991; under Prime Minister Hawke's New Federalism policy, COAG was established in 1992 as an ongoing council. Comprising the Prime Minister, the premiers and chief ministers, and the president of the Local Government Association, COAG needs to be understood as a reflection of the basic concurrent nature of Australian federalism and as signalling 'cooperative federalism in Australia' (Painter 1996, p. 101).

9 Compared to the average annual growth rate in Australian recurrent health services expenditure of 4 per cent between 1989–90 and 1996–97, expenditure in areas of state responsibility grew more slowly—3.2 per cent for public hospitals, 2.8 per cent for nursing homes, 1.5 per cent for ambulance services, and a negative growth of –5.9 per cent in public psychiatric hospitals (due to deinstitutionalisation efforts). In comparison, costs rose faster in areas of Commonwealth responsibility, principally for medical services (rising 4.9 per cent) and pharmaceutical services (rising 8.4 per cent) (Australian Institute of Health and Welfare 1999, p. 17). However, a note of caution, as growth rates may depend on the chosen timeframe.

10 Similar cuts in other areas of social expenditure reinforce the interpretation that debt reduction was taking priority over social spending. Between 1993–94 and 1997–98, real per capita expenditure on welfare decreased 19.5 per cent ($241 to $194). The cuts to aged and disabled welfare (–17 per cent, $123 to $102) are of concern, given an ageing population and the cuts to expenditure on nursing homes. The large decrease in spending on net housing (–71 per cent, $34 to $10) was due to the imposition of higher

user charges. The only area of social spending to experience a real per capita increase was law, order, and public safety (6.9 per cent, $306 to $327), with the main increase being in administration expenditure rather than in police or prisons (Hancock & Cowling 1999).

11   The areas where private health insurance makes some contribution and consumers contribute substantially to costs are those not covered by Medicare, such as private hospitals, specialist medical fees, dental services, nonmedical professional services, aids, and appliances.

12   Witnesses presenting evidence to the Senate inquiry into public hospital funding claimed in evidence that 'better dividends to the Australian community could have come about by channelling funds spent on the private health insurance rebate into the public hospital system' (Crowley 2000, p. xii).

5 Structural Reform and Cultural Transition

1   For further information see the NPHP website at <http://hna.ffh.vic.gov.au/nphp/aboutus.htm>.

2   The author is the former executive officer of the National Public Health Partnership. This chapter contains her reflections on the NPHP and its activities.

3   For a more detailed discussion of the establishment of the NPHP, see Lin and King (2000).

4   See <http://www.wkkf.org/programminginterests/health/turningpoint/default.htm>.

Index